Healthy Prostate

The Extensive Guide To Prevent and Heal Prostate Problems

Including Prostate Cancer, BPH Enlarged Prostate and Prostatitis

Ronald M. Bazar

BCom, McGill University
MBA, Harvard University

Healthy Prostate
The Extensive Guide To Prevent and Heal Prostate Problems
Including Prostate Cancer, BPH Enlarged Prostate and Prostatitis

Author: Ronald M. Bazar

Published by:
Ronald M. Bazar
PO Box 73
Mansons Landing
BC V0P 1K0
Canada

Email: **healthyprostate@ymail.com**

Website: **http://www.healthyprostate.co**

First Edition: October 2011

ISBN: 978-1466369252

Dedicated to the memory of my Mom and Dad,
Beatrice Millman Bazar and Bernard Bazar,
who gifted me with the grace of unconditional love
and who always believed in me.
May you rest in peace together.

Acknowledgements

I thank those who have helped me in this project. In particular I must mention Coreen Boucher [http://coreenboucher.com/], my initial editor, who was so essential to take all my pieces and to put them into a coherent whole. She took the load off my mind of structure, organization and flow, and allowed me to forge ahead wherever inspiration took me in my writing. She took hundreds of snippets and helped merge them into the book you see. Without you it would have been impossible! Coreen, thanks so much!

Shanaya Nelson [http://amaya-editing.com], my final editor, took my best and polished it beyond my wildest imagination into the final book you see. Her insights, suggestions and editing skills were always superb and so helpful. It was a pleasure to work with someone just so competent both at the micro level of minutiae and at the macro level of structure, design and refinement! Shanaya, I am just thrilled with all you have done!

My daughters, Namchi Bazar and Kaïma Bazar, stood their ground in battles about the title and subtitle, forcing me to bend to a will that saw the bigger picture. You know you are blessed as a Dad when your daughters can be so powerful! And they accomplished this with one having a new infant in her arms and the other about to birth. I am so proud of you both! You know how much you mean to me by your standing by me over these trying eight years. I love you bunches!

My nephew Aaron Bazar provided invaluable feedback and perspective that helped bring the book to a high level of excellence. Thanks Aaron!

My technical expert, Scott Onstott [http://scottonstott.com], has freed my mind from the difficult tasks that could have prevented me from getting the book into final format… and much more. His quiet confidence has been a blessing. His competency is what made it possible for me to self publish the book. Thanks so much Scott!

Lastly, my dear friend, Ann Mortifee [http://annmortifee.com], gifted me with hope at my darkest hour after my original diagnosis. She gave me the love, courage and faith to forge ahead, knowing I would find a way to heal myself. Ann, I am forever grateful!

May you dear reader have loved ones to support and nourish you along the healing way, as I have.

~~~~~~

Subscribe: Go here if you want to be on the subscribe list for updates, insights and news about the prostate:

http://www.healthyprostate.co/subscribe

or send an email with "Subscribe" in the Subject line to:

healthyprostate@ymail.com

Live links: Go here if you want to buy an ebook version at a 50% discount so that the links in your book can be clicked to load:

http://www.healthyprostate.co/discount

~~~~~~

Table of Contents

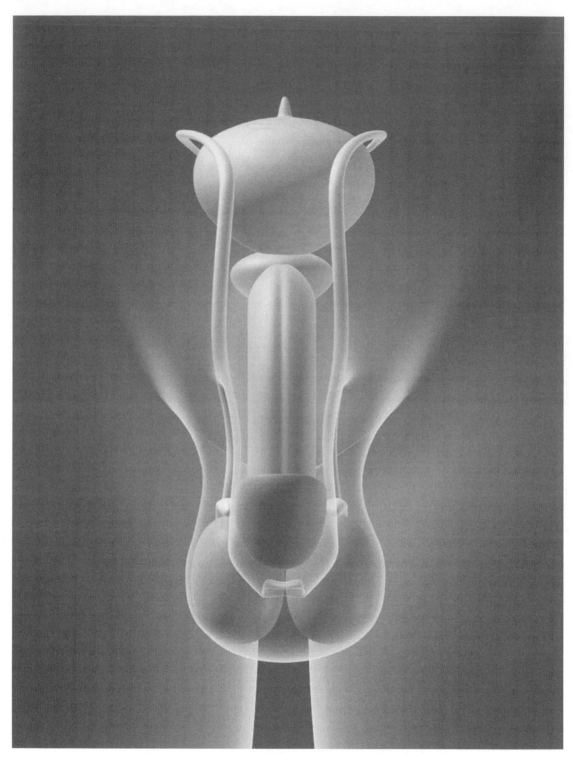

An artist's 3D image of the male "plumbing" system. That's the bladder at the top with the prostate (smaller oval) underneath and the "crown jewels" below.

Preface

Dear Reader,

Given the vast amount of information easily available to the average seeker for prostate problems, it can be overwhelming and daunting. How in the world do you sort through it all and make some sense of it?

It took me eight years. That's how I did it. I was motivated because I wanted to find solutions to my extremely enlarged prostate without the risks of conventional surgeries or drugs. I explored books, websites, and information from practitioners. Not as a scholar, for that I am not, but from a very practical aspect: I asked myself, "What works? Or what seems to be well presented and offers good ideas and solutions?"

No one person has "the answer"—including me. All I hope to achieve is to wake you up to what I believe are the real causes of the explosion in prostate disease cases. In this book, I point the way to reversing your prostate condition by giving you useful information so that you can make good choices for yourself.

This book will help you to be well armed with new insights and tools to shorten your healing journey from eight years (which is how long it took me) to months for you. You will be able to completely transform your prostate problem using an enlightened approach tailored to you.

The more I reflect on the causes of our spiraling increase in prostate problems in modern Western men, the more I realize that the root cause stems from our modern lifestyle itself.

Our lifestyle has:

- put convenience of food ahead of quality and nutritional benefit;

- refined and processed and converted once healthy foods into dangerous sources of toxins, devitalized and denatured and incapable of nourishing us;

- made corporate agendas and profits more important than the health of customers;

- stifled independent options in healthcare and monopolized control of our health into organizations that work hand in hand with both mega corporations and government agencies;

- destroyed the health of our farm land with factory farming methods that deplete our soils and poison our waters and our food with toxins that cause disease upon disease;

- allowed genetic modification of our heritage in the seeds of the earth and its patenting; and

- made us loose touch with the central importance of nutritious food as the very foundation of our health.

We have ourselves to blame for these changes. By our actions and lack of self-education we have allowed the slow devolution of our health, and now we pay the price. Prostate disease is a condition that results from the choices we make, with or without awareness.

My purpose in writing this book is to help you to see the role you have played in getting to where you are with a condition that is changing your life. If you are lucky, and you are still healthy, this book will help you act now before your life is impacted by prostate problems, something the odds say will be coming your way.

There is a lot to learn. I have done my best to make it much easier for you. I have distilled down a vast array of information that will quickly get you up to speed and offer you a choice from the mainstream options, which are to poison, cut, slice, burn, freeze or irradiate you out of your dilemma.

This book will show you that there are many options and alternatives. Surgery is only one of the paths that lie before you. This book will arm you with information, and then it will be up to you to decide which path is best for you.

I ask that you keep an open mind, be ready to learn and to see whether what I present makes sense for you. You will know if the information I offer resonates with you, if it rings a bell and urges you onwards with changes that you can make to heal yourself. Yes, I said *heal yourself* as that is precisely what I claim is possible for you… to heal your prostate.

Many links are offered for you to dig deeper if interested. **Healthy Prostate** is designed to be interactive and comprehensive, while at the same time making it easy to read, understand and learn.

To keep the book interesting and readable I have included many sources. It is impossible to do justice by summarizing everything when the source can offer much more depth. Others do far better at specific research than I do, and I link you to them. Thus you can use the book as a prostate resource guide. If a reference grabs your attention, go there to read more.

Healthy Prostate is also a quick sourcebook for many suggested items (see the Appendix at the end of the book). You can use the links or just go to your local health food store or bookstore where you may be able to find them.

It will take work if you choose the path of healing yourself. Sorry, no free lunch is offered here! Part of the process is a learning curve, learning about the prostate and causes of its diseases, and then learning what to do to cure those diseases. The benefits of doing this work are many, because healing your prostate heals all of you. Following this process will create a foundation of health and will have a bonus side effect of drastically minimizing sickness and chronic conditions that plague so many people as they get older. Improving your health will help you to lose weight, and feel younger, lighter and happier! Great and positive side effects!

Change is needed if you go down the path of natural healing. It doesn't happen just by reading! You got here by the day-to-day choices you made either with or without awareness as to the consequences. Now is the time to embrace the changes and new habits that will set you on the road to life's most precious gift of good health.

In all the many books, websites and articles that I have studied intensively for eight years on the prostate, nowhere have I found anywhere close to the breadth of information available in this book. My goal was to give you all the ammunition you need to have a great shot at healing your prostate.

My job has been to share with you what I have learned during those eight years of intensive research and practice so that you can short-cut a lot of what I went through. You will discover plenty in this book that will make you think, and it may challenge some of your viewpoints and beliefs. That is good! It means I have done my job. It then is completely up to you to decide what route you want to follow to get to the destination you want.

Change is not easy for most of us. Yet when we know we must do it, we can. We do learn and rise to the occasion.

Some will question my credentials, as I have no official background in medicine, natural alternative medicine, complementary medicine or even nutrition. I make no claim to any of those! I am self-taught by necessity of my choice not to succumb to surgery. Many decades of following a diet that is as healthy and natural as possible have made me comfortable and knowledgeable about the prostate and how to heal it.

I have a strong business background with a Bachelor of Commerce from McGill University and a Masters in Business Administration from Harvard University. Most of my career has been as an entrepreneur. Perhaps that kind of creative thinking and ability to forge ahead has served me with my prostate. For me, discovering I had a prostate disease became a mission to find a way to heal my prostate naturally.

Perhaps that, too, was born out of my years involved in the health industry: introducing ginseng to North America, running a water and air purifying business, consulting to natural food manufacturers or retailers and writing children's educational books about non-smoking, safety and the environment.

When reading this book, I ask only that you read with an open mind. I make no apologies for my point of view. I believe we are able to heal ourselves with our will and the tools to do so, and with a little help from our friends and spirit guides!

Some of the tools may seem alien to you and many will criticize them as invalid and unscientific. I know without a shadow of doubt that the tools I share in this book are both powerful and effective. Suspend your disbelief and allow yourself to learn how to heal yourself.

Perhaps my greatest gift in this book will be for you to realize your absolute uniqueness regarding your health and what is best for you. I spend a lot of time explaining food and diet choices because food is fundamental to your health. After you have read this book, you will know what foods are best for you and what to avoid. You will learn how to manifest that uniqueness into a diet of food and supplements that is perfect for you and no one else. And best yet, you will *know* that it is just right for you. You will not need to follow the dictates of someone else; you will decide for yourself what is best for you. You will learn to be your own expert and to create your own perfect diet.

I wish you the best in your journey to health. For the women reading this book, many of the recommendations are equally valid for you—simply substitute the word "prostate" for "uterus" or "breast."

A healthy prostate is good indicator of your overall health. This book will not only help you to heal your prostate, it will also benefit your whole body and substantially reduce your risks of other kinds of diseases.

May you live a long life with great pees to the end!

We all know the power of focus and concentration: If you are using a magnifying glass to light a flame and the lens is too close or too far away from the kindling, nothing happens. If you focus the beam to a tiny point, in an instant you can start a fire.

Similarly, this book can help you focus and in an instant you can stop the disease processes and begin the healing processes. You can heal your prostate!

The information in this book may seem overwhelming. If you feel confused and don't know where to start, then try this:

- *skim the book, then put it down for a while;*

- *read and absorb one chapter at a time;*

- *start with stopping the worse offenders—reduce your toxic food inputs;*

- *then focus on adding new foods and behaviors slowly;*

- *let that become a new habit;*

- *then focus on the next thing.*

The turtle wins the race with slow steady progress. You can do it! One step at a time! It only takes one new thing, one new habit, at a time. That's the way to get to regain your health and truly heal your prostate!

My Story, Part I: How I Came To Know So Much About The Prostate

Hey, I've been there! I could not pee! Not even a drop...

In late May 2003, I woke up in the middle of the night with a fierce urge to pee. I got up and went to relieve myself and nothing would come out! The pain of not being able to go soon became unbearable.

My prostate had squeezed the urethra shut tight (that's the tube that drains the bladder out through to the penis). I was in agony with a bladder filled up *(and continuing to fill up!)* and no way for the urine to come out.

I wanted to go something fierce but couldn't! Nothing would come out no matter how much I strained!

I could not believe what was happening. I was in pain from the urgency to go but not a drop of relief and I was exploding! Yikes! I started walking around and doing deep breathing but nothing changed. I kept trying but to no avail. It just got worse and worse and ever more painful as time passed oh so slowly!

For a few months, I had been waking up more often in the night to go pee, and whenever I was outside and it was cold, I had to go quite frequently. Sometimes I would sit on the seat and it would take a minute or two before urination happened, but I had <u>never</u> experienced what was happening to me in the dark of the night around 5 am! This intense pain was new, and it came out of nowhere.

By 7 am I was in severe extreme pain and starting to realize that maybe this was something serious. What would I do if I couldn't go? I was living on a remote Gulf Island in British Columbia, Canada. There was a health clinic, but it was only open 3 days a week and this awful event happened on a Saturday. I waited some more and by after 8 am I realized I desperately needed help. I was able to reach the doctor at 9 am, and she told me she would meet me at the clinic. I was in agony by now and it took a lot of control to drive the 15 minutes to the clinic. She proceeded to get ready to use a catheter after a few quick examinations. She put the catheter in and at last the urine could escape. The relief was overwhelming!

Over 800 ml came out, about 80% of a quart. I asked the doctor what she thought was happening. She said it was most likely a bladder infection. I asked her if it could be the prostate, as my Dad had had a condition of BPH (Benign Prostatic Hyperplasia) or an enlarged prostate condition. She decided to do a digital rectal exam and said the prostate was enlarged a bit but nothing abnormal for a 55 year old. She started me on antibiotics for the supposed bladder infection, tied the catheter (still in me) to my leg, attached a fluid bag and said to call her on Monday. I did and she had set up an appointment for me with a top urologist in town a few days later. I was instructed to stop at a pharmacy to buy a new catheter before the appointment.

I bought the catheter and went to the urologist's. He proceeded to remove the catheter (that was painful after 5 days inside me), put in a camera catheter to look around (that was even more painful), pulled it out (ouch!), and then opened the package of the catheter that I had bought with his sterile gloves touching the outer wrapper and without cleaning his hands or catheter from possible contaminates proceeded to put the new catheter in me! By now I was feeling awful and hurt from the pain so much!

Next came the news. He said I had BPH. I said, "What is that?" He explained it stood for extreme Benign Prostatic Hyperplasia, also known as Benign Prostatic Hypertrophy, or simply an enlarged prostate. I said, "How could that be? My doctor said it was most likely an infection, and my prostate was only normally enlarged." He said it was definitely enlarged and then did a digital rectal exam of the prostate and again said it is most definitely enlarged. I guess doing that all day made him more expert on the nuances of prostate sizes.

I was now in shock both from the painful examinations and the news. I asked him what to do about the BPH. He said surgery is the only option! This shocked and stunned me. I asked if there was any other choice. He said you could use the catheter! Well let me tell you that having that inside you is a bit of a restriction and carrying a bag of pee around is not fun and games. But surgery!

I asked him when would that happen. He said the waiting list is one year!!! (This is Canada, a country notorious for medical procedure waiting lists.) I could not believe that. A year with a catheter and a bag of pee! OH MY GOSH! He said there is an emergency list and he would try to put me on that. "How long is that?" I asked. "One month" he said. Wow, one month with a catheter!

The examination was over and I left there, got into my car and drove away. In pain and shock, I broke down. I had always been very healthy and was very fit and athletic. I had just run a marathon a year earlier and was in fine shape. I also ate a healthy diet of lots of organic foods and no dairy and meat. So I was at a complete loss. It was all I could do to make it home (a 4-hour journey involving two ferries), where I crawled into bed with my catheter and bag of pee.

This was a life-turning point. I was scared and frightened when I discovered at the urologist's office that I had BPH. I was in complete shock and tears when I drove home. My life felt shattered. I had lost my innocence and faith in myself and my health. And I was only 55 then.

Yet out of that darkness came a new beginning for me. I discovered so much that was waiting to be unearthed. I found the way to real health. I discovered what really is important in this precious gift of a life we are given.

Have faith in yourself! Have courage! For it is possible to renew and heal your prostate naturally. I wish that I had the information and resources you will find in this book back when I had my crisis. Oh, what a difference it would have made!

That is why I have gathered this material to create this book. My hope is that *Healthy Prostate* will empower you and your loved ones to open the door to a new beginning. You deserve vibrant natural prostate health without the fearful side effects of modern medicines, prostate surgery, or radiation.

I awoke the morning after my visit to the urologist who diagnosed me, still in shock from being healthy one day to being diagnosed with an extreme prostate condition, BPH.

My dear friend and neighbor Ann came over and sat with me on the porch as I told her what had happened and of my desire to find a solution. I was scared, fragile, uncomfortable wearing my catheter and bag, and I was extremely vulnerable. She hugged me and told me that she supported me and that she knew I could do it. Having that faith in me was just what I needed to have the courage to move on.

I decided then and there to find out as much as I could before I had the surgery. I began with mainstream medical sources. I soon discovered that there seemed to be several possible treatments.

My urologist had said my options were simple. Have the TURP operation or learn to live with a catheter. I had asked if there were any more options and he said, "No."

Why hadn't he told me about the pills you could take or some of the experimental laser treatments? He could have explained that there are these other options that are not known to work in my extreme condition, if that were the case. Or perhaps he could have said that the government medical plan in Canada does not cover them or that they were unproven...

His not telling me about them led me to the conclusion that he was a poor doctor, a poor communicator (definitely!), and an uninformed one-size-fits-all urologist motivated by fees from surgeries. I did not trust him and decided I had better find out a lot more and fast.

Back at home, I called my local doctor here on the island, about a week into the wearing of the catheter and told her I wanted it taken out so I could see what I could do while waiting for my surgery. I did not tell her I would not go through with the operation. On the 10th day I went to the clinic and had the catheter removed. It hurt after being in there for all that time!

I then went to a quiet lagoon on the ocean and walked slowly along until I had to pee. Would it come out? Could I pee again? Oh, what a relief— I could! At least now I could work on finding solutions from the alternative health field and heal myself!

Little did I know what awaited me!

The literature on mainstream Western medicine was quite extensive at the time, which was in the year 2003. There wasn't quite as much as there is today regarding side effects. Yet, the more I found out, the more I realized that conventional medicine was no cure-all. The side effects were real, quite extensive, and scary for me.

- Incontinence, possible diapers for life at 55! No way!

- Erectile difficulties? No way!

- Impotence! Yikes!

- Retrograde ejaculation (you feel it but it goes into the bladder and not out the urethra).

- Pills that could make you feel terrible.

- Surgeries that could lead to complications.

- Surgeries that could not be successful or would have to be repeated.

These medical options held no attraction for me at all. I just knew that I wanted to find a way to heal my prostate without radical surgery. So next began my search for non-mainstream, alternative approaches to the problem of an enlarged prostate.

This was the path that I was most comfortable with because I had an extensive background in this area. I had radically changed my diet in 1976 when I had a severe, reoccurring stomach flu with high fever—over and over again. I adopted a macrobiotic diet that worked very well for me for years.

A macrobiotic diet consists of whole foods, lots of grains, beans, sea and land vegetables, nuts and seeds, and fruit and limited sweets of only the natural type.

Over the next 30 years this diet was the foundation of my eating. I did add chicken and fish occasionally and some rare dairy, but limited amounts. Never did I know that there was an ingredient, an anti-nutrient, in my diet that was slowly weakening my prostate.

So why in the world with such a seemingly healthy diet could I find myself in such an extreme condition as to have an enlarged prostate requiring emergency surgery and wearing a catheter and collection bag of urine in the meantime?

Something made no sense at all to me. I felt healthy as I always was during these years. I was very athletic: running, swimming, hiking, climbing, skiing and all at an advanced level of expertise. I had just done a marathon in 2001. So what was causing me this condition?

I decided then and there that I would not do the surgery but would find the solutions to heal myself without pharmaceuticals or surgery. I have been successful and you can be too!

Introduction

An "extensive guide to prevent and heal prostate problems, including prostate cancer, BPH enlarged prostate and prostatitis," that's quite a promise on the by-line of the book! But that is exactly what I will share in this hands-on discourse by a 63-year old man who has had the most extreme case of an enlarged prostate himself—my case was so extreme I could not even pee!

Why the title *Healthy Prostate*? Let's face it, if a man has a healthy —prostate, then his life—especially his sex life—will have a lot more get up and go! Hey guys! We've all got one.

You see, men actually do have an extremely complex sexual plumbing system equal to or greater in complexity to women's. Yet we have been led to believe we are simple and uncomplicated critters! Get an erection, have sex. Make babies if you want.

Well, most men have no idea how amazing our plumbing is, and by plumbing, I mean our ability to pee, have sex and produce powerful sperm. The most crucial and sophisticated piece of that puzzle is the prostate.

Heck, I didn't even know what a prostate was until I was in my 50s, and always thought it was a "prostrate"! That's kind of how it will make you feel when your prostate is not working properly... you prostrate!

Well, in this book I will explain exactly what a prostate is and how crucial it is to our health and happiness. That small gland that sits just below the bladder sure has a big impact on men.

You see, there is something in our modern lifestyles that is causing an epidemic of prostate problems for men. Epidemic? Yes! It is estimated that 6.5 million American men visit doctors for an enlarged prostate every year. In 2007, another 223,000 were diagnosed with prostate cancer in the USA. In the same year, 29,000 men died from prostate cancer.

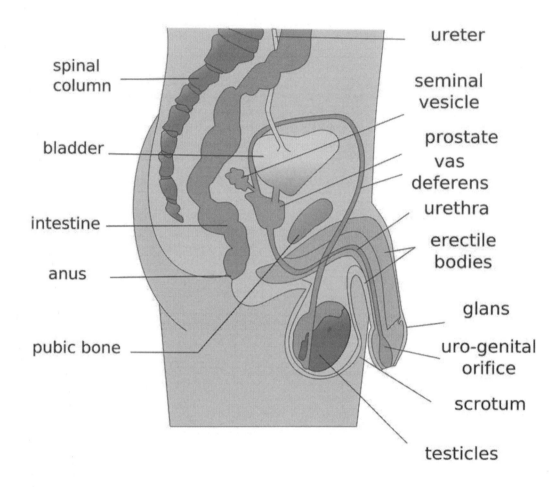

spinal column

bladder

intestine

anus

pubic bone

ureter

seminal vesicle

prostate

vas deferens

urethra

erectile bodies

glans

uro-genital orifice

scrotum

testicles

Most men will face a prostate crisis at some point in their lives, usually after age 50. Knowing this, you have a choice to consider now: should you institute preventive measures before that point? If you already have symptoms of prostate disease or have been diagnosed, there is still time for you to reverse the condition.

Healthy Prostate gives you the insights and tools you need to choose a natural method of preventing or healing your prostate problem. The good news is that these tools work. The bad news is that you have to change—change your habits that led to the disease and invest in learning new skills, techniques and diet changes.

If it is possible, take the stance that this "bad prostate news" is actually a huge blessing in disguise, as it will not only help you heal or prevent prostate problems, but it will also have the positive side effect of making you much more vital, healthy, and you'll also lose weight. Your family will also benefit if they share in the lifestyle changes.

You've heard the stories of prostate problems:

- it's so hard to pee that it hurts;
- dribbling instead of a strong stream;
- waking up many times at night to go pee;
- burning feeling when you do finally pee;
- having to wear adult diapers;
- having to go every 5 minutes for hours on end;
- complete blockage and inability to pee at all;
- needing to use or wear a catheter;
- urgency—the need to go right NOW;
- soreness and infection;
- no more sex, erections or ejaculation;
- words like Enlarged Prostate, Benign Prostatic Hyperplasia, (BPH), Prostatitis; or the more and more common Prostate Cancer.

No fun at all—that's for sure—and you have no control over the symptoms. They can leave you in a miserable state and affect your day-to-day life profoundly.

If you are like most men, you'd rather shy away from the idea of disease—avoid it and hope it doesn't happen to you. But you know the stats: virtually all North American men will have some kind of prostate problem or disease eventually, and prostate disease is striking men earlier in life than before.

The doctors say that prostate disease is the natural course of things as a man ages. In fact, doctors go so far as to say that aging is the cause! But that observation is not as causal as they claim. Correlation is not causation! Prostate diseases are *not* universal as doctors imply. If their claims were true, why is it that in traditional societies in other parts of the world there is virtually no prostate disease? Prostate diseases are extremely rare to a ripe old age in these societies.

For example, there is a remote northern Japanese island called Okinawa. The Okinawans are known for their healthy aging and longevity. The men live active lives right to a very old age… and do *not* suffer prostate ailments!

This is similar to many other Asian enclaves not touched by our Western modern lifestyles. A Western male is 30 to 50 times more likely of getting clinical prostate cancer than an Asian, Indian or African man. An American fares even worse, especially Black Americans.

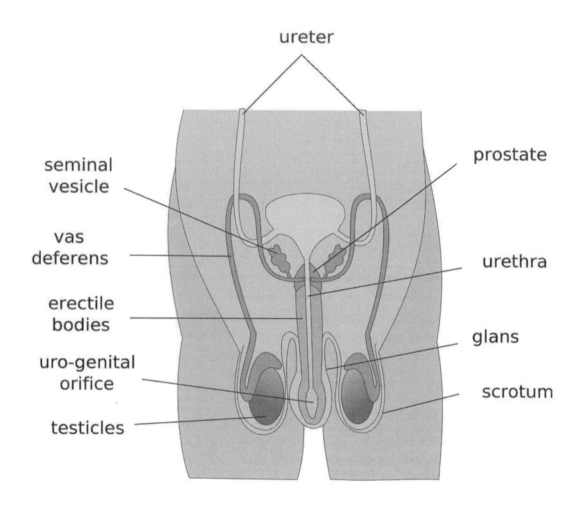

Worse, prostate diseases now happen to younger and younger men. It is not just an old man's disease anymore. We all know people who are having some kind of prostate problem. We need to examine more closely what happens to men as they get older. The Okinawans prove that old age does not cause prostate diseases. It is what we do over the course of our lives that causes our health problems.

Well, there is hope! *Healthy Prostate* provides in-depth information, far beyond what you'll receive from most health practitioners, and it also gives you a big dose of hope. This book gives you explanations that you won't find in doctors' offices or even on natural health websites. *Healthy Prostate* provides real and explicit solutions to prevent and reverse these scary symptoms.

Some of what you will learn in the book is controversial, both because it will challenge you to effect change in your life and because it will contradict many health advocates and pundits who claim they have the answers. I have some of the answers, and I share these answers with you, but more importantly I will show you *how to find your own answers.*

I call the outcome a happy prostate because a healthy prostate allows a man to be healthy and vital and sexual until very old age. And that's what we want!

The good news for women is that the ideas presented will benefit you, too—not just in having a healthy man in your life, but in avoiding many women's diseases as well.

Both men and women will find *Healthy Prostate* to be a blessing for a life of health and vigor. This book will tell you how to achieve that state. There is a catch and some of you will not like it, but I will say it anyway.

You are responsible for your prostate health and, if you so choose, you can be responsible for fixing your prostate problem, but not without effort, self-education and an investment of some time and money.

Disease doesn't just "happen" to you out of the blue. We create the conditions for disease to take place by our lifestyle, intake of toxins, and poor eating habits over many years. Do you want to submit to a life of slowly declining vitality and dependency on your doctor and the drugs your doctor prescribes with all kinds of side effects and a reduced quality of life? Or do you want to seize the moment and make the changes needed to navigate out of the crisis that is facing you now? You decide.

My intent is to show you that it is possible, that you can regain your vitality and prostate health. *Healthy Prostate* will guide you.

First, you have to educate yourself to understand the causes so that you can embrace the necessary lifestyle changes. Making these changes will lead to a far better outcome than faced by the majority of Western men. The rewards of making the effort to change are well worth the costs.

It is possible to have a vibrant and healthy prostate. It is possible to prevent prostate illnesses, and it is *very* possible to change an already existing condition.
If you want a magic bullet and are unwilling to sacrifice your day-to-day lifestyle for a healthy life, then surgery, radiation, chemo and toxic medications may be the only alternative. If you choose this path do not forget the possible incontinence and sexual difficulties that are a by-product of those medical treatments, which will be played down by the doctors.

In addition, remember that the benefits of many prostate operations do not last the rest of your lifetime. You may need treatment *again*, but with much poorer results the second time.

What I offer in this book is not for everyone because of the conscious effort it requires to improve your health and to reverse a condition that may have taken decades to create.

Many ideas here too will be dismissed by the mainstream medical and pharmaceutical sector as "radical and should not be trusted or attempted as it could risk your life." This is partly because they do not know any better (surgeons are taught to operate on people, not to heal or reverse disease through diet and lifestyle) and partly also because it is profitable for them.

If you embrace the concepts in this book, you can be healthy and vital and avoid the risks of today's invasive and ineffective approaches for long-term prostate health.

Natural Prostate Statement

To keep those in the medical field happy, ignore the following personal thoughts and proceed to the Official Disclaimer at the end.

As you know, those in the medical field and drug companies have a virtual monopoly on your health (by law).

Providing health advice is a tricky thing. To protect against liability claims, authors add a disclaimer in health books and on most health websites stating that the reader should always discuss health problems with their doctor, that all information presented is for entertainment or educational purposes only, and that the book or website has not been approved by the FDA.

The government, particularly the food and health branches of the government, assumes that people are not intelligent enough to assess for themselves what is best for them. These agencies value information provided by doctors and do not recognize procedures or information from other sources.

Doctors, sometimes through ignorance or personal financial motives and association with the pharmaceutical industry, often prescribe unnecessary surgery or over-prescribe prescription drugs. Often doctors fail to fully inform their patient of or underestimate the side effects or consequences of recommended drugs, treatments or surgeries.

Take a look at this chart on deaths induced inadvertently by a physician or surgeon or by medical treatment or diagnostic procedures (over 775,000 annually), or the annual *unnecessary* medical events (over 16 million per year). These numbers are staggering: Table Of Iatrogenic Deaths In The United States [http://bit.ly/qEh187]

The pharmaceutical industry also tries to minimize the side effects of their drugs. Pharmaceutical companies push drugs on the public with sophisticated marketing techniques and research grants to doctors and medical colleges even if the drug is harmful. This is apparent from the high number of drug recalls that happen after those side effects manifest in later years.

Your doctor's main interest may be to maximize income, not to improve your health. We have a sickness-care system, not a health-care one. Doctors believe that "prevention" means "early detection," which translates to more money for the doctors and the pharmaceutical industry, and a greater dependency on doctors and drugs. I believe it is wise to get several opinions before allowing anyone to "treat" or "diagnose" you.

In defense of well-meaning doctors, they have not been trained to determine the underlying causes, and the public has not been adequately educated about the responsibility they have for their own health through lifestyle, diet and exercise choices. There simply is a lot of ignorance around the sad state of our health.

Many patients have entrusted their health to their doctors, and doctors play the role they were trained for—diagnose and treat symptoms with the latest medical or pharmaceutical information and procedures.

Maybe there should be a disclaimer like the following on doctors' or medical association websites:

"Please be advised that the information contained herein is based on symptomatic medicine and should not be used to understand the underlying causes of disease. Since we are industry funded and influenced, many side effects of our practices, procedures and surgeries are played down; we allow many drugs to be sold that have not been properly tested for long-term effects on your health.

Please discuss with your alternative health practitioner whether the information is safe and useful to you before undergoing treatments, surgeries, radiation, chemotherapy or taking other possibly toxic drugs."

The medical field and pharmaceutical companies discourage us from using our brains! They want you to believe that alternative health information is not valid and should be taken with a big grain of salt, as it may be harmful to your health (and that their information and procedures are not). They claim that your doctor knows best and has only your interest at heart and that your doctor is truly informed about disease causes and alternative treatments.

Well, I don't believe that, yet—to play it safe—you will find a disclaimer at the end of this section, because I am required to include that statement to protect those in the medical field and protect myself against liability claims.

I do believe that people have the ability to make sense of information, learn from it, and choose what is best for their health. Of course you should check with trusted health advisers who truly have your interest foremost and are open to new ideas. This does include your doctor if he or she is one of the rare ones who look at the whole picture and see you as a whole person.

Yes, there are many bogus fast-buck alternative health sites on the web, but this does not mean all alternative health sites and books are useless or dangerous. You will find doctor-run sites and clinics that are highly promotional that claim amazing results with their latest techniques. These techniques have been shown to be no more effective than regular procedures! Being informed and learning are our right, and people can turn to certified alternative practitioners or whomever for good information and advice. In the end you are the one responsible for your health choices even if you give that right to your doctor.

My views on Western medicine may sound harsh. There is a time and a place for Western medical achievements—like emergencies or acute conditions! Sew me up! Regular doctors can be incredibly useful for traumas and injuries and corrective surgeries. I applaud them for their skills in these areas and for their dedication.

But healing chronic conditions—no way. Chronic conditions develop over time. As such they have real underlying causes. Symptomatic mainstream medicine is light years away from understanding causes and hence true healing.

Physicians are not trained to find causes; they are symptoms experts. Doctors even think that early detection is prevention, when in fact detecting early symptoms still does not address the real underlying causes of the disease or disorder.

Giving people drugs earlier is not preventing diseases and disorders. Making symptoms seemingly go away is not healing, as the underlying causes have not been addressed. In the case of prostate diseases like benign prostatic hyperplasia (BPH) and prostate cancer, surgeries not only have many undesirable side effects, but also often require another surgery later on, which is less effective.

Discover the causes. Change the conditions. Allow healing to happen. That's my formula.

This is not to say that there are not many well-meaning doctors. Some excellent ones also practice alternative healing (at the risk of being disbarred). As in anything, there are good doctors, poor ones and great ones. There are some who are in it for the bucks or feel they are a god because they are *the doctor,* and there are some who genuinely want to help, are open to other healing modalities and put you first. I have been fortunate to meet some of the latter—and it helps cancel out some of the others!

Doctors spend just a minute amount of time being trained on prevention, believing that the symptoms are the cause. For example, doctors believe that as men get older their prostates get larger; thus getting older is the cause. This is ridiculous! There are many cultures in other parts of the world where prostate disease is minimal even among older men!

Alternate views challenge the medical worldview and are not easily accepted by established medical practitioners. What this means in the case of your prostate disease is that doctors will attempt to remove prostate symptoms through medical intervention. Doctors play down the major side effects of these interventions like incontinence or erectile difficulties (bye-bye sex life!) and ignore the dangers of some of their testing procedures (e.g., biopsies that can increase your risk of prostate cancer).

On the other hand, natural healing doctors or natural health consultants like naturopaths look to find the underlying causes of the disease and change those so that the symptoms disappear as a consequence. Doesn't this make sense?

Seek out practitioners who deal with cause, provide clear information, work to prevent disease, and who address you as a whole being who has the innate ability to heal yourself. Educate yourself by reading everything you can find about your health problem, including information from outside the medical establishment. What you find may truly help you!

Now for the official disclaimer!

Official Disclaimer and Legal Notice

- IMPORTANT! PLEASE READ -

MEDICAL DISCLAIMER:

The statements in this book have not been evaluated by the Food and Drug Administration (FDA) or any other government agency of any country. Nothing in this book is intended to treat, cure or prevent any disease. The information presented is not intended to replace the advice of your doctor.

This book is for informational and educational purposes only and is not a substitute for medical advice, diagnosis or treatment provided by a qualified health care provider. It is offered as research and personal opinion to help you understand your current situation and to help you expand your knowledge as a more informed participant in your health choices. You and you alone are responsible for what you do.

Please see your physician before changing your diet, doing a cleanse or treatment, starting a new exercise program, or taking any dietary herbs or supplements of any kind, or following any of the advice or suggestions in this book. It may also be wise to seek the advice of a qualified natural health professional to supplement the advice of your doctor.

The views and statements expressed in this book represent the opinion of the author and should not be considered scientific conclusions. The author does not assume any liability for the information contained herein. Specific medical advice should be obtained from a licensed health care practitioner.

As the reader, you agree that no responsibility or liability will be incurred to the author with respect to any loss, damage, or injury caused or alleged to be caused directly or indirectly by the information contained herein. **If you do not agree to this statement, then please do not read this book!** If you have a severe medical condition, please see a licensed healthcare practitioner.

The information in this book is not intended to replace your doctor and is not to be viewed as medical advice. It is intended as a sharing of knowledge and information from the research and experience of the author. I encourage you to make your own health care decisions based upon your own research and in partnership with your physician.

This book does not give medical advice or engage in the practice of medicine. Under no circumstances do I recommend a particular treatment for your health condition and in all cases I recommend that you consult your doctor before pursuing any course of treatment.

Taking any advice described in this book should be a decision based on personal research and on: the understanding of; the advice and support of; and under the direction of a qualified natural health professional and your doctor or physician or all of them!

Whew – that was a mouthful! Hope you got the message! How ridiculous that such a disclaimer is needed. (I stretched it way out for emphasis.)

Bottom line: you decide if anything here makes sense and then seek whatever other advice and help you want, including the advice of your doctor.

Principles

We are all unique! This is a fundamental statement. There can be no one solution that works for everyone. I will point the way and give you the tools to find your own answers. You are the master, and your diet, supplements and treatments will be unique for you and will change over time as you change and adapt.

So what are the first principles?

1. You are responsible for you. Nobody else, including your doctors, alternative practitioners and well-meaning friends and family have that responsibility. You got where you are, and you will escape from it, by taking charge of your health. You only get one body. You decide how to treat it.

2. You can change what ails you. You must spend time to educate yourself. Good health is one of life's greatest blessings and can be had if you make the effort.

3. It will cost you in the short run—your time, money and effort. So if you want a magic bullet, a magic pill or easy street, then bye for now! This ain't for you! This book is talking about positive changes for a life of health and great sex.

4. If you have been compromising your health by eating the cheapest food you can buy, then you are only cheating yourself. It will cost more to buy quality food, but it will save you immensely in the end. What does it cost you if you develop prostate diseases that destroy your quality of life down the road?

5. Little by little—that's how you got here and that's how you will change. Young men feel invincible and believe that what they do and eat has no effect. Yes, that may be how you feel, but the reality is you are robbing your inner bank bit by bit. You may not notice it for a long time, but then you will find one day that your vault is empty!

6. Just like the frog in the pot who's cooked into soup because he doesn't feel the heat gradually increase and doesn't jump out—you will eventually be faced with a prostate health crisis. So deal with it NOW before it is too late!

7. The good news is that even if you already have prostate disease, there is much you can do to reverse it and turn the temperature down before you, too, become soup!

8. Prevention is best, and it is never too late to start with good, life-affirming habits and a diet that will help you thrive and lose weight.

9. There are many pundits who preach their way as gospel. I have learned from many of them. I do not prescribe to any one path or solution, and I will challenge many experts in this book and will leave you empowered and in charge of your prostate health and life.

So let's get to it!...

Chapter 1: The Prostate

The Male Plumbing System

The word prostate was originally derived from the Greek word "prohistant," meaning to stand in front of. Supposedly Herophilus of Alexandria came up with the word in 335 BC when he used it to describe an organ located in under the bladder. For about 2,300 years that was all anyone knew about the prostate. Only in the past 65 years have doctors started to determine the purpose of the prostate and discover some of the problems that occur with this important gland of the male body.

Picture a walnut, that's about the size and shape of a normal healthy prostate. It's made of muscle, gland (meaning it secretes something), and connective tissue. At birth, the prostate is pea-sized, and it stays that size until you hit puberty. At puberty your hormones cause it to grow. This is significant—I'll explain why later.

Your prostate continues to grow, but this isn't problematic until after mid-age when it can affect urination and cause all sorts of problems. For such a small part of our body, when it is unhealthy it sure can have a big effect!

Imagine the prostate that sits right behind the pubic bone, beneath the bladder, and in front of the rectum, where the combination of muscles, fibrous tissues, and glands all wrapped into one called the prostate is located. Rather than being just one gland, the prostate is actually 20 to 60 clusters of small glands called acini, and each of these connects to the urethra (the pee tube that empties the bladder out through the penis).

All of this is wrapped up in muscular tissue called the prostatic capsule. There are three zones: the peripheral zone, the transition zone, and the central zone. During a digital rectal exam (DRE), a doctor can feel the peripheral zone, which is the largest part of the prostate gland and is closest to the rectal wall. This is the area where most prostate cancers begin (perhaps in part because it is easy for the peripheral zone of the prostatic capsule to absorb toxins from the adjacent rectum).

The transition zone—the smallest area of the prostatic capsule—makes up 5 to 10% of the entire prostate and is usually the area that grows much larger as the result of Benign Prostatic Hyperplasia (BPH) or an enlargement of the prostate. This zone encircles the urethra, so enlargement causes pee problems.

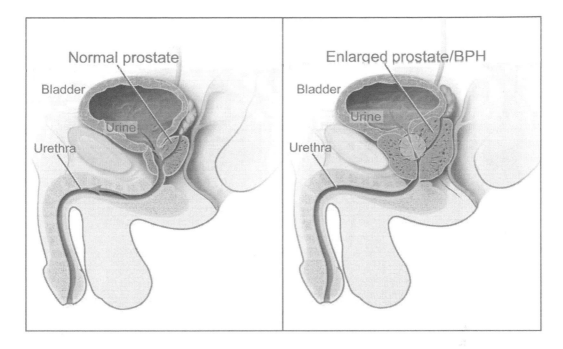

The central zone is where the seminal vesicles attach. They produce about 60% of your ejaculate. The central zone is rarely associated with any health problems, perhaps because of the flushing it gets through ejaculation.

Attached to the prostate are nerves that are responsible for controlling the erectile function of the penis. It is not something you want to tinker with unknowingly! It just might affect your sex life.

Male Sexual Reproductive Organs

Take a look at the components of the male sexual reproductive organs:

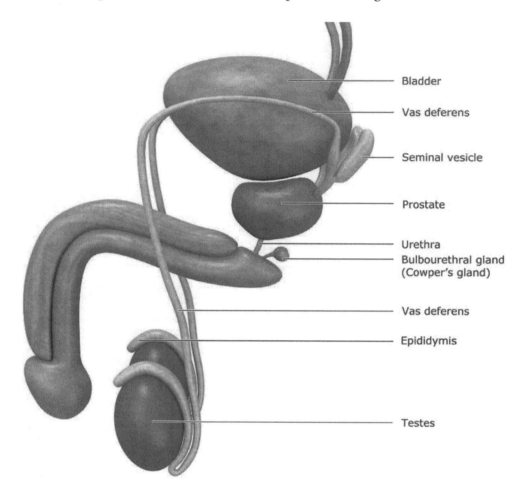

1. **Testicles or Testes - your "balls"**

   The purpose of the **testicles** or **testes** is to produce sperm cells and to hold onto them until they mature. Once matured, the sperm cells leave the testicles and enter what is known as the *epididymis*.

2. **Epididymis**

   This is a tightly coiled small tube attached to each of your testicles. It stores the mature sperm cells and it is where the sperm learn to swim (they need to know how to do this if they want to get to the innermost reaches of a vagina to impregnate an egg—they are wired for that!). Swelling of the testicles occurs during sex, and the testicles also produce fluid, which is added to the sperm cells in the epididymis. This new solution is only 5% of the eventual ejaculate. This solution moves onwards into your *vas deferens* tubes during ejaculation.

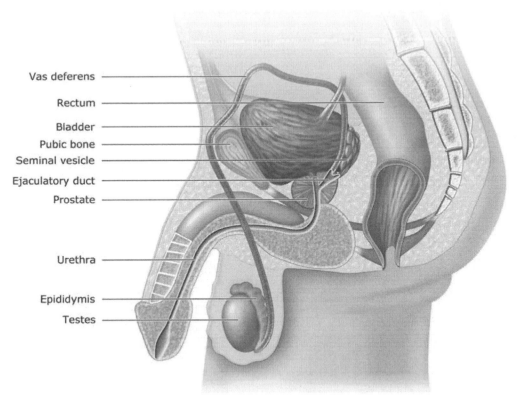

Vas deferens
Rectum
Bladder
Pubic bone
Seminal vesicle
Ejaculatory duct
Prostate
Urethra
Epididymis
Testes

3. Vas Deferens or Seminal Ducts

These two tubes (which match the epididymis and testicles) move the sperm upwards into the pelvic area before ejaculation. The tubes unite with the ducts of the *seminal vesicles* just before the *prostate gland*. By the way, these are the tubes that are cut, tied, or cauterized in a vasectomy to prevent pregnancy. No happy day at the beach for those sperm cells!

4. Seminal Vesicles

These two small glands (the seminal vesicles), located right beside the prostate, produce about 60% of the seminal fluid. During ejaculation this fluid is added to the sperm mixture from the seminal ducts and then proceeds into the prostate gland.

5. Prostate Gland

The prostate gland located below the bladder produces a thin, milky, alkaline fluid, called prostate fluid. During ejaculation, the sperm and the semen mixture from the two seminal vesicles enter into the prostate via the ejaculatory ducts and then pass through the prostate gland while the prostate fluid is added to it. Prostate fluid makes up about 30-35% of the total semen.

During ejaculation the semen is pumped by the muscles of the prostate (remember that the prostate is both a secreting gland and a muscle) through the ejaculatory ducts inside the prostate into the urethra and out through the penis. Aaaaaah! What a journey! That's why it feels so good!

Prostatic fluid is very rich in the minerals zinc, magnesium and potassium. This fluid produced by the prostate serves several functions in reproduction. Prostatic fluid:

✓ encases and protects the sperm with an alkaline fluid;

✓ energizes the sperm cells with its nutrient-rich minerals; and

✓ helps to make the vaginal canal less acidic on the way to the uterus, thereby increasing sperm survival.

6. Cowper's Glands or Bulbourethral Glands

The *Cowper's Glands* are two pea-sized glands beside the prostate deep inside what's called the perineal pouch. They secrete a clear slippery mucous to lubricate the urethra (the pee tube from the bladder) before the semen passes through it. Very helpful!

This alkaline fluid is also known as a pre-ejaculate. Its alkalinity helps neutralize any acidic urine in the dual-purposed urethra, which carries both urine and sperm—but don't worry! A little bladder sphincter blocks any urine from leaving the bladder during sexual arousal. The Cowper's Glands add the final 5% of the ejaculate volume. The Cowper's Glands are also known as the bulbourethral glands.

The urethra now carries the semen out and through the penis on its journey to wherever!

Hey, what about the penis? I didn't forget that! Surprisingly, the penis is just the delivery vehicle! It may be a sexual organ, but it is not a reproductive organ. The same holds true for the prostate erection nerves, which attach to the outside of the prostate. These nerves are responsible for erections once there is some sort of stimulus that triggers them from the brain.

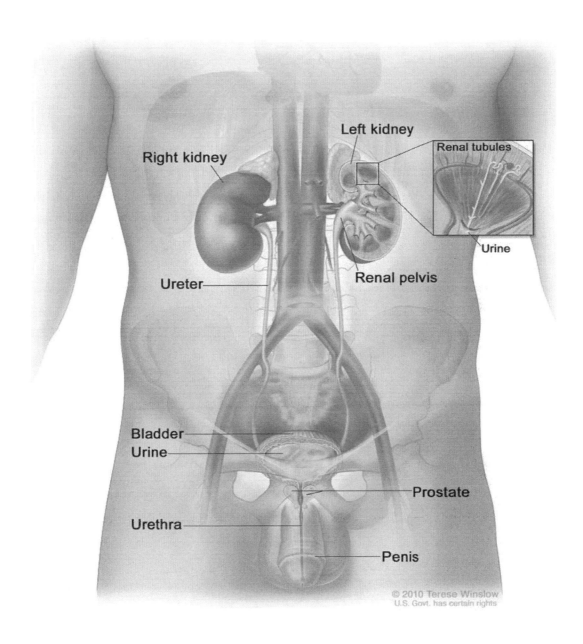

Right kidney

Left kidney

Renal tubules

Ureter

Renal pelvis

Urine

Bladder

Urine

Prostate

Urethra

Penis

© 2010 Terese Winslow
U.S. Govt. has certain rights

The Prostate's Purpose

The prostate has at least seven major functions, some of which we just mentioned:

1. The primary job of the prostate is to produce and secrete some of the alkaline seminal fluids (about 30-35% of the semen ejaculate). Being alkaline, the prostate fluid helps the sperm survive in the acidic vaginal environment. New fluids are continually being created and secreted in the prostate to get ready to transport sperm, and because of this, it is considered to be a gland, as all glands secrete something.

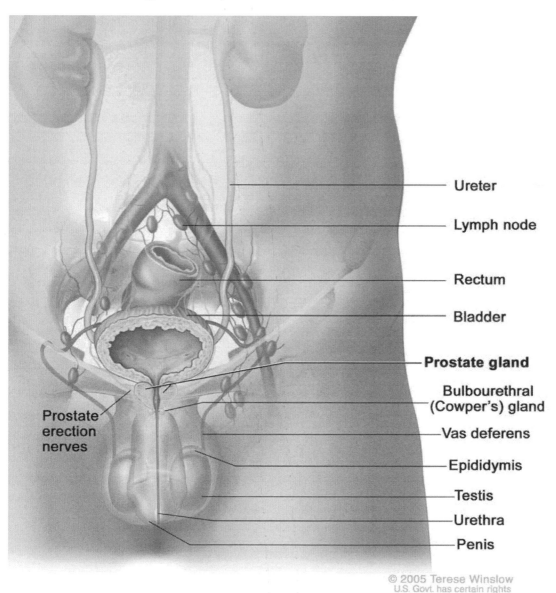

Ureter

Lymph node

Rectum

Bladder

Prostate gland

Bulbourethral (Cowper's) gland

Vas deferens

Epididymis

Testis

Urethra

Penis

Prostate erection nerves

2. The prostate then mixes that fluid with the fluids from the seminal vesicles and the sperm from the testicles. Fluid produced by the prostate and seminal vesicles are delivered into the urethra to transport sperm during orgasm. The urethra is the urine tube running from the bladder and out through the penis.

3. The prostate is also a muscle that pumps the semen out through the penis with enough force to enter into the vagina to help the sperm succeed in reaching the uterus and ensuring procreation of the species.

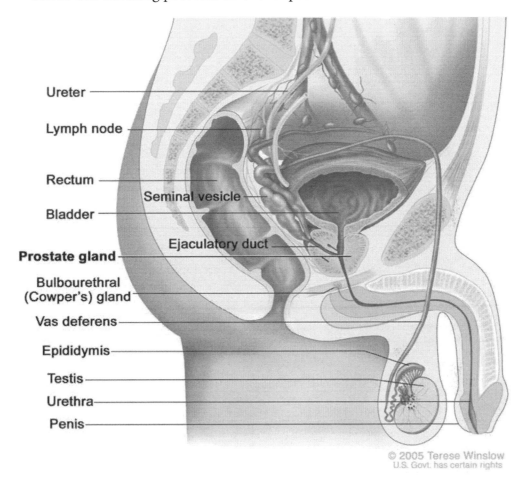

© 2005 Terese Winslow
U.S. Govt. has certain rights

4. An added bonus for males, the pumping action of the prostate sure feels good, making sex a desirable motivation, thus also helping procreation!

5. The prostate's fifth function is as the Male G-Spot. Prostate stimulation can produce an exceptionally strong sexual response and intense orgasm in males that are receptive to this sexual technique. As we will learn later, the ability to control ejaculation at the prostate can also lead to prolonged orgasms.

6. The prostate also filters and removes toxins so that the sperm are protected, which enhances the chance of impregnation and ensures that men seed with the optimum quality of sperm. This is perhaps the prostate's most important function!

7. Lastly, the prostate erection nerves are responsible for erections. If these nerves, which attach to the sides of the prostate, get damaged, then erectile difficulties are guaranteed. That is why many medical procedures (surgery and radiation) have an unwanted side effect of erectile difficulties. These nerves trigger the penis to swell and harden with extra blood flow into it, producing an erection.

Back view of prostate

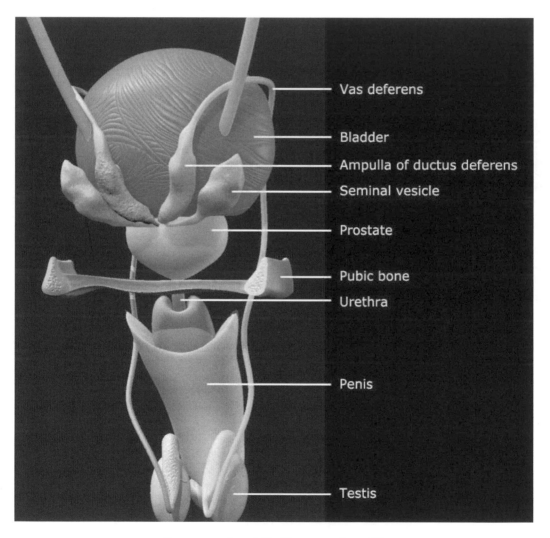

Image courtesy http://www.med-ars.it/

Toxins & Prostate Disease

It is this sixth function of toxin removal that produces such rampant prostate disease. Our prostates are overloaded with toxins because of the horrendous amount consumed in our modern societies from our poor diets, the hidden toxins in the food supply, the bodycare and household products we use, toxins in our water and air, and electromagnetic radiation.

As we age we accumulate more and more toxins, which affects our hormone levels and sensitive prostate tissues. Diseases of the prostate results in the form of enlargement (BPH), infection (prostatitis), or cancer (prostate cancer). The result is simple—an epidemic of prostate disease.

This is why it appears that aging causes prostate disease, but that is nonsense! Doctors are out to lunch on this diagnosis! Aging is not the cause! It is just an observation or correlation.

We cause prostate disease. It just appears more often as we get older because the conditions accumulate over time. But that is NOT the natural state of men. Look at other non-modern cultures that are not exposed to what we are and you will see a dramatic difference in rates of prostate disease—their rate is just a tiny percentage of ours.

Tragically, the prostate disease rates are increasing. It takes a lifetime of poor choices and exposures and, lo and behold, men are almost guaranteed to have prostate problems. No fun. It has a BIG impact on a man's life. It affects your peeing big time and your sex life drastically too.

On top of that, conventional treatments have a long list of serious side effects to take the wind out of your sails! Incontinence and impotence are real and are downplayed by the practitioners who benefit from an ever-rising market for sick prostates. Treating prostate disease is a good business to be in—and it is a huge business!

Give me a break! The conclusion here is not more surgeries, toxic drugs, radiations, and chemos! We must change the causes. We have to take charge of our health and adopt new life-enhancing and toxic-minimizing habits. Otherwise we are doomed to an unhappy ending and, if the rates of prostate disease keep going up, perhaps we threaten the very survival of our species.

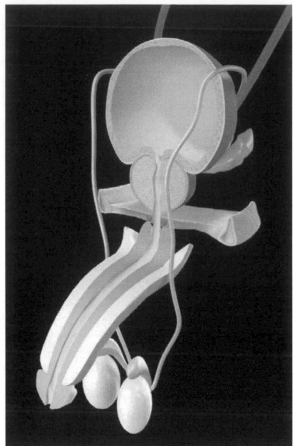

Image courtesy http://med-ars.it/

The Prostate and Peeing

The prostate also influences the urinary system. I found that out when I was unable to pee—not even a drop—because my enlarged prostate squeezed my urethra shut! An enlarged prostate will squeeze the urethra tube and make peeing difficult or even impossible. Any time the prostate is inflamed or irritated, the urethra is directly and negatively impacted. As you can see in the above diagram, the prostate is right under the bladder, and it surrounds the top of the urethra.

In addition, a recent study by the American Foundation for Urologic Diseases links ongoing urinary issues with difficulty getting an erection and enjoying healthy ejaculation. Men with urological diseases have HALF AS MUCH sex than men who are free from infection, and the number of men with an enlarged prostate causing sexual complications is double what doctors had believed. A healthy prostate is necessary to support a satisfying, energetic sex life.

The Prostate and Sex

Because the prostate erection nerves are crucial for a good erection, any intervention through radiation or surgery can easily cause serious problems to achieve this important male activity. The nerves are very delicate and can easily be damaged. Prostate enlargement puts pressure on these nerves, making them less responsive and resulting in diminished erections and erectile difficulties, one of the symptoms of BPH, an enlarged prostate.

Enlargement of the prostate also reduces the volume of ejaculate that is produced in the prostate and that wants to pass through it from the seminal vesicles. The flow can be reduced to a trickle or to none at all! We will talk more about the role of the prostate in achieving maximum sexual pleasure in a later chapter.

The Key to a Healthy Prostate

The prostate is our bellwether. It is the most powerful indicator of the health of the nation (at least the male half!). The prostate serves an important function in the health of the human species. The prostate is key to your masculinity—especially sexual pleasure and potency. The solution is obvious. Stop the causes!

> *"The prostate gland was designed to filter toxins and impurities out of the semen to produce its finest sperm product for conception and reproduction of a strong healthy species. The most common impurity in our systems today are xenoestrogens or man-made estrogen mimicking molecules. These chemicals disrupt the normal male estrogen-testosterone balance and lead to unwanted prostatic growth."*

Jockers, Dr. David. 24 February 2011. "Natural solutions help prostate problems"

www.naturalnews.com/031486_prostate_health_solutions.html [http://bit.ly/pTnXW3] (Accessed 8 May 2011)

Many herbal supplements on the natural health market are designed to ease enlarged prostate symptoms and to help reduce the size of the prostate.

However you must realize this: **Food is the most important medicine—it is the key to turning your prostate health around.**

Yes, combined with herbal supplements and other treatments, it is very possible to reverse your condition, but not without effort and change on your part.

Have you seen the ads: Miraculous Prostate Formulas or guaranteed cures with their supplement? In my opinion, these prostate supplements are oversold and hyped. Without changes to diet and your body's energy system, which addresses the causes, these supplements may be a waste of time and money.

One advantage of prostate supplements is that they have fewer side effects than drugs but there are still some potential side effects, including worsening of your symptoms, because there could be herbs in the mixture that irritate your prostate no matter how great their properties sound.

That is why you must personally test everything you take to see if it is harmful. I will show you how to do that later on. I speak from experience here because I have had negative reactions to many supposed healthful herbs and supplements. That was before I knew how to test them. With the ability to test food and herbal remedies, your diet, lifestyle, and herbs can be very effective, and you can avoid medical treatments that can have serious consequences.

Chapter 2: Toxic Chemicals and Bioconcentration

One hundred years ago the chronic diseases we have today were extremely rare. Now, with tens of thousands of chemicals in the environment—on our soil, in our food, in our bodycare and cosmetic products, in the air, and in the water—it is no wonder we suffer so many ailments.

Today we eat artificial foods that have had the life force stripped from them and toxic chemicals added in when the food was grown or when it was processed, and usually both. Those toxins work there way into our bodies, eventually causing serious disease. In the case of the prostate, we get enlargement, infection, and cancers.

Bioconcentration occurs when toxins—hormones, pesticides, herbicides and antibiotics—accumulate up the food chain. Cows eat grains that were sprayed with pesticides and herbicides and drink water with leached runoff toxins. These toxins start to concentrate in the bodies of the cows as they grow older. If the cows are also fed genetically modified (GMO) grains like corn or soybean products that have genes alien to the animals added into the grains, then more toxins are produced as the cows try to assimilate the GMO food. Hormones are often given to cattle to fatten the cows up. The estrogen in the hormones fed to cows are one of the causes of prostate enlargement and "man boobs." Too much estrogen is dangerous.

By the time we drink the milk or eat the dairy products, the food is laden with serious chemical residues that start the same bioconcentration in us! The same happens when we eat the meat. We become toxic ourselves, and cancers can easily find a home. Cancer is the body's reaction to the toxins.

Antibiotics fed to cattle also concentrate in the milk as well as the meat. These antibiotics strip our intestines of good bacteria and cause bloating and weight gain, as we are unable to digest properly the food that we eat. Obesity results. Our livers get filled with toxins and we become a host for disease.

Commercial milk and dairy have high levels of insulin-like growth factor (IGF-I), which can significantly increase your risk of prostate cancer.

We also ingest estrogen-mimicking pesticides and residues on the sprayed foods we eat. These estrogen-mimicking chemicals arc also present in bodycare and household products. These chemicals cause prostate problems and male breast enlargement. They weaken the body, reduce sex drive, and cause weight gain.

If you think the chemicals in your detergents and bodycare products arc harmless, think again! Your skin is the body's largest organ and will absorb what is put on it. Many of the ingredients in these products are toxic soups of cancer-causing chemicals. Yes, when you are young or gifted with a strong constitution you may not notice the effects until years later, but it will happen, and then you will wonder why!

Harvard University's Environmental Health Perspectives published results in January 2011 showing that 99% of all pregnant women in the USA test positive for multiple neurotoxic and carcinogenic substances, many banned for years. Sadly this toxic load is passed on to their newborns. In all women tested, the concentrations were higher for most chemicals than considered safe.

Bisphenol-A (BPA) is a chemical that mimics the female sex hormone estrogen and is used to make all kinds of products from plastic baby bottles to the linings of tin cans. So watch what you eat. BPA was recently banned in Canada because of its toxicity. Exposure to BPA is known to cause hormone imbalance and endocrine disruption, infertility, sperm destruction, heart disease, diabetes, and cancer, as well as obesity.

It seems that governments will only act after the evidence is overwhelming, but in the meantime decades pass while we poison ourselves until we have chronic diseases and sick prostates!

> *"Toxins are everywhere—from household cleaning products to plastics in our kitchen-ware, phthalates and Bisphenol-A in our plastic water bottles, and even in our tap water and air supply. We live in a sea of toxins, and a large body of growing evidence shows that these toxins are, in part, responsible for the epidemic of disease we see in the twenty-first century. Toxic exposures affect the health of all brains, young and old. We must also deal with all the by-products and toxic metabolic wastes created by our own bodies."*

> Hyman, Mark MD. The UltraMind Solution: Fix Your Broken Brain by Healing Your Body First [http://amzn.to/nmMElp]

Well listen up, change now or pay the price down the road. Prostate disease develops slowly and won't be detected until symptoms develop. Time is its ally. That is why at midlife men often face prostate ailments. Prevention is so much easier than reversing the damage. **Proper prostate nutrition is crucial**. It is never too early to start or too late to reap the benefits.

Is the solution to prostate disease to take mainstream medicine? Can you counter the toxins in your body by adding more toxins in medical drugs, chemo, or radiation? For me, that is insane.

The solution for too many bioconcentrated toxins is to change your inputs, not to have surgeries or to take more toxic chemicals in pills for your prostate. Stop using toxic products and eating contaminated food. Yes, I use the word "contaminated"— it is a crime that we have government inspectors who pass on this food as safe. Eat better food and cleanse the toxins out of your body, and give your body a chance to heal.

Diet is everything. It is the foundation, and *everything else* is an add-on. Get your diet together and *everything else* will fall into place. Replace the bad food with good food. Eat real food and avoid manufactured, adulterated factory foods. Eat food as nature intended. We'll talk a lot more about this later on. Yes, it will cost more to protect your health, but it will be a lot less in the long run when you are free from prostate diseases. **It costs more... but it saves you money and just may save you!**

Chapter 3: Diseases of the Prostate

There are three basic prostate diseases or problems: enlargement, infection, and cancer. The technical names for these are:

- Enlarged prostate, BPH, or benign prostatic hyperplasia

- Prostatitis

- Prostate cancer

Think about it for a moment—do you really think disease just strikes out of the blue? Or do we play a huge part in the:

- choices we make daily (e.g., food, bodycare and household products and cooking methods)

- toxins we ingest from our contaminated food supply

- emotional stresses on our minds and bodies

- inoculations, antibiotics, and pharmaceuticals we have taken over a lifetime

- quality of the water we consume every day

- bad health habits and lack of exercise we accumulate over time

- and many other daily decisions we make that impact us whether we are aware or not of their health consequences?

Well, if you think it just strikes you and "woe is me," then this book will challenge your viewpoint.

If you do accept the premise that you play a huge part, then you have taken the first big step. You are on the path to acceptance and responsibility, excellent starting points for the blessings of a health challenge. I call it a blessing because, if embraced, you will be able to renew and revitalize yourself.

This book will help you learn about your health and really transform yourself, leaving you stronger and healthier than ever before, shedding years as your body finally becomes nourished from the inside out, instead of poisoned from the outside in.

Illness can be a blessing if you look for the gifts of increased awareness and self-growth through the acceptance of your ultimate responsibility for your health. Now you have a chance to change the conditions that caused your prostate problem and heal.

It is your choice to either embrace the blessings of your symptoms or go the route that will leave you with serious side effects with a possible reoccurrence of disease.

So enter the dragon and learn what your prostate has to teach you!

Disease and Illness

Chronic disease, in general, is something that is created over years and decades. There is a widespread belief among mainstream consumers that it is something that just strikes spontaneously *without any real cause*. This view is reinforced by conventional Western medicine. The fact is most of us are creating disease every day of our lives. To live healthy and to live longer we simply need to stop creating disease.

Most of us are not in tune enough with our bodies to know if we are facilitating the conditions for disease or not. Disease and its contributing factors are controllable. These include what you eat, what chemicals you expose yourself to, how much exercise you get, your prevalent state of mind, and what supplements you take or don't... just as I have already documented.

To be specific, nutritional deficiencies such as lack of calcium or vitamin D can trigger disease. Dietary excess of any particular food or food group can cause an imbalance. Toxins will wreak havoc throughout your body. Emotional states such as stress, anxiety, and anger will spread into tissues and create *dis-ease* in the physical body.

There is plenty of literature about this. Dr. Thomas Lodi, a brilliant cancer doctor in Arizona, wrote a book called "*Stop Making Cancer*" [http://bit.ly/nbAJB5] and Dr. Gabor Mate in Canada has a well-researched and insightful book called "*When the Body Says No.*" [http://amzn.to/r4a5ic] Somehow, the mainstream media still isn't getting the message.

Cancer, diabetes, heart disease and Alzheimer's are all examples of some of the most common degenerative diseases around today. Diseases take many years to grow and expand. A malignant tumor can quietly grow inside a woman for a whole decade before being picked up in a mammogram.

Similarly, prostate problems don't just appear one day. Even though it seemed that way to me when I woke up in the middle of the night completely unable to pee, I know now that it was brewing inside for quite a while. That night was like a left hook from somewhere, and I didn't even know I was in a fight!

Even if you think you don't have a problem now, it could be building if you are not following good prostate habits and good health habits in general. The earlier you can adopt healthy prostate habits, the much greater the chances of avoiding conditions later on. I discuss these later in this book.

The troubling thing is that prostate problems are happening to more and more men and at an earlier age than before. Men in their 40s and 50s are now demonstrating prostate problems, and this was very rare a generation ago.

So why do doctors tell their patients, "There was nothing you could have done to prevent this"? It may be because doctors don't want to give people the idea that, ultimately, they have the ability to control their own health. Perhaps even more often, doctors don't believe that people can control their health.

The medical industry creates the dependency—of us on them—by implying that disease is random, spontaneous, and that the medical authorities have control over health, disease, and treatment.

Well, dear reader, look into the mirror. You are the one responsible, and you can be the one who changes course to healing and prevention.

Let's take a look at the conventional medical insights and treatments of prostate problems as our starting point. If you visit your doctor or urologist, this information will help you understand their recommendations. Just remember that conventional treatments are not the only way to change your condition. My insights and views on natural medicine will follow.

Benign Prostatic Hyperplasia – BPH - Enlarged Prostate

What is BPH?

BPH is a non-cancerous growth of the prostate gland. This now bigger prostate squeezes the urethra pee tube that it surrounds, causing a whole range of symptoms from very mild to extreme.

As the prostate grows larger, it presses against the urethra like a clamp on a garden hose. The bladder wall becomes thicker and irritated. The bladder begins to contract more often even when it contains small amounts of urine, causing more frequent urination. As the prostate grows, it applies more pressure to the urethra. Eventually, the bladder weakens and loses the ability to empty itself, and so begins a whole range of uncomfortable to painful symptoms.

The extreme version is called *acute urinary retention*—when you are unable to pee at all. It is the most painful of the symptoms and can be relieved by the insertion of a catheter. If acute urinary retention is unaddressed, death can result in about two days.

It is possible to have prostate enlargement and prostate cancer at the same time, but having BPH does not increase your chances of developing prostate cancer. It is very rare to have both conditions.

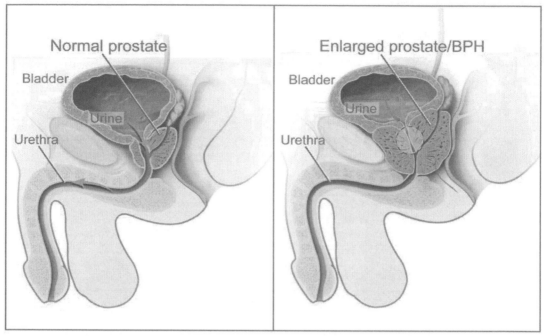

This video by MedlinePlus about the enlarged prostate gland [http://1.usa.gov/pFnvHd] provides a fairly standard medical outlook on BPH. Most men with BPH have minor symptoms initially, but with time the symptoms can and do get worse. Here is what you should look out for:

✓ Dribbling at the end of urinating

✓ Inability to urinate (acute urinary retention)

✓ Incomplete emptying of the bladder

✓ Unable to voluntarily control urination (incontinence)

✓ Needing to urinate two or more times per night (nocturia)

✓ Pain with urination or bloody urine (can be infection)

✓ Slowed or delayed start of the urinary stream

✓ Very frequent urination

✓ Straining to urinate

✓ Strong and sudden urge to urinate

✓ Weak urine stream

The effects of BPH and its symptoms can vary from minor to major on a man's lifestyle, especially when away from the easy convenience of your bathroom. As the condition worsens it will also impact your sex life. It can make it harder (!) to get an erection ☹ and can result in much lower semen ejaculation to none at all. Prostate cancer is the leading form of male cancer, but an enlarged prostate (or BPH) is the most common prostate disorder, and it impacts your quality of life greatly.

What Causes BPH?

One conventional theory of the cause of BPH is that it results from a decline in the production of testosterone, the body's main male hormone. Interestingly, castrated men don't get BPH.

As men age, production of male hormones is reduced, but not production of estrogen, which is believed to be responsible for the enlarged prostate tissues (although others think it is the testosterone that causes it... we'll discuss this later). This is similar to how women have a higher ratio of testosterone to estrogen when they go through menopause. In a sense, BPH could be seen as part of a man's version of menopause.

This change in hormones, and therefore prostate enlargement, is strongly correlated to aging. By age 40, the prostate in many men is the size of an apricot, much bigger than a walnut, the normal size. At this larger apricot size, the prostate is just starting to press on the urethra and bladder. The symptoms may go unnoticed. By 60, the enlarged prostate is the size of a lemon! More than half of Western men ages 60 and over will have BPH. After age 80 BPH goes up to 90%.

Solution on wish list—don't get older! But that wouldn't work because the biggest misconception of all is that aging causes prostate disease. Of course, if we are doing things that accumulate slowly and cause prostate conditions, time and/or aging will make it apparent. But aging is NOT the cause! We know this because 90-year-old men in rural Asia have a very low rate of prostate disease.

So beware of a lot of the information that comes next because believing prostate disease is a natural part of the aging process is a commonly held view. Later I will explain what I believe are the true underlying causes—not just the symptoms.

Many of these so-called mainstream causes are not really causes, instead they are observations couched as causes. For example, it's generally accepted that hormones are related to BPH. However, no one can absolutely say with confidence why hormones lead to prostate enlargement.

What has been observed in Western men is this:

- The male hormone, testosterone, peaks during adolescence.

- Testosterone production decreases dramatically by about 55.

- The decline of testosterone causes other hormones like estrogen to be released, which then stimulates further production of hormones.

- Hormones like estrogen can't prevent drops in testosterone.

- An increasing ratio of female estrogen hormones to male testosterone hormones can result in an increase of di-hydro-testosterone or DHT. DHT can irritate and inflame the prostate sometimes causing the prostate to enlarge.

So what causes these changes? Is BPH inevitable and universal across all men worldwide? No, it isn't! Many remote cultures have virtually no prostate disease. Rural Asians in particular have a dramatically lower incidence of prostate disease. Here are some common medical viewpoints or facts about prostate enlargement:

- The likelihood of developing an enlarged prostate increases with age. (Mostly in Western societies.)

- BPH is so common that it has been said all men will have an enlarged prostate if they live long enough. (Mostly in Western societies.)

- A small amount of prostate enlargement is present in many men over age 40 and more than 90% of men over age 80. (Again, mostly in Western societies.)

- Genetic predisposition, environment, diet and lifestyle are also factors of BPH.

  MedlinePlus. "Prostate Diseases"
  www.nlm.nih.gov/medlineplus/prostatediseases.html
  [http://1.usa.gov/qmTmva] (Accessed 28 June 2011)

BPH Symptoms

Most Western men will experience an ever-enlarging prostate. How will you know when it's happening to you? Your peeing will show you. Difficulties ensue as the prostate starts to grow and presses up against the bladder. The enlarged prostate starts to squeeze the urethra, eventually restricting the flow out from the bladder.

This decreases your ability to empty the bladder. Retained urine makes an environment ripe for bacterial growth and infection. Urine can back up into the kidneys further spreading infection. More severely, the infection can spread into the blood. A complete inability to release urine is known as acute urinary retention, which is life threatening and extremely painful.

Another symptom of prostate disease is the decline in sperm count. Toxins are entering our sperm and cannot be removed fast enough by our ailing prostates. Sperm count has dropped about 50% over the past 50 years.

So what happens from the perspective of a man with an enlarged prostate? In layman's terms, here are some prostate problem signs:

- ✓ You have to go pee again and again, frequently, because your bladder just doesn't seem to empty enough and it constantly feels full.

- ✓ Your sleep suffers because you wake up at night more and more often to pee.

- ✓ Sometimes you have to pee so bad, but it is hard to start.

- ✓ Once you do finally pee it sometimes stops and dribbles until it starts again.

- ✓ You obsess about where to find the next bathroom once you leave home.

✓ Sometimes your pee feels burning hot while you go because you have to go so badly, but only a little comes out   it hurts so much you could scream!

✓ Other times, the urge comes so suddenly and powerfully and is almost impossible to hold back for very long—you hope you get to the can in time!

✓ When you have sex, ejaculation hurts and/or only a tiny amount of semen comes out.

✓ The ejaculate does not have the normal creamy white color—it is clear and there isn't much of it.

✓ Drops of blood appear in your semen or when you pee.

✓ You find yourself uncontrollably dribbling into your underwear.

✓ You suddenly find yourself needing to go urgently, desperately, but nothing comes out! Yikes this is the worst!

✓ Sadly, these symptoms result in erectile difficulties in some men and reduced sex drive, limiting your ability to have and sustain an erection and have ejaculations

☹ Sad is how you feel at best!

Men with partial blockages will find that certain environments or activities inhibit the urethra or bladder from relaxing and releasing pee, such as cold temperatures or a long period of not moving. Taxi drivers and truck drivers are examples of professions with higher risk of enlarged prostates. Add office workers to the list! Sometimes the opposite can happen—the cold temperature makes you go pee even more often.

Some men will not know they have an enlarged prostate because they are unaware of these symptoms. Then it comes as a surprise when they have an examination by a doctor. Some men will not experience any enlarged prostate symptoms at all... until they suddenly find it hard or impossible to go pee. This condition, called acute urinary retention, can be triggered by taking over-the-counter medicines for colds and allergies, excessive drinking, cold temperatures, or prolonged periods of sitting.

If you sit a lot all day, make sure you get up to move every hour and if you can't, you must do prostate exercises while you sit. See Chapter 19 for information on prostate exercises.

Dealing With the Symptoms of BPH

In one-third of the cases of mild BPH the prostate heals itself without treatment. The other two-thirds of the cases require treatment at some point.

For those who experience the whole gamut of symptoms, you will find some of these symptoms are manageable while others can be painful, embarrassing, or outright scary. For example, blood in the urine is caused by pushing or straining to pee—and it is alarming!

Serious conditions can result if symptoms are left to progress: bladder and kidney damage, infections of the urinary tract, bladder stones, acute urinary retention, incontinence, and erectile and ejaculatory dysfunction.
Welcome to the world of men's prostate problems!

Each man will experience BPH differently. We all have our own unique combination of symptoms. It is important to recognize symptoms early and to start changes to prevent the symptoms from worsening, heal your body, and reverse the damage. Ignore all the fear mongering around the prostate.

The message is clear—your health is your wealth—and prostate health is the key to your functioning as a vital man who is able to have a full life and a great sex life into old age.

There is a lot to learn, particularly about diets, because most so-called "healthy" diets may still lead to diseased prostate conditions. In fact, that is exactly what happened to me! Every person is different, and you need to learn how to tell what foods are right for you. I will show you how to test foods so that you can know what foods are right for you to eat.

In the meantime do the following:

- ✓ Drink less after supper so that you need to pee less during the night. Avoid caffeine, as it is a diuretic that will make you go pee.

- ✓ Pee when you have to. Try not to wait.

- ✓ Drink less alcohol, which increases urine production.

- ✓ Stop taking decongestants. They can cause the muscles that control urine flow from the bladder into the urethra (the urethral sphincter) to tighten, making peeing more difficult. In fact it can trigger complete blockage all of a sudden in men with BPH.

- ✓ Exercise regularly. Inactivity causes the bladder to retain urine. Just do a few bursts of intense exercise for 30 seconds, like walking as fast as you can, doing some push-ups, or running a sprint.

- ✓ Do kegel exercise while sitting. Squeeze the pubococcygeus or PC muscle (more on this later). This massages the prostate. Stand more and move more!

- ✓ Keep warm in the winter. Cold weather can either lead to urine retention or increase your urgency to pee or both.

- ✓ Wear loose underwear or boxer shorts. Excess heat in the scrotum is not good for the prostate.

- ✓ Eat more vegetables especially cruciferous vegetables such as cabbage, broccoli, and cauliflower. These veggies help to reduce excess estrogen.

It is crucial for men to become informed about prostate symptoms so that they can take preventative actions earlier on. It is also important to have regular checkups with your doctor, including a prostate exam and urinary flow tests.

BPH Conventional Treatments

This section is all about the world of conventional treatments so you can understand that viewpoint. Read on to decide if that approach makes sense for you. Talk to your doctor and even take a list of possible treatments with you to your doctor's appointment so that you are informed and can ask questions. Several conventional treatments are available. Educate yourself so that you can find the treatment or solution that's best for you.

Watchful Waiting: This is described in other parts of the book with other prostate diseases. If your symptoms are manageable, you may choose to live with them rather than take pills every day or have surgery. To make sure your condition isn't getting worse, schedule regular check-ups with your doctor. With watchful waiting, you can be ready to choose a treatment as soon as you need it.

Medicines: There are several medicines to shrink or relax the prostate to keep it from blocking the bladder opening.

- Alpha 1-blockers (doxazosin, prazosin, tamsulosin, terazosin, and alfuzosin) relax the muscles of the bladder neck and prostate. This allows easier urination. Most people treated with alpha 1-blocker medication find that it helps their symptoms.

- Finasteride and dutasteride lower levels of hormones produced by the prostate, which reduces the size of the prostate gland, increases the urine flow rate, and decreases symptoms of BPH. It may take 3 to 6 months before you notice much improvement in your symptoms. Potential side effects related to the use of finasteride and dutasteride include decreased sex drive and impotence.

  Enlarged Prostate: MedlinePlus Medical Encyclopedia [http://1.usa.gov/pS8Bwq]

Nonsurgical Procedures:

Doctors can now remove parts of the prostate during nonsurgical day procedures, which means no overnight stay, in a clinic or hospital. Thin tubes are inserted through the urethra to deliver controlled heat to small areas of the prostate. A gel may be applied to the urethra to prevent pain or discomfort. Several transurethral procedures (sticking a catheter instrument up your penis) are available for BPH:

- **TUMT** (transurethral microwave thermotherapy) destroys prostate tissue by using a probe in the urethra to deliver microwaves.

- **TUNA** (transurethral needle ablation) destroys excess prostate tissue with electromagnetically generated heat by using a needle-like device in the urethra.

- **Prostatic Stents** used occasionally to keep the urethra open.

- **TUVP** (transurethral electrovaporization) uses an electrical current to sculpt out part of the prostate.

- **WIT** (water-induced thermotherapy) uses hot water to destroy the tissue blocking the urethra to open the channel.

- **ILC** (interstitial laser coagulation) uses a laser to destroy tissue and reduce the size of the prostate.

- **HoLEP** (holmium laser enucleation of the prostate) uses a special laser wavelength that is highly absorbed by water and can cut soft tissue. This treatment can be used for very large prostates that would normally require surgery.

Surgical Procedures:

- **TUIP** (transurethral incision of the prostate) widens the urethra by making a few small cuts in the bladder neck, where the urethra joins the bladder, and in the prostate gland itself.

- **TURP** (transurethral resection of the prostate) is the procedure used for 90% of all prostate surgeries for BPH—it is the standard operation. With TURP, an instrument called a resectoscope is inserted through the penis to remove the excess tissue. It is less traumatic than open forms of surgery.

  TURP has a high risk (80%) of retrograde ejaculation, which is when semen works its way back into the bladder instead of coming out the tip of the penis. Other risks: impotence, incontinence, blood loss, and urinary tract infection. This procedure is now available using lasers. Read more here: Transurethral resection of the prostate: MedlinePlus Medical Encyclopedia [http://1.usa.gov/rlEp8D]

- *Simple or Partial Prostatectomy* is the removal of the inner portion of the prostate through an incision in the lower abdomen. This is an invasive surgery used for very large prostate glands to remove the enlarged part of the prostate gland. This procedure is open surgery performed while the patient is under general anesthesia. (This surgery should not be confused with a radical prostatectomy, in which the entire prostate gland is removed for men with prostate cancer.) Read more about BPH and medical procedures here:

  Enlarged Prostate: MedlinePlus Medical Encyclopedia [http://1.usa.gov/pS8Bwq]

  Benign Prostatic Hyperplasia - Symptoms, Treatment and Prevention [http://bit.ly/pWEEBh]

- Read these industry-funded sites that explain all the different procedures in greater depth. *Buyer beware* as despite the claims to being superior, many of these private "state of the art" procedures have not been proven over time to be superior to the standard TURP:

www.ProstateDiseases.org

BPH Treatment Options [http://bit.ly/pd1mII5]

All of these procedures have serious potential side effects that can impact your life as much as or more than your existing symptoms. Doctors downplay these side effects, as they have a vested interest in the procedures AND are not informed about any alternative methods. (Do not be surprised if your doctor dismisses alternative treatments as useless.)

Conclusion: get castrated... no more prostate problems! Too bad there are other side effects like no more sex.

The Side Effects of Conventional Treatment

If you think that BPH operations are harmless, think again. In my experience, side effects are not fully explained and are minimized. Why? Because doctors:

- think they are providing the best treatment based on what they know and what they have available to offer,

- often directly benefit financially from the procedures, and

- are unaware of any other options.

If they do know of alternative options, they could risk losing their medical license by offering those alternative treatments.

All of the conventional treatment options I mentioned in this chapter have consequences of: major discomfort to pain; possible incontinence to impotence and sexual difficulties, including retrograde ejaculation (no ejaculate comes out the penis—it goes back into the bladder); and often the treatment will need to be repeated at a future date with scarring occurring with each attempt, which makes each procedure less successful and exacerbates the side effects.

Fun, fun, fun till Daddy took the T-bird away!

If you follow your urologist's advice, he will play down the side effects of BPH medications like Flomax, Avodart, and Finasteride (trademarked by Merck under the name Proscar). So what aren't they telling you? Just take a look at the list of side effects.

Partial list of side effects of BPH drugs (from standard medical literature):
- ✓ breast enlargement or tenderness
- ✓ abnormal ejaculation or none
- ✓ decreased sex drive
- ✓ dizziness
- ✓ headache
- ✓ fatigue
- ✓ impotence

- ✓ no erections
- ✓ diarrhea
- ✓ back pain
- ✓ sore throat
- ✓ decreased libido
- ✓ itching
- ✓ hives
- ✓ difficulty breathing or swallowing, wheezing
- ✓ unexplained skin rash
- ✓ erectile dysfunction

Finasteride is prescribed on the belief that it reduces the incidence of prostate cancer by 25%, yet the Norris Cancer Institute showed that patients taking Finasteride had an increased risk of getting the aggressive and fatal form of prostate cancer by 300%!

Another study showed that Proscar/Finasteride increased the chance of getting male breast cancer by 34%.

The Food and Drug Administration panel of cancer experts voted 17-0 with one abstention stating that <u>the risks of Merck's Proscar outweighed its benefits</u>. In a similar vote, the panel voted 14-2 with two abstentions against GlaxoSmithKline PLC's Avodart. <u>Both drugs are already approved to treat enlarged prostate</u>.

FDA panel rejects drugs to prevent prostate cancer [http://yhoo.it/nSN6jA]

Why are these drugs allowed to be sold? Because they are profitable.

Many people accept the risks and try these conventional procedures. It was not my choice. I decided it was much more important to address the causes and make changes so that my overall health improved and my prostate symptoms eased as a result.

This is a major choice for you dear reader! How do you want to live? Do you want to surrender to the medical profession that pays no attention to other modalities and alternative ways of healing, writing them off as valueless?

My intention in writing this book is to educate you about your prostate, give you mainstream information and treatment options so you can evaluate those options, and then offer you alternatives so you can evaluate those options as well. I then provide you with a roadmap that you can customize for your own optimum prostate health.

If you want to boggle your pee brain (pun intended!), then you can read some mainstream literature here: PubMed [http://1.usa.gov/qaw7q3]

Try searching under BPH and see what you get, or search for prostate cancer, and you'll find thousands of articles on each search!

To read more about natural insights and treatments for the prostate, then visit the NaturalPedia website links below.

Prostate – NaturalPedia Search Results [http://bit.ly/oIlsW8]

BPH – NaturalPedia Search Results [http://bit.ly/oIlsW8]

International Prostate Symptom Score

The International Prostate Symptom Score (IPSS) is an international questionnaire. The IPSS questions will help you assess the severity of your prostate symptoms. Answer each question honestly, and then total your score at the end.

1. Incomplete emptying: Over the past month, how often have you had the sensation of not emptying your bladder completely after you have finished urinating?
0 = not at all
1 = less than 1 time in 5
2 = less than half the time
3 = about half the time
4 = more than half the time
5 = almost always

2. Frequency: Over the past month, how often have you had to urinate again less than 2 hours after you finished urinating?
0 = not at all
1 = less than 1 time in 5
2 = less than half the time
3 = about half the time
4 = more than half the time
5 = almost always

3. Intermittency: Over the past month, how often have you stopped and started again several times when urinating?
0 = not at all
1 = less than 1 time in 5
2 = less than half the time
3 = about half the time
4 = more than half the time
5 = almost always

4. Urgency: Over the past month, how often have you found it difficult to postpone urination?
0 = not at all
1 = less than 1 time in 5
2 = less than half the time
3 = about half the time
4 = more than half the time
5 = almost always

5. Weak stream: This past month, how often have you had a weak urinary stream?
0 = not at all
1 = less than 1 time in 5
2 = less than half the time
3 = about half the time
4 = more than half the time
5 = almost always

6. Straining: Over the past month, how often have you had to push or strain to begin urination?
0 = not at all
1 = less than 1 time in 5
2 = less than half the time
3 = about half the time
4 = more than half the time
5 = almost always

7. Nocturia: Over the past month, how many times did you most typically get up to urinate from the time you went to bed until the time you got up in the morning?
0 = never
1 = once
2 = twice
3 = thrice
4 = 4 times or more
5 = 5 times

Enter your total score here _____

Results are classified as:
0 - 7 (mildly symptomatic)
8 - 19 (moderately symptomatic)
20 - 35 (severely symptomatic)

An additional question is how bothersome are your symptoms?
Bother score: This helps assess your perceived quality of life due to your urinary symptoms, and the score ranges from 0 (delighted) to 6 (terrible).

How would you feel if you were to spend the rest of your life with your urinary condition just the way it is now?
0 = Delighted
1 = Pleased
2 = Mostly satisfied
3 = Mixed
4 = Mostly dissatisfied
5 = Unhappy

The IPSS is used globally and is based on both the presence and severity of symptoms. Its purpose isn't to be used alone. In combination with other tests, the IPSS can help determine the stages of BPH for patients. These stages are:

1. Patients do not need immediate treatment, as they don't have any bothersome symptoms or significant urine obstruction. Their physicians will observe them closely over time.

2. Bothersome symptoms are present, but no significant urine obstruction. At this stage, symptoms are treatable with medication.

3. There is significant urine obstruction of less than 10 ml of urine released per second (ml/s) and persistent residual urine of more than 100 ml. A TURP (transurethral resection of the prostate) surgery may be recommended by the physician.

4. Complications of BPH are present, such as chronic retention of stones in the bladder. In this case a TURP would definitely be required.

Prostatitis

Prostatitis is essentially an infection and/or inflammation of the prostate gland. There are several varieties of prostatitis, which fall into four categories.

Current belief is that BPH (an enlarged prostate) and prostatitis do not increase your risk of getting prostate cancer or any other kind of prostate or kidney disease, although little research has been done. There is a lot less information available on prostatitis than other prostate conditions.

Although many of the symptoms of prostatitis resemble that of BPH, it is known to occur in men of any age. One thing that differentiates prostatitis from BPH is pain in the perineum, testicles, lower back and abdomen.

These are the four types of prostatitis:

1. Acute bacterial prostatitis
2. Chronic bacterial prostatitis
3. Chronic prostatitis/chronic pelvic pain
4. Asymptomatic inflammatory prostatitis

You may have discovered that you have prostatitis in various ways. For example, you may have discovered it in a complete physical exam, a digital rectal exam (aka DRE) and/or other prostate tests. Personal and/or family history may have played a role.

When it comes to diagnosis, the most crucial test is a urinalysis. Your doctor will use this to figure out which kind of prostatitis you have. All kinds of other tests might include the cystoscopy—in which a camera is inserted up the penis to see the bladder and prostate, a CT scan, an ultrasound, an X-ray and a blood test.

You may find the Prostatitis Foundation's website [**http://bit.ly/qz8XIU**] to be a very useful resource.

Symptoms of Prostatitis

You'll see by the following list of symptoms that there are many similarities to BPH, and there are also differences to watch out for:

- Frequent peeing throughout the day, but also at night
- Difficulty urinating, which is characterized by dribbling or hesitation
- Pain or burning feeling when peeing
- Urgency to urinate
- Pain in the abdomen, groin or lower back
- Pain in the perineum

- Pain in the penis or testicles
- Painful ejaculations

These symptoms may be present across the board for the four types of prostatitis, but each one comes with its own set of more individual, possible symptoms. Let's take a look.

Acute Bacterial Prostatitis

Acute bacterial prostatitis may be due to bacteria, a virus or a sexually transmitted disease (STD). Men with acute bacterial prostatitis will likely suffer the classic symptoms of infections such as fever and chills, nausea, vomiting and an overall feeling of malaise or yuckiness. They'll have to urinate frequently, which will be painful and not very satisfying because it will be a weak flow. Prostatitis can also have quite the opposite effect, infrequent urination. They may experience lower back pain as well.

Chronic Bacterial Prostatitis

Chronic bacterial prostatitis is much less common and can be due to a bacterial condition or an inflammation of the prostate. It is considered chronic because it is an ongoing condition characterized by bacterial infection located in the prostate. Symptoms could include:

- frequent urinary tract infections that are mild or flare up into bladder infections
- occasional or frequent bladder infections that are minor to acute
- frequent urination
- persistent pain in the lower abdomen or back

Chronic Prostatitis or Chronic Pelvic Pain

This most common type of prostatitis is known by several names and accounts for 90% of all cases. It may be known as chronic prostatitis without infection, chronic nonbacterial prostatitis, or chronic pelvic pain syndrome.

Why men get chronic prostatitis is not well understood, but it's thought to be related to stress and irregular sexual activity. It may also be linked to activities like operating heavy machinery, driving a truck, or other activities that expose the prostate to strong vibrations, which may cause an inflamed prostate. Cycling and jogging may also cause irritation to the prostate gland. Symptoms range from mild to painful, or remain the same over a period of time, and can include:

- recurrent pelvic, testicle/genital pain
- rectal pain

- painful urination or ejaculation
- erectile difficulties

Asymptomatic Inflammatory Prostatitis

Lastly, if it's found that your prostate is inflamed while you are undergoing a test for other reasons, and you have no other symptoms of prostate issues, your case will be labeled as asymptomatic inflammatory prostatitis.

According to the medical profession, bacterial infections similar to those found in bladder infections are the main cause of bacterial prostatitis, while possible causes of chronic prostatitis/chronic pelvic pain may include: stress, immune problems, infections, injury and prostate stones, a food allergy, or a virus.

Conventional Prostatitis Treatments

Prostatitis is usually treated with antibiotics. In some cases it is treated with BPH meds or surgeries with all the risks described in the BPH section of this chapter. In the case of nonbacterial prostatitis, treatments may include anti-inflammatory medications or muscle relaxants, hot baths, sitz baths, drinking extra water, relaxing when urinating (easier said than done when pain is present), and ejaculating frequently to remove toxins from the prostate (the most fun treatment so far!).

My take on prostatitis is that as with any infection, if the host is weak, then bacteria can take hold causing infection. The best course is to build up the immune system by avoiding poor quality foods and other toxic inputs. Cleanse, improve the diet and exercise more to increase circulation. A strong immune system will make it very hard for infectious bacteria to find a home in the prostate.

As with BPH, the pain of prostatitis can be quite severe at times. Antibiotics will weaken your immune system, may not solve the problem, and could lead to different conditions and further antibiotic attempts. In addition, after taking antibiotics the condition may easily reoccur. If you do take antibiotics for your prostatitis condition, then be sure to make changes to also rebuild your immune system so that your prostatitis does not become chronic.

As with all prostate diseases, the message your body is sending is that something is not right! One of the best ways of treating prostate infection is by making some serious lifestyle changes, especially in your diet (see Chapters 5, 6, and 7 for more info on diet).

Changing your habits and lifestyle will bring permanent relief. While this may seem daunting at first, the benefits to your overall health and energy are worth the changes. There are also many hidden benefits, and I describe them further on in the book.

To read a ton of information about prostatitis and natural insights and treatments, then go to the NaturalPedia website:Prostatitis - Naturalpedia Search Results [http://bit.ly/oJc08q]

For books on prostatitis: Prostatitis Books [http://amzn.to/nBPuCh]

The following list is from the Prostatitis Foundation [www.prostatitis.org]

"Alternative medicine recommendations for prostatitis.

1. *Use medicinal herbs with antibiotic and anti-inflammatory properties such as Echinacea, Goldenseal, and Garlic, to help reduce inflammation and knock out infection.*

2. *Begin a daily regimen of vitamin and mineral supplements that include antioxidants, vitamins A, C, E, Beta-carotene and Selenium. Also take 60 mg of Zinc Picolinate if symptoms are present, otherwise 30 mg would be sufficient.*

3. *Cranberry juice has properties that dislodge bacteria from the bladder wall so that loose invading bacteria are washed away. Cranberry juice may help to prevent infection from spreading to the bladder from the prostate and vice versa. Can be taken as a juice, or as chewable tablets. Take 1 tablet 3X/day.*

4. *Hydrotherapy, or water therapy, helps increase circulation in the prostate while helping to relax and open the urinary tract. Sit in a tub full of the hottest water you can tolerate for 15-30 minutes. Cold soaks may also be therapeutic, and should be alternated with hot soaks. Also recommended are hot and cold packs applied to the prostate area (between the scrotum and anus), the hot to cold ratio should be 4:1, 2-3X/day. *NOTE* Hot soaks are not recommended for acute infection or inflammation.*

5. *Relax and try to reduce stress. Learn stress management techniques and employ enjoyable exercise. Use herbs like Valerian, Crampbark, and Scullcap to help relax muscles.*

6. *Eat lightly. Whole grains, steamed vegetables, fresh fruits, herb teas and tinctures, such as Saw Palmetto and Siberian Ginseng, are good for the male reproductive system. Buchu, Saw Palmetto and Pipsissewa are great genito-urinary tonics and astringents that help strengthen and heal, as well as having anti-microbial actions. Couch Grass, Watermelon Seed and Pipsissewa are natural diuretics that help flush urine, prevent urine build-up, and provide support for other preventive methods. Echinacea and Siberian Ginseng are immune-system enhancers that help the bodies natural defense system build resistance. Comfrey, Couch Grass and Marshmallow have demulcent properties to help sooth and protect.*

7. *Last, but not least, do you Kegel exercises faithfully.*

8. *Massage and prostate massage may help."*

"Prostatitis Alternative Medicine FAQ"
www.prostatitis.org/altmedfaq.html [http://bit.ly/p4CkxW] (Accessed 8 May 2011)

Note: See the section on personal testing to know which of these herbs may be helpful.

Prostate Cancer

These words scare many men. Why? Because prostate cancer is the second leading cause of cancer death and men hear more and more stories about it. According to MedlinePlus, the U.S. National Institute of Health, men who are most at risk are:

✓ African-American

✓ Men older than 60

✓ Men who have prostate cancer in the family

Specific environmental factors increase your chance of having prostate cancer. You are at higher risk if you:

- Have been exposed to agent orange

- Abuse alcohol

- Are a farmer and are exposed to pesticides and herbicides

- Eat a diet high in fat, especially animal fat

- Are a tire plant worker

- Are a painter

- Have been exposed to cadmium

MedlinePlus also states that the lowest number of cases occurs in Japanese men living in Japan, unless a previous generation in your family has lived in the U.S., and are even lower in the Okinawan region. Those who are vegetarian are also at lower risk.

Miller, S. 23 September 2010. "Prostate Cancer." www.nlm.nih.gov/medlineplus/ency/article/000380.htm [http://1.usa.gov/nOzNrm] (Accessed 29 March 2011)

African-American men should take special note of what research is revealing. They have the highest prostate cancer incidence in the world. Not only do they develop prostate cancer twice as frequently as Caucasian men, they are twice as likely to die from prostate cancer as other American men.

Although genetics may play a role, diet is clearly a major factor. Eating food containing a lot of animal fat is linked to prostate cancer. On average, African-American men eat 2 to 3 times more fried, broiled and grilled meats. Preparing meat in these ways produces a carcinogenic substance known as heterocyclic amines.

If you're an African-American man or care about someone who is, the best way to lower the risk of prostate cancer is to limit intake of fried, broiled, and grilled meat. Before we jump into the quagmire and try to make sense of all this info, let's first step back and look at it from a different perspective.

Prostate cancer is a relatively new disease, as are most cancers. Any explanation that does not address this fact may easily miss crucial information. There is something that we started doing in the past 60 years that is new and deadly.

Secondly, prostate cancer is primarily a Western disease. It is rare in rural Asian and other non-Western communities, as is BPH or enlarged prostate. We will examine true causal factors later.

So, what does the medical establishment say about prostate cancer? Let's critically review that info, keeping the above factors in mind, as we assess it.

Symptoms of Prostate Cancer

In its early stages, prostate cancer does not usually cause symptoms, but eventually some of these symptoms will most likely occur. The symptoms listed below can occur with prostate cancer, but more often are symptoms related to other non-cancerous prostate problems like BPH:

- Needing to urinate frequently, especially at night
- Difficulty starting urination or holding back urine
- Inability to urinate
- Weak or interrupted flow
- Straining when urinating, and retention of urine in the bladder
- Painful or burning urination
- Difficulty having an erection
- Painful ejaculation
- Blood in the urine or semen
- Frequent pain or stiffness in the lower back, hips, or upper thighs when the cancer has spread

The first four are also seen in cases of prostate enlargement, in which there is no cancer. The other symptoms may also be caused by infections or prostatitis. It is not easy to diagnose prostate cancer from symptoms alone. In some prostate cancer cases, few if any symptoms are present.

How is Prostate Cancer Diagnosed?

A diagnosis of prostate cancer can be confirmed only by biopsy. During a biopsy an urologist (a doctor who specializes in diseases of urinary and sex organs) removes prostate tissue samples, usually with a needle. This is generally done in the doctor's office with local anesthesia. Then, a pathologist (a doctor who identifies diseases by studying tissues under a microscope) checks for cancer cells.

"Biopsy results are reported using something called a Gleason grade and a Gleason score.

The Gleason grade is how aggressive the prostate cancer might be. It grades tumors on a scale of 1–5, based on how different from normal tissue the cells are.

Often, more than one Gleason grade is present within the same tissue sample. The Gleason grade is therefore used to create a Gleason score by adding the two most predominant grades together (a scale of 2–10). The higher the Gleason score, the more likely the cancer is to have spread beyond the prostate gland:

- *Scores 2–4: Low-grade cancer*

- *Scores 5–7: Intermediate (or in the middle) grade cancer. Most prostate cancers fall into this category.*

- *Scores 8–10: High-grade cancer (poorly-differentiated cells)*

- *There are two reasons your doctor may perform a prostate biopsy:*

- *Your PSA [prostate-specific antigen] blood test is high, see also PSA [http://1.usa.gov/o7cRfw]*

- *A digital rectal exam may show a large prostate or a hard, irregular surface.*

Because of PSA testing, prostate cancer is diagnosed during a rectal exam much less often. The PSA blood test will also be used to monitor your cancer after treatment. Often, PSA levels will begin to rise before there are any symptoms. An abnormal digital rectal exam may be the only sign of prostate cancer (even if the PSA is normal).

Men may have blood tests to see if the cancer has spread. Some men also may need the following imaging tests:

- *Bone scan: A doctor injects a small amount of a radioactive substance into a blood vessel, and it travels through the bloodstream and collects in the bones. A machine called a scanner detects and measures the radiation. The scanner makes pictures of the bones on a computer screen or on film. The pictures may show cancer that has spread to the bones.*

- *Computerized tomography (CT) scan: An x-ray machine linked to a computer takes a series of detailed pictures of areas inside the body. Doctors often use CT scans to see the pelvis or abdomen.*

- *Magnetic resonance imaging (MRI): A strong magnet linked to a computer is used to make detailed pictures of areas inside the body."*

Miller, S. 23 September 2010. "Prostate Cancer." www.nlm.nih.gov/medlineplus/ency/article/000380.htm [http://1.usa.gov/nOzNrm] (Accessed 29 March 2011)

Conventional Cancer Treatments

In terms of conventional medical treatment, your doctor may recommend one or more forms of treatment depending on your type of cancer and the risk factors. Older patients may just continue with monitoring using prostate-specific antigen (PSA) tests, possibly biopsies. For others, your doctor may suggest several options, including surgery and radiation.

Surgery

A thorough investigation as to the benefits and risks of surgery will evaluate whether or not surgery should be done. If you're a healthy man who may live another 10 years or more, the mainstream medical approach suggests you may want to consider surgery.

Over-treatment is a growing trend. Once any cancer is detected by urologists, more and more often, doctors recommend the complete removal of the prostate. If done, a "radical prostatectomy" will remove the entire prostate and possibly some surrounding tissue to treat the cancer if it hasn't spread beyond the prostate gland.

The surgeon, although in some places it can be done with robotic surgery, will also remove the seminal vesicles while trying not to damage nerves and blood vessels. These are the two small fluid-filled sacs next to the prostate that produce about 60% of the semen.

Then the surgeon will reattach the urethra to the bladder neck which is part of the bladder, and remove lymph nodes to check for spread of cancer while in there. It's possible that a drain will be left in your belly to help extra fluids be released after surgery, as well as a catheter to help drain the bladder of urine through the urethra.

A cautionary note regarding robotic surgeries: "Johns Hopkins research shows hospital websites use industry-provided content and overstate claims of robotic success."

"Hospitals Misleading Patients About Benefits of Robotic Surgery, Study Suggests" [http://bit.ly/nKyi50]

As with any surgery, there are risks, which include blood clots, respiratory problems, infection, blood loss, heart attack or stroke and reactions to prescribed meds.

Post-surgery side effects may develop such as erectile dysfunction or problems with controlling urine or bowel movements. Additional risks of this operation include rectal injury and tightening of the urethra at the point where scar tissues develop.

Radiation Therapy

As with other forms of cancer, radiation therapy may be used after surgery if there's a risk that some cancer cells are still present. A machine that looks like a normal x-ray machine directs high-powered x-rays at the prostate gland to kill cancer cells. It can also be used for pain relief if cancer has metastasized (spread) to the bone.

Radiation therapy lasts 6 to 8 weeks, 5 days/week, and is administered at an oncology unit. It is usually a painless procedure. However, the list of side effects is long. These include:

- ✓ impotence
- ✓ incontinence
- ✓ appetite loss
- ✓ fatigue
- ✓ skin reactions
- ✓ rectal burning or injury
- ✓ diarrhea
- ✓ bladder urgency
- ✓ blood in urine

Another type of radiation therapy is prostate brachytherapy, often used for a smaller, slow-growing cancer that is discovered early.

Tiny radioactive seeds are inserted into the prostate gland through the skin behind the scrotum by a surgeon using small needles. The seeds may be temporary or permanent. Side effects may include:

- ✓ pain
- ✓ swelling or bruising in your penis or scrotum
- ✓ red-brown urine or semen
- ✓ impotence
- ✓ incontinence
- ✓ chronic diarrhea
- ✓ painful defecation

Proton therapy, which is another type of radiation, beams protons directly onto a tumor with less damage to the surrounding tissue.

Keep in mind that radiation reduces your natural immune system and can leave untreatable lifelong internal scarring and pain. In some cases, it leads to other conditions or even further cancer in surrounding glands.

In terms of prostate cancer, <u>no evidence</u> has been presented that proves that the chance of dying from prostate cancer is reduced by radiation if that cancer is present only in the prostate. The likelihood of dying of prostate cancer is the same with or without radiation. It is good to know that it seems best to <u>not</u> undergo radiation treatments given there is no benefit as far as life expectancy!

Hormone Therapy

This form of therapy is primarily used to help alleviate symptoms for men whose cancer has spread beyond the prostate. Because prostate tumors need testosterone to grow, hormonal therapy treatments decrease the effect of testosterone on prostate cancer and can prevent further growth and spread of cancer.

Hormone therapy is sometimes advocated not only for prostate cancer but also prostate enlargement. The theory is that testosterone causes the disease and reducing it by administering excess estrogen (the female hormone) will make you better.

This has been proven to be ridiculous in study after study but the mistaken notion seems to persist. Common sense says that if high testosterone were the cause then young men should be replete with cancer as they have the highest levels of testosterone.

Roger Mason in *The Natural Prostate Cure* [http://amzn.to/prm90b] cites study after study to disprove the connection of high testosterone to prostate disease. In addition to being ineffective, hormone therapy has risks and side effects including impotence.

There are two types of drugs used for hormone therapy. The primary drug is LH-RH. Possible side effects include:

✓ nausea and vomiting

✓ hot flashes

✓ anemia

✓ lethargy

✓ osteoporosis

✓ reduced sexual desire

✓ decreased muscle mass

✓ weight gain

✓ impotence

LH-RH is given with another drug, called androgen-blocking drugs, which has these possible side effects:

✓ erectile dysfunction

✓ loss of sexual desire

✓ liver problems

✓ diarrhea

✓ enlarged breasts

Another kind of hormonal treatment is the surgical removal of the testes, called orchiectomy, which produces much of the body's testosterone. However, this is rarely done.

At some point, some prostate cancers may no longer respond to hormonal treatment. An oncologist will recommend chemotherapy and immunotherapy, a single drug or a combination of drugs.

Now, if you're talking about prostate cancer that has spread, then there are drugs to reduce testosterone levels or have your testes surgically removed, or chemotherapy (which almost sounds nice after that thought!)

Phew! Exit stage right! None of these procedures are harmless. The side effects or consequences of any of these treatments are risky at best and can be life-changing very easily... incontinence leads to wearing diapers! Or say good-bye to your sex life with impotence in many cases, and more problems, and many of these side-effects can worsen over time.

Bottom line? Conventional medical treatments for prostate cancer do not improve life longevity and can leave you with greater problems.

Clearly what you just read is completely symptomatic medicine. It assumes there is only one way to go: to choose from a list that poisons, radiates, slices and dices or some combination of these. So, let's take a look at another possibility being promoted in the mainstream.

Active Surveillance

Doing nothing seems to be your best solution according to a new study on prostate cancer!

> *"Study Weighs Comparative Effectiveness of Low-risk Prostate Cancer Treatments*
>
> *When it comes to the treatment of low-risk prostate cancer, a new comparative effectiveness study* [http://bit.ly/pOO7ae] *has concluded that the various approaches—including active surveillance, surgery, and radiation therapy— result in similar overall survival and tumor recurrence rates. However, compared with the immediate treatment options, active surveillance yields both a comparable net health benefit and more quality-adjusted life years for men age 65 and older, according to the economic model used in this study."*
>
> National Cancer Institute. 12 January 2010. www.cancer.gov/aboutnci/ncicancerbulletin/archive/2010/011210/page3 [http://1.usa.gov/qTvryV] (Accessed 10 May 2011)

Here is a book written in 2010 by Dr. Manson, who has a very go-slow approach to prostate cancer:

Invasion of the Prostate Snatchers: No More Unnecessary Biopsies, Radical Treatment or Loss of Sexual Potency [http://amzn.to/oxkJl8]

This is the Random House synopsis of the book:

> *"Every year almost a quarter of a million confused and frightened American men are tossed into a prostate cancer cauldron stirred by salespeople representing a multibillion-dollar industry. In this flourishing business, the radical prostatectomy is still the most widely recommended treatment option. Yet a recent and definitive study in the New England Journal of Medicine concluded that out of the fifty thousand prostate operations performed annually, more than forty thousand are unjustified. But this is no surprise given that 99 percent of all doctors treating this disease are surgeons or radiation therapists. <u>The appalling fact is that men are still being rushed into a major operation that rarely prolongs life and more than half the time leaves them impotent.</u> Invasion of the Prostate Snatchers is a report on the latest thinking in prostate cancer therapy: close monitoring–active surveillance rather than surgery or radiation–should be the initial treatment approach for many men...*
>
> *[This book] provides convincing evidence that this noninvasive approach can be crucial in preventing tens of thousands of men from being overtreated every year. Invasion of the Prostate Snatchers serves as an indispensable map through the medical minefield of prostate cancer."*

Yikes! According to these doctors, 80% of radical prostate surgeries are unnecessary!

So if you do have a prostate cancer diagnosis, *doing nothing* may well be your best solution according to both Dr. Manson's book and the study by the NCI.

My Conclusion

Changing the conditions in your body by cleansing, diet enhancements, supplements and other strategies in this book may well help rid your prostate of the cancer.

Prostate cancer is a relatively new disease (surfacing mostly over the last 60 plus years at an increasing rate despite all the "wars" against cancer) and is rarer in other parts of the world, so the obvious conclusion is we are doing something that causes this cancer. I submit it is our environmental toxins and food supply. If so, we should be able to stop those, cleanse the body by detoxing and rebuilding our health and immunity with healthy alternatives. That way, the cancer will no longer have a host to grow in.

Another tragic situation is that doctors are not free to promote alternative ideas for treatment as they could lose their license! They are not allowed to offer them.

If you want to read a ton about prostate cancer and natural insights and treatments, search NaturalPedia's site for the term "Prostate Cancer": Prostate Cancer – NaturalPedia Search Results [http://bit.ly/qBeG83]

Unconventional / Alternative Medicine Prostate Cancer Insights

Early screening for prostate cancer is not prevention. Real prevention happens when we make changes to our diet and nutrition by our life-enhancing choices and becoming aware of what causes prostate cancer. It is misleading to say that early screening equals prevention.

All early screening does is force men down the road to risky, unnecessary and side-effect-filled surgeries and medications that benefit the sickness industry of the big pharmaceutical and health maintenance organization (HMO) companies. Real prevention is not at all profitable to pharmaceutical companies—but it is profitable for you!

Rather than submit to life-changing medical practices that studies show are no better than doing nothing at all, learn how to heal yourself! And do it without all the major side effects. Real prevention has untold benefits, not just for prostate cancer but also for your overall health and well being.

The prostate seems to react to hormone levels: both to "male" hormones like testosterone and to "female" hormones like estrogen. In truth, men and women have both types in different amounts. It is their relative balance that influences our health.

This relative balance—between testosterone and estrogen—is affected and influenced by aging, diet and the ability of the liver and intestines to detoxify, amount and type of exercise, smoking and exposure to hormone-like chemicals in food and from the environment.

Andreas Moritz, an amazingly insightful writer and well-known alternative health practitioner, has lots to say about cancer in his books. If you have prostate cancer, I recommend reading his material in depth.

> *"The following statement... is very important in the consideration of cancer:* ***"Cancer does not cause a person to be sick; it is the sickness of the person that causes the cancer."*** *To treat cancer successfully requires the patient to become whole again on all levels of his body, mind and spirit. Once the cancer causes have been properly identified, it will become apparent what needs to be done to achieve complete recovery...*
>
> *Standard cancer treatments may lower the number of cancer cells to an undetectable level, but this certainly cannot eradicate all cancer cells. As long as the causes of tumor growth remain intact, it may redevelop at any time and at any rate.*
>
> *Curing cancer has little to do with getting rid of a group of detectable cancer cells. Treatments like chemotherapy and radiation are certainly capable of poisoning or burning many cancer cells, but they also destroy healthy cells in the bone marrow, gastro-intestinal tract, liver, kidneys, heart, lungs, etc., which often leads to permanent irreparable damage of entire organs and systems in the body. A real cure of cancer does not occur at the expense of destroying other*

vital parts of the body. It is achievable only when the causes of excessive growth of cancer cells have been removed or stopped...

Cancer, like any other disease, is not a clearly definable phenomenon that suddenly and randomly appears in some part(s) of the body like mushrooms popping up out of the ground. Cancer is rather the result of many crises of toxicity that have as their common origin one or more energy-depleting influences... all hinder the body in its effort to remove metabolic waste, toxins and 30 billion dead cells each day. When these accumulate in any part of the body, they naturally lead to a number of progressive responses that include irritation, swelling, hardening, inflammation, ulceration and abnormal growth of cells. Like every other disease, cancer is but a toxicity crisis and marks the body's final attempt to rid itself of septic poisons and acidic compounds that result from not being able to properly remove metabolic waste, toxins and putrefying dead cells in the body...

Prostate Cancer and Its Risky Treatments

There is, indeed, enough scientific evidence to suggest that most cancers disappear by themselves if left alone. A 1992 Swedish study found that of 223 men who had early prostate cancer but did not receive any kind of medical treatment, only 19 died within ten years of diagnosis. Considering that one third of men in the European Community have prostate cancer, but only one percent of them die (not necessarily from the cancer), it is very questionable to treat it at all. This is especially after research has revealed that treatment of the disease has not decreased mortality rates. On the contrary, survival rates are higher in groups of men whose "treatment" consists merely of watchful waiting, compared with groups undergoing prostate surgery... Far from being a safe procedure, one study found that a year after the surgery, 41% of men had to wear diapers because of chronic leakage, and 88% were sexually impotent.

Even the screening procedure for prostate cancer can be dangerous. According to a number of studies, more men who are screened with the PSA (prostate-specific-antigen) screening test die from prostate cancer compared to those who are not tested. A recent editorial in the British Medical Journal sized up the value of the PSA test with this comment: "At present the one certainty about PSA testing is that it causes harm."...

Another serious problem with PSA tests is that they are notoriously unreliable... In fact, doctors at the Fred Hutchinson Cancer Research Center (FHCRC) in Seattle estimated that PSA screening may result in an over-diagnosis rate of more than 40 percent...

If men learned how to avoid a buildup of toxins in the body, prostate cancer could perhaps be the least common and the least harmful of all cancers. Aggressive treatment of early prostate cancer is now a controversial issue, but it should be controversial for every type of cancer, at whatever stage of development."

Moritz, Andreas. *Timeless Secrets of Health and Rejuvenation*
[http://amzn.to/nmUh4Y]
Also by the same author (read the reviews while there)
Cancer Is Not A Disease - It's A Survival Mechanism [http://amzn.to/rbKt9l]

Researchers conducted a study on prostate cancer diagnosis and treatment and determined that after the introduction of (PSA) prostate antigen screening tests in 1986 there has been an over-diagnosis of prostate cancer in the US. This means that many men in the US are being diagnosed and treated for prostate cancer when they have no health problems whatsoever.

Welch and Albertsen's Journal of the National Cancer Institute article [http://bit.ly/mScXtT]

> *"Rather than catching or curing disease, aggressive cancer screenings and unnecessary biopsies are actually spreading deadly 'superbugs' among patients… As much as five percent of prostate biopsies develop infections from the procedure—or about 50,000 Americans every year, and an equal number in Europe. Nine out of 10,000 men whose tests were negative for prostate cancer died within a month from sepsis and other complications, according to a recent study in the Journal of Urology…*
>
> *A 2004 study from the John Wayne Cancer Institute in California indicates that if you do have cancer, getting a needle biopsy may increase the chance that the cancer will spread by as much as 50 percent compared to patients who receive the more traditional excisional biopsies (or 'lumpectomies')."*
>
> Alliance for Natural Health USA. 24 May 2011. "Conventional Medicine Runs Amok: Prostate, Breast, and Colon Screenings" www.anh-usa.org/conventional-medicine-runs-amok-prostate-breast-and-colon-screenings [http://bit.ly/od9lMW] (Accessed 30 May 2011)

Causes of Prostate Cancer

Prostate cancer is the second most common cause of death in men of all ages. In men over 75, it is *the* most common cause of death from cancer. It's rare, but not unheard of, that a man younger than 40 will be diagnosed with prostate cancer.

There is so much convincing evidence on the role of diet in prostate cancer that suggests that prostate cancer may be considered a "nutritional disease." If you spend just a bit of time searching the Internet, you will find a huge amount of information on prostate cancer, from government-run sites to cancer organizations, from Western medical points of view to alternative practices.

Both Western and alternative medical research identifies the following factors as contributing to a higher risk for prostate disease and cancer:
- ✓ high blood pressure
- ✓ diabetes
- ✓ high insulin levels
- ✓ being overweight or having a beer belly
- ✓ sedentary lifestyle and professions like long distance truck driving
- ✓ diet high in fat, especially saturated fat
- ✓ excessive intake of calcium, especially from dairy

- ✓ history of STDs (sexually transmitted disease)
- ✓ exposure to heavy metals especially cadmium and mercury
- ✓ high exposure to agricultural pesticides and herbicides
- ✓ high red meat consumption (especially grilled and broiled meats which create carcinogens from the fat burning on the flames)
- ✓ low intake of fruits and vegetables
- ✓ low selenium usually due to depleted soil
- ✓ low vitamin E and other antioxidants
- ✓ getting older
- ✓ low levels of vitamin D

Chapter 4: Prostate Exams and Tests

Digital Rectal Exam (DRE) or Prostate Check

All men should have an annual Digital Rectal Exam or Prostate Check during their annual physical exams. It is an important step to know the health of your prostate.

Your doctor may scare you with his views on what to do if he finds a prostate problem during this prostate exam. Do not succumb to your doctor's point of view. That's how they see the world. Doctors see symptoms and do not understand root causes. Remember you are in control of your body! Use this information as a launching pad for finding your own solutions to heal yourself naturally. But first you need to understand the prostate to know how to heal it.

While not a man's favorite to say the least, the Digital Rectal Examination or DRE will give you and your health practitioner some idea of the state of your prostate gland. Your doctor will insert a lubricated, gloved finger up your butt (rectum).

The doctor will feel the surface of the prostate *through* the thin rectal wall. The prostate is right next to the rectum and is easy for your doc to feel it. Size, shape and consistency can all be assessed. Healthy prostate tissue is soft like the tissue at the base of the thumb, palm-side. If malignant tissue is present, your doctor will feel something firm, hard and often asymmetrical.

It is quite possible for him to feel your prostate gland and to determine its general health and condition in less than a minute. Enlarged prostates, cancerous growths or lesions, lumps or irregularities, can be felt by the digital rectal exam.

Unfortunately, most practitioners need some training to take a little more time for the rectum to relax before pushing the finger in. The best way is for the finger to first touch the rectum gently so that the muscles can relax. Insertion then becomes easier if done slowly. Ask your practitioner to take their time so that the digital rectal exam is more comfortable.

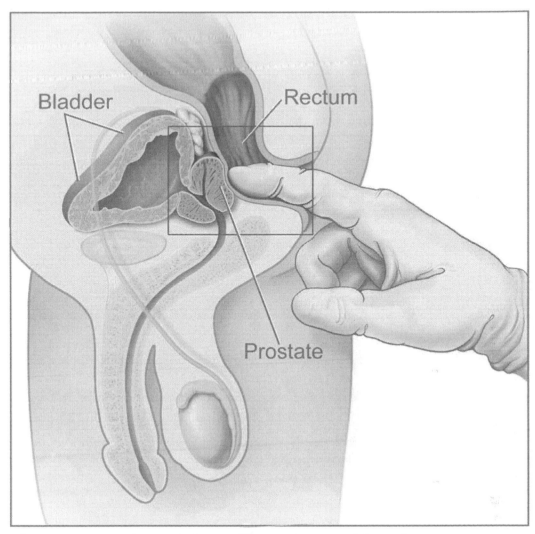

Digital Rectal Examination: side view of the male reproductive system and urinary anatomy, including the prostate, rectum, and bladder.

Family doctors can easily misdiagnose an enlarged prostate because they are not a specialist who does this prostate check countless times. So seeing an urologist may be a good idea because urologists have an expertise and skill your general practitioner lacks.

I remember my general practitioner diagnosing that I had an infected bladder and not an enlarged prostate or BPH when I first came in after being unable to pee. She just did not have enough experience to diagnose an enlarged prostate. To my doctor, my prostate did not feel abnormal for a man of my age; however, several days later the urologist did the same test and knew immediately that I had an enlarged prostate.

After a DRE has been done, there are other prostate examinations that your doctor can do to investigate further.

Cystoscopy Prostate Examination

The urologist may also insert a camera catheter to do a prostate check or prostate examination if they suspect a serious problem. In this procedure the camera allows the doctor to see the inside of the prostate and bladder. An enlarged prostate can cause problems in the bladder, and a cystoscopy prostate examination can enable your doctor to see what's going on inside your prostate and bladder.

This procedure enters not through the rear as in a normal DRE but the front—down the penis inside the urethra through the prostate gland and into the bladder.

Yup, this one can hurt especially if done fast, as my urologist did! The catheter and camera size are not small. They do use a local anesthetic, but it did not make much difference to me. Years later a new urologist did the same procedure in the hospital and it was not painful. So request a painless procedure for your comfort.

I will talk a lot more about male catheters and catheter insertion as well as how to use them safely when instant relief is required (see the "Catheters" section in Chapter 13 for more info).

PSA Testing

Prostate-Specific Antigen or PSA is a protein discovered by Richard Ablin, a research professor of immunobiology and pathology at the University of Arizona College of Medicine. Both normal and cancerous cells produce PSA, which is a marker of inflammation. Because PSA is found in blood, the PSA test is done with a standard blood sample, which is then measured in a laboratory. The same doctor invented the PSA Test, the most popular tool for detecting prostate cancer. In 1994, this test was approved by the Food and Drug Administration (FDA).

The PSA Controversy

There is a lot of controversy surrounding the PSA test. Does the test actually save lives? The resounding answer is "No." This conclusion is really important for you to know because your doctor or urologist will recommend procedures that could be hazardous to your health based on a PSA test!

Be well informed because doctors will use the PSA test to request a biopsy just to "be sure," but biopsies are NOT harmless and can cause a quiet prostate cancer to become much more active and to spread.

The funny thing about the prostate is that *less is best*. And if you follow the suggestions later in the book you can prevent prostate problems and even reverse them if you have one. Time is on your side no matter what your doctor says. If he thinks you have an extreme case (as mine did... I was put on the emergency surgery list), he will want to rush you into conventional procedures.

I suggest that you **do not rush this**. Reverse the conditions in you, the host, because you gave birth to them, and save yourself from awful side effects. Doctors play down the side effects because they do not know any other way to help you, because they can lose their license to practice medicine if they suggest natural health alternatives, and sometimes because it is profitable for them to do so.

Increased PSA levels don't necessarily mean cancer is present, and most statistics suggest that the PSA test doesn't even lengthen the life of prostate cancer patients. The New York Times reported on two studies from the *New England Journal of Medicine*, one involving 182,000 men in Europe and the other involving 77,000 men in the US:

> *"Prostate test found to save few lives*
>
> *Dr. Peter B. Bach, a physician and epidemiologist at Memorial Sloan-Kettering Cancer Center, says one way to think of the data is to suppose he has a PSA test today. It leads to a biopsy that reveals he has prostate cancer, and he is treated for it. There is a one in 50 chance that, in 2019 or later, he will be spared death from a cancer that would otherwise have killed him. And there is a 49 in 50 chance that he will have been treated unnecessarily for a cancer that was never a threat to his life.*
>
> *Prostate cancer treatment can result in impotence and incontinence when surgery is used to destroy the prostate, and, at times, painful defecation or chronic diarrhea when the treatment is radiation…*
>
> *The benefits of prostate cancer screening, he said, are 'modest at best and with a greater downside than any other cancer we screen for.'"*
>
> Kolata, Gina. 18 March 2009.
> www.nytimes.com/2009/03/19/health/19cancer.html [http://nyti.ms/oPxSon] (Accessed 5 May 2011)

And read this article as well:

> *"New Finding Suggests Prostate Biopsy is Not Always Necessary*
>
> *PSA picks up any prostate activity, not just cancer," said lead investigator Gary G. Schwartz, Ph.D., M.P.H., … 'Inflammation and other factors can elevate PSA levels. If the levels are elevated, the man is usually sent for a biopsy. The problem is that, as men age, they often develop microscopic cancers in the prostate that are clinically insignificant. If it weren't for the biopsy, these clinically insignificant cancers, which would never develop into fatal prostate cancer, would never be seen.'"*
>
> Wake Forest Baptist Medical Center. 8 June 2010.
> www.wakehealth.edu/News-Releases/2009/New_Finding_Suggests_Prostate_Biopsy_Is_Not_Always_Necessary.htm [http://bit.ly/q8bCuB] (Accessed 5 May 2011)

BPH, the state of having an enlarged prostate, also has higher levels of PSA. So, someone with BPH could be diagnosed with cancer because of "false-positive" results, which could lead to more invasive tests. In fact, there are many other reasons why PSA can be high. These include:

- prostatitis
- infection
- certain factors can disturb the prostate and temporarily increase PSA
- riding a bicycle/motorcycle
- digital rectal exam
- prostate massage
- over-the-counter drugs (such as Ibuprofen)
- having an orgasm within the past 24 hours
- urinary tract infection
- insertion of a urinary catheter
- a prostate biopsy or urinary tract surgery
- African-American men have higher normal PSA levels
- some people naturally produce more PSA
- levels go up with age
- high stress levels

Many doctors swear by the PSA test even though research and evaluation continue to show that PSA testing does not lower the rate of death by cancer, and in fact increases the incidence of over-diagnosis.

Even Richard Ablin, who invented the test, now retracts its utility saying it is not effective! Yet it is still the most-used diagnostic test. In a New York Times article, Richard Albin publicly declared the PSA test "a hugely expensive public health disaster... hardly more effective than a coin toss."

www.nytimes.com/2010/03/10/opinion/10Ablin.html [http://nyti.ms/qLNROo]

One of the main concerns is the fact that there is no specific normal or abnormal PSA level. PSA levels vary and fluctuate, and are influenced by many things. Beware of your doctor urging you on based on results of your PSA test! The theory they are currently working with now is that one abnormal test doesn't require further testing, but if PSA rises over time, then perhaps more tests are needed.

Most doctors are using the following ranges with slight variations:

- 0 to 2.5 ng/ml is low

- 2.6 to 10 ng/ml is slightly to moderately elevated

- 10 to 19.9 ng/ml is moderately elevated

- 20 ng/ml or more is significantly elevated

An estimated two-thirds (2/3) of men who show an elevated PSA level (> 4 ng/ml), according to UK cancer researchers, but do not have prostate cancer, will end up suffering the anxiety, discomfort and risk of follow-up investigations.

I let them do all these tests because I had passed such a big volume of blood clots and my doctor was worried. I knew I didn't have cancer. However, I wasn't sure what I was going to do because I had not yet discovered the triggers that were causing my prostate to block and shut down my urination. I was at the end of my rope and, at that time in my life, I didn't know what you are now learning!

If your doctor suspects that your PSA test results could hint at cancer, it could easily lead to a biopsy—even if the higher PSA levels aren't a big deal at all. Large numbers of men are regularly referred for biopsies only to discover that they don't have cancer.

I had the biopsy done because the CT scan showed how massive my prostate was. My very friendly and competent urologist said I had a prostate "the size of Texas"! The biopsy results showed that I didn't have cancer.

A needle biopsy is currently the only test that can reliably indicate whether cancerous cells are in the prostate. It is done when your doctor suspects cancer from a DRE or PSA test (which is so unreliable).

Needles are inserted into the prostate gland and small samples of tissue are removed for testing. The biopsy may or may not find cancer depending on how well they sample the different areas of the prostate.

The microscopic examination of the tissue tries to determine if cancer is present and to what level. There are some real potential problems with a biopsy. Not only can a biopsy be very harmful to the prostate, it can lead to painful, long-lasting infections that are difficult to treat. It can easily add bacteria from the bowel into the prostate (usually the biopsy is done through the rectum). If cancer is present, watch out!

The biopsy needles can spread the cancer to other parts of the prostate, release cancerous cells into the bloodstream, and may spread the cancer to other organs or glands nearby, making a relatively benign form of cancer highly fatal. Metastasis is the term used to describe the spreading of the cancer outside the prostate. Metastasic prostate cancer often results in prostate cancer death but not from inside the prostate capsule itself!

It is clear that PSA screening may do more harm than good, leading often to biopsies! The potential harms of a screening program outweigh any benefits. Because the test is notoriously unreliable, most public health agencies are not even recommending the test any longer.

Knowing now what I do, I would never have allowed my urologist to do a biopsy! In the UK, the National Screening Committee's experts now recommend <u>against</u> a regular screening using PSA tests. After weighing all the evidence, they say it's not advisable. It's contentious there because of concerns of over-diagnosis. PSA testing usually leads to biopsies, which are harmful and may possibly spread cancer cells to nearby tissues and organs if they are present.

Basically, over-diagnosis is this. Imagine you're diagnosed with cancer and it is left untreated. Yet, you would never experience any symptoms. This happens with slow-growing, non-spreading cancers. You're more likely to die of other causes before noticing or being affected by symptoms. Why increase the risk with biopsies?

> *As many as 50 percent of all prostate cancer diagnoses may be cases of over-diagnosis, according to a study published in the British Medical Journal.*
>
> *Over-diagnosis refers to the detection of a cancer that, if left untreated, would never have any negative effects on a person's life. This happens with cancers that grow slowly and do not spread to other organs, so that a patient dies of other causes before ever experiencing any symptoms.*
>
> BBC. 6 December 2010. "Experts scrap prostate screening proposal". www.bbc.co.uk/news/health-11930979 [http://bbc.in/njDfqC] (Accessed 5 May 2011)

The idea behind cancer testing is to increase the life span of the patient. This is why biopsies do not make sense for diagnosing prostate cancer. Most prostate cancers are slow growing and show up later in life. It's so slow that most men will die of other causes before exhibiting symptoms of prostate cancer. Or another way to look at it, cancer "survivors" would have enjoyed the same lifespan with or without treatment (and with fewer complications!).

Dr. Ablin, the researcher who first developed PSA testing, said,

> *American men have a 16% lifetime chance of receiving a diagnosis of prostate cancer, but only a 3% chance of dying from it... In other words, men lucky enough to reach old age are much more likely to die with prostate cancer than to die of it.*
>
> Albin, R. J. 9 March 2010. "The Great Prostate Mistake" www.nytimes.com/2010/03/10/opinion/10Ablin.html [http://nyti.ms/qLNROo]

There is also no way to tell in early stages if the cancer is "normal" or "aggressive." Or, as Ablin put it, which of the two types of cancer—the one that will kill you or the one that won't. Jennifer Stark, research fellow at Harvard School of Public Health, led a study that was published by the *British Medical Journal* in 2009. It was clear from her findings that PSA tests are unreliable.

Jennifer Stark said,

"PSA cannot differentiate between indolent and lethal prostate cancer... Before PSA testing is performed, men should be... informed that the test cannot tell whether they have a life-threatening cancer."

Reinberg, S. 25 September 2009. "Studies Find PSA Screening Unreliable." news.healingwell.com/index.php?p=news1&id=631343 [http://bit.ly/nZcAn5] (Accessed 30 July 2011)

Now look at this study!

*"...**elevated PSA measurements are not necessarily potential signs of prostate cancer at all.** Instead, they can simply be caused by a hormone normally occurring in healthy bodies.*

According to a study just published in Cancer Epidemiology, Biomarkers and Prevention, the researchers discovered that parathyroid hormone, which the body produces to regulate blood levels of calcium, can raise PSA levels in healthy men who do not have prostate cancer. Unfortunately, elevated PSA levels currently set off alarm bells in the mainline medical establishment, leading many men to be biopsied and then treated unnecessarily with surgery, chemo, radiation, and/or emasculating hormones."

Baker, Sherry 23 November 2009, "Scientists Find Prostate Cancer Biopsies Often Not Needed" www.naturalnews.com/027552_prostate_cancer_biopsies.html [http://bit.ly/rcVRGC] (Accessed 5 May 2011)

An American study published in 2008 revealed that PSA screening did not reduce the death rate in men 55 and over. In other words, guys, early detection usually offers at best only minor benefits!

These days, nearly all men who receive a cancer diagnosis end up doing the conventional, symptomatic approach (surgery, radiation, microwave, hormone treatment and/or toxic drugs including chemotherapy), which attacks only the superficial symptoms.

Even worse, conventional treatments can lead to unnecessary personal harm, such as bacterial infection, relapse of symptoms, and the unintentional spreading of cancerous cells to the bloodstream or other organs and glands. The two most common side effects of these aggressive approaches are impotence and incontinence. Fun, fun, fun!

Lastly, Dr. Otis W. Brawley, MD, who is the chief medical officer for the Cancer Society is "against telling people that [PSA testing] works or that it saves lives when the evidence that supports those statements simply does not exist."

Leading authorities on the subject, such as Ablin and Brawley, are not alone. The American Cancer Society warns all to use increased caution when using PSA screenings. The American College of Preventive Medicine outright refuses to recommend the screening on a routine basis. Even the Preventive Services Task Force, a federal panel evaluating screenings, is against screenings for men 75 years and older.

Isaacs, T. 4 August, 2009, "Prostate Screening Can Lead to Unnecessary Treatment and Risks 95% of the Time". www.naturalnews.com/026766_Prostate_cancer_screening.html [http://bit.ly/qe5feA] (Accessed 29 March 2011)

Study after study discredits PSA testing. So why are 30 million men still being screened for PSA? After learning all of this, what are we left with?

Harmful Diagnosis and Biopsies

There are three immediate negative impacts on the patient from PSA screenings:

- stress and anxiety

- financial expense

- false readings leading to unnecessary biopsies

The last one proves to be the real issue. If high levels of PSA are found in the test, a snowball effect ensues, usually leading to biopsies. There are many possible negative consequences of biopsies:

- psychological stress

- pain

- fever

- bleeding

- infection

- the spread of cancer cells to surrounding tissues

The last item is the worst one—the biopsy test itself can cause cancer cells to escape the prostate into surrounding tissues and spread the cancer that was once contained in the gland. Most prostate cancers are contained.

If any signs of cancer are present in the biopsy results, doctors keep the ball rolling. Conventional treatments vary, but all are damaging, as mentioned earlier. For example, three adverse side effects of prostate surgery or radiation therapy include:

- depression

- urinary incontinence

- erectile dysfunction

Now consider this: the findings from a 2009 European study indicate that 70 percent of diagnosed men have cancers that will cause them no harm whatsoever if left untreated. The study showed that just 1 out of 50 men would be saved through PSA screenings. The other 49 men would receive surgery with no benefit whatsoever, but *likely suffer impotence or incontinence because of the treatments!*

A study conducted by Dr. Martin Sanda at the Beth Israel Deaconess Medical Center says, "Men diagnosed with low-risk tumors who deferred treatment were still doing fine an average of 8 years—and up to 20 years—following their diagnosis."

As I was researching PSA testing, it didn't take me long to figure out what is truly going on. In the words of Dr. Ablin, who discovered PSA testing:

> *So why is it still used? Because drug companies continue peddling the tests and advocacy groups push "prostate cancer awareness" by encouraging men to get screened….*
>
> *I never dreamed that my discovery four decades ago would lead to such a profit-driven public health disaster. The medical community must confront reality and stop the inappropriate use of P.S.A. screening. Doing so would save billions of dollars and rescue millions of men from unnecessary, debilitating treatments.*

> Ablin, R. J. 9 March 2010. "The Great Prostate Mistake"
> www.nytimes.com/2010/03/10/opinion/10Ablin.html
> [http://nyti.ms/qLNROo] (Accessed 30 July 2011)

PSA screenings bring in huge profits. Over-screening is a long-established source of revenue with one out of three men over the age of 75 getting tested annually. Advocacy groups funded by drug companies promote prostate cancer awareness and push the test, yet no one is educating individuals of the limitations and uselessness of being tested over the age of 55.

Dr. Brawley, the chief medical officer for the Cancer Society, stated, "Several of the leading prostate cancer survivor organizations that do a lot of the pushing of screening are funded by the makers of the PSA screening kits."

Lastly, Dr. Ablin states that rather than being prescribed to the entire population of men over 50, the PSA test does have limited use if utilized wisely. For example, regular testing of individuals who have a family history of prostate cancer makes sense. Or, if regular testing shows that the PSA levels go up and up and up, then there is a chance of cancer.

> ***"Bottom line: the researchers conclude that many men with prostate cancers detected by PSA screening are most likely undergoing treatment for clinically insignificant cancers that pose little if any threat to their lives."***

> *Baker, S.L. 15 October 2009. "Men not being informed about low benefits and high risks of PSA prostate cancer screening"*
> *www.naturalnews.com/027246_Prostate_cancer_screening.html*
> *[http://bit.ly/runEjR] (Accessed 8 May 2011)*

In the end, it all comes back to each of us being responsible for educating ourselves and being proactive in our own health and disease prevention. The bottom line is that we must all be very wary of PSA tests and what your doctor recommends. Some other tests that you may encounter if you have any prostate problems include:

Urodynamic Testing

This takes place in your doctor's office. It is used to measure the amount of urine in the bladder, pressure and flow evaluation. For patients with BPH or suspected BPH, the uroflowmetry, pressure-flow studies, and post-void residual test, and other tests (all described below) are useful for analyzing sphincter deficiency and the severity of incontinence.

Uroflowmetry

First, let's look at uroflowmetry, which is used to evaluate and record urine. Patients with a full bladder will pee into a device that measures the volume of pee, how long it takes and the rate of flow. It also evaluates the obstruction. You can try this at home. Use a standard measuring cup (a 2-cup measure is best) and a wristwatch with a second hand or digital timer. Drink lots of water, wait as long as you possibly can before peeing, then see how long it takes you to eliminate 200 ml (3/4 of a cup). A study done in 2002 by H. L. Leporet al. came up with following average rates of flow:

Client	Age (yrs)	Quantity (ml)	Time (seconds)	Rate (ml/s)
Healthy man	40 – 60	200	11	18
Healthy man	60+	200	15	13
Man with BPH	n/a	200	20 – 40	n/a

Pressure-Flow Studies

The most accurate way of detecting and evaluating urinary blockage is to measure the pressure of the bladder while urinating. The not very fun part of this test is that a catheter is inserted into the penis, through the urethra and up into the bladder. There is a rare chance of urinary tract infection as a result.

Post-Void Residual Test

The purpose of the Post-Void Residual (PVR) test is to measure how much pee is left after urination. Residual urine is determined by either catheterization or ultrasound. For example, if you have "PRV less than 50 ml," then you have healthy bladder emptying abilities. Anywhere between 100 to 200 ml or even higher is indicative of blockage. Don't be surprised if your doc asks you to repeat the test— this is common as stress or anxiety can affect the results. Use deep, slow breathing before the test to try to prevent a repeat.

Other Tests:

Urine Test

While standard urine tests may help diagnose prostate problems by screening for blood or infection, chemical urine tests will also check for liver, diabetes or kidney disease.

Hyperplasia Intravenous Pyelogram

Hyperplasia intravenous pyelogram (IVP) involves an intravenous dye that is injected into major veins. This dye enables pictures of organs to be taken with a CT scan while the dye moves around. This test may be useful for men who have an enlarged prostate, as it looks for abnormalities in the kidneys, bladder and ureter tubes, which drain the kidneys.

Bladder Ultrasound

A bladder ultrasound is a non-invasive procedure that doesn't require a hospital visit. Its purpose is to determine if and how much urine is left after urination, which in turn may indicate an enlarged prostate.

Prostate Ultrasound

A prostate ultrasound can estimate the size of the prostate and is important if a biopsy is being recommended.

Radionuclide Bone Scan

If staging reveals that the prostate cancer has spread into the lymph nodes, then bone cancer often follows. A radionuclide bone scan is only used if PSA levels are above 10 ng and the patient experiences bone pain.

Computed Axial Tomography

If cancer looks aggressive or if the patient has a high PSA level, then a computed axial tomography (CAT) is used to see if cancer cells are present in other parts of the body or "metastasized".

Magnetic Resonance Imaging

If the prostate cancer hasn't spread, it's unlikely this test would be necessary. An MRI uses a strong magnet linked to a computer to take detailed pictures of the prostate gland (as well as other organs and tissues in the body).

Pelvic Lymph Node Dissection

This test is used as a final confirmation of whether or not the prostate cancer has spread. It can be done either in open surgery or, more commonly, is done with a fiber optic probe inserted through a tiny incision in the abdominal area.

Biopsy

As I mentioned in the cancer section, the prostate biopsy is the only test that can confirm the presence of cancer.

Doctors can recommend that many samples are taken during the biopsy. Even then, biopsies aren't foolproof and have been known to miss some cancers.

A pathologist looks for the abnormal cells under a microscope, seeking out those that change in appearance, are misshapen and irregular. If cancer is found, the pathologist will "grade" each tissue sample in order to determine how far along the cancer has developed. It also allows the physician to get a look at the tumor's behavior.

As I have already mentioned, a biopsy risks the spreading of the cancer outside the prostate and usually leads to surgeries that are not needed.

New Prostate Procedures

There are new, heavily-marketed, high-tech prostate procedures that claim wonderful results, such as Laparoscopic or keyhole surgery, often using the highly promoted da Vinci robotics system and other robotic methods.

Don't believe all the claims; these procedures are still damaging. Yes, you may leave the hospital sooner but a recent study in the Journal of the American Medical Association [http://bit.ly/p4Ycdi] found more problems later on (30 days to 18 months):

> "Conclusion: Men undergoing MIRP vs RRP experienced shorter length of stay, fewer respiratory and miscellaneous surgical complications and strictures, and similar postoperative use of additional cancer therapies **but experienced more genitourinary complications, incontinence, and erectile dysfunction.**" (Accessed 5 May 2011)

Common Prostate Medications

In this section I provide information for common medications prescribed for prostatitis and BPH (or enlarged prostate).

Prostatitis

Antibiotic treatment for bacterial prostatitis includes the use of tetracycline, trimethoprim-sulfamethoxazole (TMP-SMX [Bactrim, Septra]) or quinolone. Men at increased risk for sexually transmitted disease might benefit from Trimethoprim-sulfamethoxazole (Bactrim, Septra), Doxycycline (Vibramycin), Ciprofloxacin (Cipro), Norfloxacin (Noroxin) or Ofloxacin (Floxin).

Other medications that are used for treatment of prostatitis include carbenicillin (Miostat), cefazolin (Ancef), cephalexin (Keflex), cephradine (Velosef) and minocycline (Minocin).

BPH (Enlarged Prostate)

Pharmaceutical treatments are available. Here's some of what the makers say about them:

Finasteride (brand name: Proscar) and dutasteride (brand name: Avodart) block a natural hormone that makes the prostate enlarge, but these drugs do not help all patients. Another kind of medicine, called alpha blockers, also can help relieve the symptoms of BPH. Some of these drugs are terazosin (brand name: Hytrin), doxazosin (brand name: Cardura), tamsulosin (brand name: Flomax) and alfuzosin (brand name: Uroxatral). Alpha blockers have been used for a long time to treat high blood pressure, but they can also help the symptoms of BPH, even in men who have normal blood pressure.

If you think these medications are harmless, think again. They can easily affect your sex life: reduced libido and erectile difficulties are the price you pay. The pills affect your hormones, and as such can contribute to prostate cancer. Over time, you go from reducing your enlarged prostate to the end of sex as you knew it to the increased risk of prostate cancer!

Both pharmaceuticals and doctors promote these pills because they are profitable, not because they will heal your prostate condition. Doctors will advise you to take the pills, saying that they work. (The heck with risks, as they are minor in their opinion.)

What about surgeries? Removing or zapping your prostate with surgeries or even with laser or infrared techniques does not work in the long run and has big risks of incontinence (no control of peeing) and hence the need to wear adult diapers. The commercials on TV make that appear like a normal easy thing, like for babies. These may be good in some situations—but they are not a first choice solution for most men!

How could it *not* affect your sex life? I don't know about you but I want that part of my life to continue until I am much older. Surgeries often result in impotence or incontinence. Or both! (Yikes!)

Conventional Approaches Concluded

Now that we have examined the conventional medical literature on prostate conditions, their treatments and the variety of testing, what can we conclude?

1. Prostate disease is a major health concern for men because of the three types of conditions: enlargement, infection/inflammation, and cancer. Most Western men will experience some form during their life.

2. The symptoms can be minor to major and can have a profound effect on day-to-day functioning and lifestyle, especially the frequent urge to urinate and the difficulties when peeing.

    urologyhealth.org/adult/index.cfm?cat=05&topic=250 [http://bit.ly/r6bWmq]

3. Detection through the PSA test is very controversial because it can often lead to biopsies and to prostate cancer procedures that most often have no greater success than "watchful waiting."

    The American Urological Association published this:

"It is not known with certainty that the use of PSA testing decreases the risk of dying of prostate cancer. Screening with PSA does result in identifying more cancers than would be detected without the use of PSA. However, many of these cancers may be small and very slow growing. Such cancers may not pose a threat to them men who have them. This is sometimes called over-detection.

If men who have such cancers are uniformly treated, many men may suffer the side effects of treatment without the benefit of a longer life (called over treatment). Prostate biopsy is associated with a small risk of side effects such as bleeding or infection. A limited number of men may find the biopsy very painful. All men considering biopsy should understand the risks of the biopsy itself as well as the risks of over detection and over treatment."

American Urological Association Foundation. January 2010, "PSA & Prostate Center Screening". www.uropartners.com/conditions/condition.php?id=28 [http://bit.ly/oVaVlE] (Accessed 29 March 2011)

4. The medical treatments from meds and surgeries to radiation and chemotherapies all have major side effects as a consequence: incontinence, erectile difficulties, ejaculation problems and more.

5. Even some of the newer procedures like robotic surgeries still have side effects and no differences in outcomes, but can be promoted aggressively as a very profitable method for the medical practitioners offering them.

    "Results are similar for men with prostate cancer whether they have open surgery or laparoscopic surgery, a new study has found...

    Currently, open radical prostatectomy (ORP) is considered the standard treatment, but the use of laparoscopic radical prostatectomy (LRP), with or without robotic assistance, is becoming more widespread..."

    Preidt, R. 22 February 2010. "Two Surgical Methods Equally Successful for Prostate Cancer". www.cancerissues.com/ms/news/636190/main.html [http://bit.ly/pPzlnJ] (Accessed 29 March 2011)

6. The understanding of the causes of prostate diseases are very limited, and the American Urological Association goes as far as to say that the causes of prostate cancer are unknown. They do list some possibilities, but they are not shown as methods of prevention or healing.

7. If you live in the U.S. you have the highest incidence of prostate problems in the world (10-100 times greater than some rural Asian traditional societies whose diets are not yet Westernized) and, if you are dark-skinned, then you have twice the rate as white-skinned men.

8. Prevention is almost non-existent and early detection is marketed as prevention, when in fact it is a way of scheduling more and more tests, often leading to very aggressive biopsies that can worsen the condition or spread it.

9. Another tragic situation is that doctors are not free to promote alternative ideas for treatment, as they could lose their license! They are not allowed to offer them.

The Risks of Conventional Treatments

Let's look further at some of the assumptions of today's medical diagnoses. We must re-examine the progression that medical diagnosis takes. A DRE may or may not be done, and if done it may be inconclusive. Prostate cancer feels different than an enlarged prostate in that it can have a spongy feeling during a DRE. Then a PSA test is done. If the PSA levels are elevated, doctors recommend a biopsy even though a high PSA level can indicate many things and not necessarily cancer. It could be that ejaculation happened in the last 48 hours, or higher stress, or some infection or medication taken.

The PSA test is just too unreliable. You can have a healthy prostate and a high PSA or a low PSA and a cancerous prostate.

A biopsy is the only way to know if cancer is present in the prostate. If it is, then the outcome will be one of the procedures outlined earlier if you subscribe to conventional medical practice. Keep in mind that the biopsy itself can lead to the spread of cancerous cells throughout the body. Biopsies also increase urination difficulties and erectile dysfunction.

Here's the problem: medical prostate treatments have not been proven to reduce prostate-related fatalities! Statistically it has now been shown that actively not treating the prostate disease and cancer has the same or better result than conventional treatments! So why in the world should you try a conventional approach?

You would be much better off trying *unconventional approaches,* as they could have a much better chance of turning the corner!

There are awful side effects for conventional medical treatments. Impotence is almost guaranteed and incontinence highly likely. Look at the explosive growth of adult diaper usage. I remember working in my Dad's pharmacy as a teen. We never had adult diapers. It would have been unheard of in the early to mid 60s!

Doctors downplay these side effects and tend to promote the success of their treatments. (It may be because they are not fully informed with the latest information or perhaps because of how they get paid; very likely it is because of liability if they do not aggressively go after cancer.)

In terms of hormone treatment, where prostate cancer patients are treated with female estrogen hormones to reduce testosterone levels, this is a mistake! In Roger Mason's massive review of worldwide literature on studies using testosterone-reducing therapies, doctors all follow one popular yet flawed study that grabbed attention and persists in its false premise. For more info on this, see Roger Mason's book *The Natural Prostate Cure* [http://amzn.to/rdZS1M].

Estrogen hormone treatment changes your body at a very base level, stripping away your masculinity. Estrogen can make you less assertive, more placid, acquire body fat, develop breasts and get hot flashes like a menopausal woman. In addition to that, forget libido. Erectile dysfunction and impotence are common consequences, as with the other treatments.

Hormone treatment increases the risk of:

- a fatal heart attack by a massive 28%

- fracturing bones within 2 years by 57%

- getting intestinal cancer by 19%

And, unfortunately, if you think it's still worth it all to cure your prostate cancer, you'll likely discover that the chance of being cured is about the same as if you did nothing at all.

Let's review some interesting results from a study done by the Cancer Council of NSW Australia. The researchers wanted to examine the quality of life 3 years after prostate cancer diagnosis for men who had localized disease and for a population control group.

One eye-grabbing sentence in the results says,

> *"Of the 1642 men with localized disease we found that in general their overall physical and mental function at three years was no different to population controls."*

> Smith, D.P. et al. 27 November 2009, "Quality of life three years after diagnosis of localised prostate cancer: population based cohort study". www.cancercouncil.com.au/editorial.asp?pageid=859&fromsearch=yes [http://bit.ly/nbgGYF] (Accessed 28 March 2011)

These researchers go on to add that although no difference was found there, there was a difference in sexual function, stating that it was worse for the men treated!

With regards to impotence: 21% of men who had a radical prostatectomy were impotent before their diagnosis, and **3 years after treatment 77% were impotent!** Those who underwent the radical prostatectomy had a poorer urinary function than those who didn't undergo the treatment.

Three years after external beam radiotherapy, men treated with a radical prostatectomy experienced the most compromised bowel function.
Just as I have written before, the lead doctor of the study, Dr. Smith, reaffirms this point: "Clinicians tend to under-estimate side-effects following prostate cancer treatment and invariably are surprised when they learn of the extent and duration of impotence following treatment."

There is further proof of no benefit of standard procedures from the National Cancer Institute, which studied the comparative effectiveness of low-risk prostate cancer treatments. The conclusions of this study state that when investigating the various approaches such as active surveillance, surgery and radiation therapy, the overall survival and tumor recurrence rates are similar.

Many prostate cancers advance slowly and aren't always life-threatening, so "watchful waiting" (aka active surveillance) is a viable strategy, especially for older men with a shorter life expectancy. Watchful waiting is advantageous since it avoids the pain and possible side effects of immediate medical intervention such as surgery or radiation, and it allows you time to make positive lifestyle changes to reduce the cancer.

The National Cancer Institute study continues on to say that active surveillance, as opposed to immediate treatment options, has a "comparable net health benefit" with a more quality-adjusted life for men 65 and older.

On the other hand, men younger than 65 or who have another 20+ years life expectancy, active surveillance produces "mortality outcomes not substantially inferior to radical prostatectomy." In other words, no treatment ("active surveillance" or "watchful waiting") gives virtually the same outcome in terms of life expectancy BUT with higher quality of life advantages!

ICER. 2010, "Management Options for Low-Risk Prostate Cancer". icer-review.org/index.php/mgmtoptionlrpc.html [http://bit.ly/pOO7ae] (Accessed 29 March 2011)

For me, it is clear that doing nothing gives a better quality of life than undergoing conventional treatments. The side effects avoided are a huge benefit to your quality of life.

The best solution then is to prevent prostate cancer in the first place, and if you suspect you may have it from a DRE or a rising PSA test, then follow the recommendations in this book—avoid a biopsy and instead heal your prostate naturally! Healing your prostate naturally is far better than conventional treatments and quite likely better than doing nothing.

My personal view on this is that it is better to assume that cancer is present and immediately take those natural precautions described in the next chapters that can slow down or even stop the cancer.

According to the autopsy study "All Men Get Prostate Cancer: What Are You Going Do About It" [http://bit.ly/o86xOb], 70% of men aged 60 have latent prostate cancer (contained by the immune system). What this means is that the cancer cells are there but not enough to trigger full-blown cancer.

Given that info, part of my calculation is that prostate cancer is generally a very slow developer, and only rarely is it fatal.

The best solution is real prevention and healing through nutrition and changes in exposures to toxins.

I will leave you with a crucial question for you to ponder. All of the risks of biopsies and medical prostate cancer treatments (often they cannot get all the cancer cells) that can cause the spread of the cancer beyond the prostatic capsule—can these themselves be a big part of what is referred to as prostate cancer deaths? Are men really dying from the prostate cancer or is it *the spreading of the cancer beyond the prostate* that results from these actions? I have never seen an answer to this question, but I would not rule out these medical procedures themselves as a major cause of the increase in deaths from "prostate cancer."

Chapter 5: Real Possible Causes

Statistically, the United States has been ranked the 37th healthiest nation in the world, as was published by the World Health Organization. This seems very low for a nation as advanced in science and technology as the USA. How has this discrepancy been created?

Too easily—through poor nutrition and lack of sufficient exercise. In general, Americans place their physical well being after their "personal, financial, social and ego-based gains." But truly, if you don't have good health, then you don't have anything at all because how can you enjoy these gains if you're not well?

Mason, Dennis 12 April 2011 "Real Health Care Begins with You." www.naturalnews.com/032040_health_care_responsibility.html [http://bit.ly/qgwgBL] (Accessed 12 April 2011)

Let's assume that we agree on putting health and fitness first. I will now move on to specifically provide a full understanding of preventing and healing the prostate from disease.

To me it is no mystery why we have such sky-high rates of prostate conditions. We have, by design and negligence, allowed our food and environment to become so toxic that disease is the body's healthy response to the onslaught!

Disease happens when the body tries to protect itself from further damage by concentrating toxins and pollutants and other excesses in a less vital organ or area of the body so that the body can still carry on.

The prostate is a deep-inside organ that is vulnerable to toxins just like the breast or uterus. The concentration of toxins in the prostate can result in any of the prostate diseases. Add to this the unhealthy habits of eating poor quality foods, little to no exercise and our sedentary lifestyles and you have a clear understanding of causes.

Each man who reads this book faces a major choice: use your new insights to change your habits and remove the causes so your body can start to heal or submit to the conventional stream with all its unfortunate side effects and consequences.

Taking Responsibility

Conventional medicine misses the boat entirely by not focusing on the causes of prostate problems:

- ✓ the massive toll of stress in our lives;
- ✓ our sedentary lifestyle combined with lack of enough exercise;
- ✓ terrible diets of chemicalized denatured non-nutritious toxic foods;
- ✓ the everyday use of toxic bodycare and household products;
- ✓ exposure to excessive environmental toxins from conception onwards; and
- ✓ lack of sunlight and vitamin D.

It then adds insult to injury by prescribing medications, treatments and procedures that further weaken the body and create unnecessary serious side effects.

We've got it all backwards! And we have bought into it as par for the course. We even go so far as to view doctors as the health givers and health providers when in fact they are a cog in a wheel that promotes symptomatic solutions they call "cures". Give me a break! Curing involves changing the causes.

You can heal your prostate. You don't need ineffective conventional medicine. You need to change the causes and your body will heal itself as a natural course of events. That is the solution and the rationale for this book.

Some of what is presented from here on in will challenge your viewpoints. Please have an open mind to the natural healing processes of the body to bring you back to better health. Like when you get a cut, and we do that all the time—lo and behold—repaired. Healing takes longer with a chronic condition, but the results are just as powerful. See if any of this prostate info makes sense to you. If it does then you will find a wealth of valuable info to help you heal your prostate problems.

We create the causes by not realizing the price we pay for our bad habits, our inattention to health and not being responsible for our own life choices. Our bad choices are easy to get away with when we are younger, when we think we are invincible.

We create disease by eating junk foods, not getting enough sun and Vitamin D, using toxic bodycare products and household products, and by not understanding that the majority of food found today in supermarkets and fast food outlets is poisonous. You may not be able to feel that everyday foods are toxic because you are toxic already. Over time, the toxins work their way deeper into your organs.

Time is your enemy. Our bodies are battling the chemicals in food, the toxins in our diets and water, artificial additives and preservatives, super-manufactured and processed products, sugars and artificial sweeteners and horrible manufactured fats, the lack of vital nutrient-rich natural foods, toxic medicines and pills, artificial supplements and synthetic ingredients, hormones added into our foods, toxins in the meat of animals that are force-fed unnatural feed and receive huge doses of antibiotics to keep them alive, pasteurization of our dairy foods, poisoning of our water, and the accumulation of cancer-causing chemicals in our medicines, foods, cooking products and containers.

Hey, you'd be lucky to survive let alone thrive!

Disease is a result of these choices. Add to that our intense stress levels, bombardment of electromagnetic fields from Wi-Fi and cellular towers, the use of toxic inoculations that weaken our immune systems, the lack of exercise in our daily living to get the blood to move and the body able to eliminate its toxic loads—we have become so toxic that it is no wonder that as we age, we get sicker and sicker.

Hey America, we're now at about "50" in world life expectancy and dropping fast! And yet we spend more and more on "disease care." Look at the old folks (over 75) around you and see that the majority are in a sad state of health, kept going by operations and prescription after prescription. But where is the vitality until very old age?

Look at our old age homes and nursing homes. We do not age well. Compare that to traditional cultures where the old worked until late in life and were strong and healthy. Look to the Hunzas and Okinawans to see wonderful examples of longevity and vitality today. Why shouldn't we be like them?

For you, how important is your health? Do you want to have pee problems and have to wear diapers or have sex problems and say goodbye to sex possibly forever?

If you think that doctors can save you, then the natural healing process is not for you. Most doctors do not fully understand the real causes of prostate diseases at all. So, they advocate for their treatments, which have side effects—serious ones in many cases—and do not cure the problem. You may get some temporary relief, but you will find that soon enough health problems will be back! Whether found in the prostate again or in another part of your body.

Curing means going to the source, finding the real causes and changing them. So listen up and embrace change if you want a healthy life and a vital prostate. The good news is that most prostate conditions are reversible and can be cured once you understand the underlying causes.

The following list of causes is not all-inclusive, which you will see as we get deeper into the issues. Understanding the causes empowers you to make the changes that will restore your natural prostate health. Remember the body can heal naturally when you remove the causes and start to nourish it with vital foods.

This is so obvious that it bears repeating: stop the causes, cleanse, change your diet and allow healing to happen.

So here is a more complete list of causes of prostate diseases and prostate problems:

✓ Inherited weaknesses and disposition—how our constitution and condition will affect us.

✓ Our diets—this is so major... food is your medicine and is the core factor to making yourself healthy.

✓ Poor stress management—it is proven that stress impacts our health and may affect our hormone balance.

✓ Improper acid/alkaline balance

✓ Our lifestyle and lack of exercise—do nothing and you get something! We were born to move, not stagnate.

✓ Harmful habits

✓ Sitting for too long—we need to move. Sitting too long congests the prostate

✓ Toxicity—toxic build up from the environment and foods has a huge impact on our health.

✓ Not enough sunlight—this is a leading cause of prostate cancer. In northerly climates there are fewer sunlight hours and more exposure is needed. If you don't get enough sun, then you are very vulnerable to prostate cancer. Both white and black men are chronically low in Vitamin D, often called a hormone. Black men even more so, which is one of the main reasons for their twofold rate of cancer incidence compared to white American men, whose rates are already amongst the highest in the world. Dark skin needs a lot more sunlight to build up safe levels of Vitamin D.

✓ Not enough oxygen—our cells are depleted and lack oxygen due to pollution and not enough exercise.

✓ Vaccines, medications and too many antibiotics—these weaken the body's immune system and make us more and more susceptible to disease.

✓ Microwaved food—this unnatural heating method damages food. You save time, and you get diseased.

✓ Hormone imbalances and natural hormonal changes—hormones from poor diets and lifestyle effects can cause many prostate problems.

✓ Too much sex or not enough sex—prostatitis can result from too much, and prostate enlargement from not enough due to the build up of toxins because ejaculation flushes out toxins from the prostate.

✓ Poor water quality and air pollution—toxins again.

✓ Poor sleep and not enough sleep.

✓ Poor, depleted soil that diminishes the nutrition in our food—since the invention of modern agri-business, there has been a huge decline in our soil's vitality. The lack of vital nutrients starve the body of its necessities, in particular selenium, magnesium, and other crucial minerals. You think you are eating healthy foods when in fact they are nutrient poor.

All of these causes of prostate disease play a crucial role in whether or not you will suffer from an enlarged prostate, prostatitis or prostate cancer. We will discuss each one of these factors and why they cause prostate diseases. The reality is that most of them can be avoided if you make a conscious effort.

Andreas Moritz offers the clearest description of cancer, in my opinion, that looks at it from a causal point of view. Here's an excerpt from his book, *Cancer Is Not A Disease - It's A Survival Mechanism* [http://amzn.to/rbKt9l], which explains the root causes of cancer and how to eliminate them for good.

"Cancer has always been an extremely rare illness, except in industrialized nations during the past 40-50 years. Human genes have not significantly changed for thousands of years. Why would they change so drastically now, and suddenly decide to kill scores of people? The answer to this question is amazingly simple: Damaged or faulty genes do not kill anyone. Cancer does not kill a person afflicted with it! What kills a cancer patient is not the tumor, but the

numerous reasons behind cell mutation and tumor growth. These root causes should be the focus of every cancer treatment, yet most oncologists typically ignore them.

Curing cancer has little to do with getting rid of a group of detectable cancer cells. Treatments like chemotherapy and radiation are certainly capable of poisoning or burning many cancer cells, but they also destroy healthy cells in the bone marrow, gastrointestinal tract, liver, kidneys, heart, lungs, etc., which often leads to permanent irreparable damage of entire organs and systems in the body. A real cure of cancer does not occur at the expense of destroying other vital parts of the body.

Each year, hundreds of thousands of people who were once 'successfully' treated for cancer die from infections, heart attacks, liver failure, kidney failure and other illnesses because the cancer treatments generate a massive amount of inflammation and destruction in the organs and systems of the body. Of course, these causes of death are not being attributed to cancer. This statistical omission makes it appear we are making progress in the war against cancer. However, many more people are dying from the treatment of cancer than from cancer. A real cure of cancer is achievable only when the causes of excessive growth of cancer cells have been removed or stopped.

If you have been diagnosed with cancer, you may not be able to change the diagnosis, but it is certainly in your power to alter the destructive consequences that it (the diagnosis) may have on you. The way you see the cancer and the steps you take following the diagnosis are some of the most powerful determinants of your future wellness, or the lack of it.

The indiscriminate reference to 'cancer' as being a killer disease by professionals and lay people alike has turned cancer into a disorder with tragic consequences for the majority of today's cancer patients and their families. Cancer has become synonymous to extraordinary suffering, pain and death. This is true despite the fact that 90-95 percent of all cancers appear and disappear out of their own accord. There is not a day that passes without the body making millions of cancer cells. Some people, under severe temporary stress make more cancer cells than usual and form clusters of cancerous cells that disappear again once they feel better. Secretions of the DNA's anticancer drug, Interleukin II, drop under physical and mental duress and increase again when relaxed and joyful. Thus, most cancers vanish without any form of medical intervention and without causing any real harm.

Right at this moment, there are millions of people walking around with cancers in their body without having a clue that they have them. Likewise, there are millions of people who heal their cancers without even knowing it. Overall, there are many more spontaneous remissions of cancer than there are diagnosed and treated cancers.

The truth is, relatively few cancers actually become 'terminal.' However, once diagnosed, the vast majority of all cancers are never even given a chance to disappear on their own. They are promptly targeted with an arsenal of deadly weapons of cell destruction such as chemotherapy drugs, radiation and the surgical knife. The problem with cancer patients is that, terrified by the diagnosis, they submit their bodies to all these cut/burn/poison procedures that, more likely than not, lead them to the day of final sentencing, 'We have to tell you with our deepest regret there is nothing more that can be done to help you.'

Cancer cells are not part of a malicious disease process. When cancer cells spread (metastasize) throughout the body, it is not their purpose or goal to disrupt the body's vital functions, infect healthy cells and obliterate their host (the body). Self-destruction is not the theme of any cell unless, of course, it is old and worn-out and ready to be turned-over and replaced. Cancer cells, like all other cells, know that if the body dies, they will die as well. Just because some people assume that cancer cells are there to destroy the body does not mean cancer cells have such a purpose or ability.

A cancerous tumor is neither the cause of progressive destruction nor does it actually lead to the death of the body. There is nothing in a cancer cell that has even remotely the ability to kill anything. What eventually leads to the demise of an organ or the entire body is the wasting away of cell tissue resulting from continued deprivation of nutrients and life force. The drastic reduction or shutdown of vital nutrient supplies to the cells of an organ is not primarily a consequence of a cancerous tumor, but actually its biggest cause.

Why would the immune system want to collaborate with cancer cells to make more or larger tumors? Because cancer is a survival mechanism, not a disease. The body uses the cancer to keep deadly carcinogenic substances and caustic metabolic waste matter away from the lymph and blood and, therefore, from the heart, brain and other vital organs. Killing off cancer cells would in fact jeopardize its survival. Cleansing the body of accumulated toxins and waste products through the various cleansing methods advocated in my book Timeless Secrets of Health and Rejuvenation (www.ener-chi.com) removes the need for cancer.

Cancer is not a disease; it is the final and most desperate survival mechanism the body has at its disposal. It only takes control of the body when all other measures of self-preservation have failed. To truly heal cancer and what it represents in a person's life we must come to the understanding that the reason the body allows some of its cells to grow in abnormal ways is in its best interest and not an indication that it is about to destroy itself. Cancer is a healing attempt by the body for the body. Blocking this healing attempt can destroy the body. Supporting the body in its healing efforts can save it."

You face a choice, a fork in the road of major size! Use your healing powers to heal yourself much like a cut does when we allow the healing to unfold using the body's wisdom, or to submit to medical procedures that ignore the "why" of the disease and the logical process of healing.

I believe one day soon, we will look back on these conventional medical procedures as primitive, outdated and unenlightened, as the ones we look at today like bloodletting and surgeries with filthy instruments and hands from the 17th, 18th and 19th centuries.

You only get one body. The better your choices, the more you reduce the chances of prostate problems. Is it too expensive? What price would you pay for your health if you had a serious diagnosis? Reduce your other choices: fancy runners, coffees, gizmos and gadgets and put your "dollars" into your **Bank of Health**, the best investment on Earth!

Cancer Panel on Carcinogens

Here is a progressive analysis by the President's Cancer Panel that took courage to publish, as it goes against the mainstream. This analysis shows the dangerous effects of toxins on the nation's health and indicates that toxins are a major cause of cancers. This obvious conclusion is denied by most cancer agencies and businesses, yet is a major breakthrough at the government level.

The analysis even cites the danger of excessive CT scans and the like as a cause of cancer! It is worth reading: "2008-2009 President's Cancer Panel Report: Reducing Environmental Cancer Risk - What We Can Do Now" **[http://bit.ly/r9kMex]**

Here are some of the highlights of that report:

"• *In 2009 alone, approximately 1.5 million American men, women, and children were diagnosed with cancer, and 562,000 died from the disease.*

• *Approximately 41 percent of Americans will be diagnosed with cancer at some point in their lives, and about 21 percent will die from cancer.*

• *With nearly 80,000 chemicals on the market in the United States … exposure to potential environmental carcinogens is widespread…. Bisphenol A (BPA), is still found in many consumer products and remains unregulated in the United States, despite the growing link between BPA and several diseases, including various cancers.*

• *Some scientists maintain that current toxicity testing and exposure limit-setting methods fail to accurately represent the nature of human exposure to potentially harmful chemicals… These data fail to take into account harmful effects that may occur only at very low doses.*

• *Only a few hundred of the more than 80,000 chemicals in use in the United States have been tested for safety.*

• *Women often have higher levels of many toxic and hormone-disrupting substances than do men. Some of these chemicals have been found in maternal blood, placental tissue, and breast milk samples from pregnant women and mothers who recently gave birth. Thus, chemical contaminants are being passed on to the next generation, both prenatally and during breastfeeding.*

• *The entire U.S. population is exposed on a daily basis to numerous agricultural chemicals... Many of these chemicals have known or suspected carcinogenic or endocrine disrupting properties. Pesticides (insecticides, herbicides, and fungicides) approved for use by the U.S. Environmental Protection Agency (EPA) contain nearly 900 active ingredients, many of which are toxic.*

- *Many of the solvents, fillers, and other chemicals listed as inert ingredients on pesticide labels also are toxic, but are not required to be tested for their potential to cause chronic diseases such as cancer.*

- *The use of cell phones and other wireless technology is of great concern, particularly since these devices are being used regularly by ever larger and younger segments of the population.*

- *Americans now are estimated to receive nearly half of their total radiation exposure from medical imaging and other medical sources, compared with only 15 percent in the early 1980s.*

- *Numerous environmental contaminants can cross the placental barrier … babies are born "pre-polluted". There is a critical lack of knowledge and appreciation of environmental threats to children's health.*

- *Many known or suspected carcinogens are completely unregulated. Enforcement of most existing regulations is poor…. Regulations fail to take multiple exposures and exposure interactions into account."*

Leffal, L. D., and Kripke, M. L. April 2010. "Reducing Environmental Cancer Risk". deainfo.nci.nih.gov/advisory/pcp/annualReports/pcp08-09rpt/PCP_Report_08-09_508.pdf [http://bit.ly/r9kMex] (Accessed 29 March 2011)

Clearly we are the victims of exposures to toxins that do us harm. Is the solution for prostate cancer to add to the body's burden by submitting to the recommended additionally toxic procedures?

Take a look at this list of carcinogens put out by the American Cancer Society. Many are found in the food supply, common household products, drugs and medicines, and scores of manufactured items. Why in the world are they not banned? No wonder cancer is epidemic. It is not our "genes" that are the cause. It is what we eat and are exposed to daily. Educate and protect yourself: Known and Probable Human Carcinogens [http://bit.ly/orEVyy]

To ensure you are best equipped for prevention, let's take a further look at the causes of an enlarged prostate, prostatitis (an infection of the prostate) or cancer of the prostate.

Real Possible Causes of Prostate Diseases: An In-depth Look

Before expanding on the causes, take a look at these differences in approach:

Conventional Medicine	Natural/Alternative Medicine
The doctor is responsible	Individuals heal themselves
Treats the symptoms	Treats the causes
Uses synthetic remedies with pharmaceutical ingredients	Uses natural remedies with earth-based ingredients
Involves surgeries and radiation, chemo or drug treatments	Involves time-tested, safe, traditional or natural treatments
Possible dangerous side effects	Minimal side effects
Creates dependency	Empowers individuals
Focus on intervention	Focus on prevention
Sees parts of the person, not the whole	Holistic—sees the whole person
Based on the medical and drug industrial complex	Based on smaller scale, real-healing modalities

Read this recent article about Conventional vs. Alternative Medicine that critiques an article in the Economist that tries to debunk Alternative Medicine: "Alternative Medicine Is Valid" [http://bit.ly/n8CXbq]

Remember no one has a monopoly on understanding what causes illness and what creates vibrant health and a vital healthy prostate!

The choices I made to deal with my prostate disease were certainly *un*conventional and took courage—courage because I didn't succumb to harassment and fear that my health would get worse if I took the time to find the natural treatments that were right for me.

You can do this, too! Your prostate *can* be healed if you are willing to learn and are open to changing the causes. You do have time to make your choices. Take your doctor's fear that you will get worse unless you act now with a BIG grain of salt. Time is on your side if you make life-affirming choices.

Inherited Weaknesses and Disposition

When we are born, we come into the world with a unique gift from our parents. We inherit a constitution and our basic fundamental health core that combines the DNA of both parents. The quality of their health determines our health foundation. You can have a strong constitution or a weak one and everything in between.

We see this in people all the time. Some are gifted with strong healthy physiques and constitutions while others are less well off and must fight to maintain good health.

Lifestyle and stress conditions and the quality of food consumed by our mothers while we were in the womb all play a big part in our overall health. These factors are important in determining our constitution: whether we are blessed with a gift or burdened with a challenge.

From Conception

It is no mystery to me why we have so many health problems. From conception to deception, we adopt health-limiting practices.

In the wisest of ancient days, prior to conception, one cleansed the body fully by fasting, sweating and purifying before making babies. The quality of the sperm and egg had to be the best. This was not common practice, but the wise ones knew how important it was for future generations.

Then when the woman was pregnant she was encouraged, as much as possible, to be calm and peaceful while being active and fit.

No medications, no junk food, no artificial sugars, no manufactured non-foods, no chemical foods, no toxic bodycare products… and the list goes on and on.

Breastfeeding and Milk

In the past, natural birthing was the norm and it took place without the interventions we have today. Today, c-sections are the norm, so Mum and Doctor can schedule to ensure they don't miss the latest fav TV show or scheduled doctor holiday! The baby then misses out on the important stimulation provided by coming down the birth canal and the stimulation that helps Mum produce milk.

To Deception

For many children in the baby boomer generation, breastfeeding was bypassed. Instead of nature's perfect food for babies, we were fed formula or milk from cows with a completely different fat-to-protein profile. We were born for Mum's milk—not cow's and not chemical concoctions filled with sugars!

Pure, natural milk is suitable for older kids after they've finished breastfeeding, but cow's milk that is adulterated from its naturally good content is not suitable for anyone. Milk today is pasteurized, which kills all the good enzymes that make milk fully digestible, and then it is homogenized. Cow's milk simply has too much protein for a new baby to digest, which creates many problems.

Cows in North American feedlots are fed grain instead of natural grasses; they are confined in small quarters and dosed with antibiotics and more. Over time the cow's body becomes toxic from alien inputs and creates a contaminated food source. Due to how we treat the cows, extra estrogen is produced in the milk. Increased estrogen in our food supply is one of the many reasons North American male and female estrogen levels are too high.

Estrogen weakens the male body, creating man breasts and inflamed prostates. Lo and behold, as we age we get BPH. Hallelujah!

Being breastfed as infants—as breast milk is the ideal food for babies, not cow's milk, which is meant for a calf—is an important factor in determining our early condition and disposition to disease.

Daily Habits

Our day-to-day diets and habits determine our health condition. If a weak constitution is combined with weak health conditions created by our choices as we move onwards in life, then the body is ripe for many chronic diseases, often very serious ones. This is especially true for prostate diseases because of the accumulation of toxins in the prostate.

Some people have a strong constitution and seem to never get sick. A man like this can abuse his body for decades with a poor diet and unhealthy lifestyle choices. This type of man, when he is in his 40s or 50s, may suffer a massive heart attack or sudden prostate cancer. His daily condition will finally overcome his powerful gifts of a strong constitution.

Therefore, what we were given from our parents and what we do with it creates our health conditions, our disposition to disease in general and to prostate disease in particular.

In the case of the prostate, men can inherit a weak constitution in that area of the body. This does not mean that men with a weak constitution are doomed to prostate diseases. It just means that these men are more susceptible than others and will have to make changes to maintain prostate health.

My father had an enlarged prostate or BPH, and I got that too, but much earlier in life than he did. For me, it was a combination of weaker constitution and a poor diet for many decades, some of the key causes of an enlarged prostate.

Our Lifestyle and Lack of Exercise

Is the price tag worth it? We have become so disconnected from nature with our big city living that we have lost our connection and ability to relax and rejuvenate in nature. This is not the way for natural health. Many of us suffer from TVitis or gameitis or internetitis, we watch or play 6 hours a day or more and do not get any exercise.

A simple tip: Add daily exercise to your life and your prostate will be happy.

A big tip: By now I hope you are beginning to understand a bit about what causes prostate problems. Knowledge is power, and making better life choices can reverse our health problems. Just start where you can with what you can. Then add more healthy lifestyle choices as you go along—choose to do it. Regain your natural prostate health!

To conclude, use your daily habits to create a stronger health condition and a healthy natural prostate. In time, good habits will affect your constitution and make you healthier. We replace all our cells every seven years. You can rebuild your body over time at the cellular level to give you real health by the daily choices you make. You have control over your health.

Our Diets

If you ask people how well they eat, the answer from most is that they eat a healthy diet. Well, if this were actually true, then why do we have an epidemic of prostate diseases and such poor life quality as we age? Why are so many elderly people so unhealthy and reliant on drugs? Why has chronic disease and the loss of functional mobility become so rampant among the elderly? Why are we not vital until old age like the Okinawans of Japan who live and work to a very old age with none of the awful health problems of most of our elderly?

We eat far too much poor quality food. And we pay a very high price for this cheap, yet devitalized food. Of course this insight is not in the interest of the companies that produce these foods or the pharmaceutical industry that gives us medical concoctions that have devastating side effects to fix us good once we have a chronic health condition.

We have bought into the "miracle" of fast and convenient cheap food and we've also bought into the medical profession, which supposedly has the answers! We are to blame for playing our part by not being conscious and conscientious of what we are doing to our bodies.

Yes, it appears that the food we eat has no immediate effect. However, the cumulative result of poor food choices adds up over time and takes its toll. We cannot discharge all the toxins quickly enough, and as a result we develop health problems as we age. It is clear what causes prostate diseases.

These prostate problems are rare in cultures that eat traditional natural foods. Men's prostate health requires natural healthy food choices.
Poor prostate health results *not* from the fact that we live longer as the medical profession would have you believe, but from accumulating toxins from our modern devitalized non-food products (e.g., chips, commercial dairy and meat, and instant foods).

Time and repetition of poor food choices takes its toll. Guaranteed. That's why we have an epidemic of prostate disease in the West.

How the West's Food Industry has Changed in the 20th Century

While diets in Asia tend to include more vegetables and smaller portions of meat, we have to be careful in concluding that meat, dairy and saturated fats therein are the causal factors of prostate disease, as many health advocates claim. It may not be the dairy and meat itself, but rather the fact that the meat and dairy we consume today is no longer the natural, healthy meat and dairy of yesteryear.

During the 20th century, our agricultural practices changed dramatically. These include a huge increase in:

- ✓ insecticides, pesticides, and herbicides
- ✓ hormones fed to animals
- ✓ contaminants and chemicals in our water supplies
- ✓ using grains to fatten animals for increased milk and meat production
- ✓ pasteurization and homogenization of milk and dairy products
- ✓ chemicalized production of vegetable oils
- ✓ consumption of denatured grains like white breads, cakes, and cookies
- ✓ consumption of trans fats and hardened fats like margarine
- ✓ sugar consumption, especially deadly artificial sugar consumption
- ✓ medications of all kinds
- ✓ harmful vaccines
- ✓ fluoridation and chlorination of our water supplies
- ✓ feeding animal by-products to grass-fed and plant-fed livestock
- ✓ bioconcentration of toxins up the food chain
- ✓ chemical fertilizer use, herbicides, and pesticides
- ✓ factory farms in which animals are confined to tiny spaces and are kept from developing severe diseases only by extensive antibiotic use
- ✓ using city sewage (sludge) for farms as fertilizer with concentrations of residues and toxins from all kinds of manufactured products and medical discards
- ✓ the use of only a few seed types, which diminishes our variety and the trace elements found in a diverse food supply
- ✓ monoculture crop methods over the last century that depletes the mineral content of the soil, as this farming method relies on petroleum-based chemical fertilizers that deplete soil of vital minerals, including zinc and selenium, both of which are crucial to prostate health

✓ Genetically Modified (GMO) Foods, something that is so alien and unknown to our bodies, now found in almost all soy, sugar beet, and corn products that make up the bulk of our fast foods and supermarket foods

All of these changes impact the quality of our food, denatures it and leads to disease, especially when combined with other Western lifestyle choices.

While profitable to industry, the change to feeding grains to livestock in order to increase weight and milk production (from a normal 6 liters per day to 30!) alters omega fatty acids (omega 3s and 6s) such that a food—once beneficial—is now dangerous to consume.

When added to the other practices above, we create the conditions for our diseases by our daily consumption of these foods. Time is the critical factor here. While one meal will not have a high impact or effect, decades of meals will ultimately lead to chronic disease, which is now considered epidemic in the West.

The above list of recent changes to agricultural approaches does not include the food manufacturing practices that are even more toxic:

✓ adding high fructose corn syrup in most prepared foods and soft drinks
✓ using artificial sweeteners that are alien to the body and not metabolized properly
✓ using MSG and its derivatives like hydrolyzed protein, which are carcinogenic
✓ adding all kinds of toxic preservatives and chemicals to our food
✓ stripping nutrients from our grain products by removing the hulls and more to make them "white"
✓ drastically increasing the sugar content in our food
✓ adding artificial flavorings and colorings
✓ using chemicals and high heat in manufacturing vegetable oils
✓ using margarine and trans fats in food preparation

You know all these things! If not, you have been totally asleep at the wheel and either have been relying on a strong constitution to temporarily avoid disaster or have bought into the medical symptomatic view of the world that disease just "happens." As I have said before, you can change this. Disease is not inevitable.

Pesticides

I've shared a lot of information with you about what is wrong with the foods we normally eat. Pesticides are a key piece that needs further exploration. The pesticides in our food are powerful endocrine disruptors. They directly affect our hormones. In the case of men, pesticides in our foods result in excess female estrogens and weaken the prostate gland that relies on healthy levels of testosterone to be in optimum shape.

Pesticides also affect body weight and mood, increase your risk of prostate cancer, and lower your sperm count. No wonder so many couples cannot conceive naturally today!

Most Americans eat over a gallon of pesticides and health-destroying chemicals each year!

Although many of these toxic chemicals are excreted, our immune system eventually becomes compromised. Over time chronic conditions develop and we find sky-high rates of prostate disease. We know the enemy now—from government to agri-biz to mass processed food manufacturers, from fast food chains to our supermarkets and restaurants—and finally us who consumes them! We are our own worst enemy!

The Environmental Working Group studied the amount of residues of pesticides found on 47 fruits and vegetables, and 87,000 tests were made between 2000 and 2007, leading to a classification of the most to the least contaminated and toxic produce.

Here is a list of the worst pesticide foods—the higher the number the worse the food:

Food Item	Pesticide Load
Peach	100
Apple	93
Sweet Bell Pepper	83
Celery	82
Nectarine	81
Strawberries	80
Cherries	73
Kale	69
Lettuce	67
Grapes (imported)	66
Carrots	63
Pear	63
Collard Greens	60
Spinach	58
Potatoes	56
Green Beans	53
Summer Squash	53
Pepper	51

Food Item	Pesticide Load
Cucumber	50
Raspberries	46
Grapes (domestic)	44
Plums	44
Oranges	44
Cauliflower	39
Tangerines	37
Mushrooms	36
Bananas	34
Winter Squash	34
Cantaloupe	33
Cranberries	33
Honeydew Melon	30
Grapefruit	29
Sweet Potatoes	29
Tomatoes	29
Broccoli	28
Watermelon	26
Papaya	20
Eggplant	20
Cabbage	17
Kiwi	13
Sweet Peas (frozen)	10
Asparagus	10
Mango	9
Pineapple	7
Sweet Corn (frozen)	2
Avocado	1
Onion	1

Note. 100 = worst pesticide load; 1 = least pesticide load.

It is in your best interest to switch to organic versions of anything over 25. The others you could get away with regular produce if need be, but the food would still lack optimum nutrient density because of the depleted soils. The non-organic produce may look the same and for some it may even taste the same, but it is deficient in selenium and a host of other minerals essential for your health. Read more on pesticides in produce here: www.foodnews.org/reduce.php [http://bit.ly/pcXMuB]

Learn to Read Labels on Produce

You will see a series of numbers on produce like an orange, usually 5 numbers in a row (e.g., 94046). The first number is the key to knowing how it was grown:

#9 = Organic (selenium and nutrient rich)

#8 = GMO foods (genetically modified genes and enzymes, also containing pesticides and herbicides)

#4 = Conventional produce (contains pesticides and herbicides)

It is time to wake up! Make changes to your food intake to maintain your health and vitality if you still think you have it or regain your health and vitality it if you've lost it.

The Health Revolution Petition [http://bit.ly/nu3L2v] is worth reading and signing to see a well thought out alternative to our current restrictive and toxic health system.

Vitamin and Mineral Content of Food Plummets

Let's take a look at how depleted our food has become from the use of pesticides and chemical fertilizers in commercial farming. This short list of the US Department of Agriculture indicates the nutritional values for fruits and vegetables versus what they were in 1975:

Fruit or Vegetable	Nutritional Value Change since 1975
Apples	Vitamin A is down 41%
Sweet Peppers	Vitamin C is down 31%
Watercress	Iron is down 88%
Broccoli	Calcium and Vitamin A are down 50%
Cauliflower	Vitamin C is down 45%; Vitamin B1 is down 48%; and Vitamin B2 is down 47%
Collards Greens	Vitamin A is down 45%; Potassium is down 60%; and Magnesium is down 85%

Wow! The vitamin and mineral content of our food has dramatically plummeted. Our food has been designed to look good and store well in transit to supermarkets. Eating conventional foods is a quick way to rob your body of essential nutrients! No wonder organic foods have been growing at a compound rate of 25% per year for well over a decade. People are cluing in—we are learning that we are healthier and happier if we eat whole non-toxic foods.

"Why your food is nutrient deficient

Trace minerals like zinc and selenium are absolutely crucial to the proper functioning of your body. And yet, nearly all trace minerals are widely depleted in the soils that grow our food.

That's because conventional agriculture extracts these minerals from the soils, year after year, while replenishing none of them. Conventional fertilizers contain virtually no trace minerals, so after just one decade of growing crops through conventional methods, the soils are depleted of crucial trace minerals that your body needs to function. Conventional agriculture, it turns out, is almost like a strip mining operation that pulls valuable minerals out of the soil and carries them away in the food, ultimately leaving the soils depleted."

Adams, Mike. 18 February 2011. "Why you should get your selenium and zinc from foods, not synthetic vitamins" www.naturalnews.com/031397_MegaFood_zinc.html [http://bit.ly/r5NFR4] (Accessed 6 May 2011)

Many consumers have realized the price of conventional food is sky high in terms of its deleterious effect on our health. The higher price of organics is well worth the health benefits.

Some may think that taking a vitamin and mineral supplement is all that is needed to stay healthy while continuing to eat conventional, toxic, and depleted produce. These people are mistaken! They have bought into another industry myth that health is found in a pill. Our bodies just can't absorb vitamins and minerals that way. In fact, so-called health supplements may actually be quite harmful to your health. (Sorry to put a damper on your "good health practices"!) I'll explain this in further detail in Chapter 9.

The bottom line is that mineral deficiency is another key cause of disease. There is just not enough nutrition in the food we eat. Guess what? Your prostate relies on lots of high-quality zinc, magnesium, and selenium to stay healthy, and you ain't gettin' it in your Standard American Diet (SAD) of denatured foods!

A healthy prostate contains a higher level of zinc than any other organ in the body. Zinc seems to protect the prostate from prostate diseases by keeping hormone levels in balance, preventing the over-production of DHT (a testosterone derivative) and inhibiting 5-alpha reductase (an enzyme involved in steroid metabolism), which helps to shrink the prostate. As a bonus, zinc also boosts the immune system by destroying free radicals and bacteria.

"Semen, the secretion product of the prostate gland, contains large amounts of zinc and the prostate gland concentrates this nutrient. In animal studies, zinc deficiency results in complete sterility. In addition, zinc is a cofactor in many reactions involving our immune system. Zinc deficiency is often associated with immune dysfunction, resulting in a number of disease conditions, from chronic viral infections to cancer. Zinc deficiency is also related to prostate enlargement. Many researchers believe that chronic zinc deficiency results in gradual enlargement of the prostate in much the same way that chronic iodine deficiency results in enlargement of the thyroid gland.

The decline in soil fertility translates into lower mineral content in our food, and the substitution of vegetables oils for animal fats has robbed the developing male of the fat-soluble vitamins (vitamins A and D) that he needs to make testosterone out of cholesterol. In addition, the vegetable oils are invariably rancid, causing irritations and inflammation in the arteries. The trans fats in margarines and shortenings used in processed foods also interfere with the production of testosterone."

"Man in the Iron Mask: The Holistic Treatment of Men's Diseases" fourfoldhealing.com/2010/06/08/man-in-the-iron-mask [http://bit.ly/r8fqnw] (Accessed 8 May 2011)

This does not mean that you should over supplement with zinc, which needs to be balanced with some copper. The best way to get zinc is by eating foods rich in zinc like oysters (best), wild salmon, liver (also contains copper), wheat germ, Brazil nuts, egg yolks, sesame and pumpkin seeds, lamb, sea salt (not commercial salt), dark grades of maple syrup and very dark chocolate. Make sure the meat and eggs are from grass-fed animals not conventionally fed ones.

Endocrin Disruptors and Neurotoxins

Now add to the mix the dangers of BPA found in some plastics used for water bottles and holding liquids, and lining the cans of canned food, and you have an even greater burden! BPA is an endocrine disruptor that mimics estrogen. It is linked to imbalanced hormone levels and decreased testosterone. Just what your prostate needs!

If we add toxins in our diet whether knowingly or not we automatically stress our prostate and deposit toxins in it. Lo and behold, one day prostate disease strikes, seemingly out of the blue. Well, now you know the real cause and the solution is obvious—change your inputs!

Neurotoxins are added to many manufactured and restaurant foods as taste enhancers. This is true of many healthy sounding chemicals, including many organic ones. These ingredients often cause serious health reactions over time, adding to the body's toxic load, causing food addictions and weight gain. We need to educate ourselves to read labels. There are just too many deadly, manufactured additives hidden in packaged and restaurant food.

As reported in NaturalNews.com [http://bit.ly/pqoXSB]:

> **"A Hundred Health Sapping Neurotoxins are Hidden in Packaged and Restaurant Food**
>
> *Monosodium glutamate (MSG) is probably the best known of the neuro-toxins. However, there are many other names for these protein additives... Even the pleasant sounding term natural flavors can mean the presence of additives toxic to the brain and nervous system....*
>
> *When the word "spices" is used, it is the tip-off that toxic additives are hidden in the product. If you're wanting to avoid neuro-toxic additives, you need to know that there is a lot more to it than just looking for it on the label....*
>
> *Even if products say "No MSG" or call themselves "all natural" or "organic," it is almost a certainty that neuro-toxic additives are in that product. There is no way to know unless you are willing to take the time to read the label."*

Minton, B.L. 11 May 2009. "A Hundred Health Sapping Neurotoxins are Hidden in Packaged and Restaurant Food". www.naturalnews.com/026244_food_MSG_neurotoxins.html [http://bit.ly/pqoXSB] (Accessed 29 March 2011)

Some Common Neurotoxic Chemical Food Additives:	
Aspartame	Nutrasweet
Beef flavoring	Protein concentrate
Bouillon	Protein extract
Caseinate	Seasoned salt
Chicken flavoring	Seasoning
Flavoring	Smoke flavoring
Glutamate	Soy extract
Hydrolyzed ingredients	Soy protein ingredients
Milk solids	Spice
Monosodium glutamate	Textured vegetable protein
Natural flavor	Yeast extract

Inform yourself! Make changes or fall victim to the insanity that has happened to our food supply. We are overfed nutritionless food and stuffed full of toxins! Remember what was noted back in the beginning of this book about the male plumbing system? The prostate filters toxins from the semen. Now do you wonder why prostate disease is so common? We put so many toxins into our systems that our prostates are overwhelmed in their filtering job.

It is time to get back to our roots. Simpler food has to become the priority in day-to-day living, not an afterthought. Yes, it will cost you more in time and effort and price, *but* it will save you in terms of health vitality and peace of mind. Your health is your wealth, and you will discover how priceless it is if you should wake up one day with prostate disease.

If you want to ensure that prostate disease does not devour you later in life, then you must change your food and health practices to ensure your vitality and health.

Chronic Conditions and Allergies

Further along the same line, let's take a look at sensitivities and allergies. It isn't any secret among practitioners in the natural health field that most patients who come to them with a long-term or chronic issue suffer from one or more allergies. What exactly is an allergy? Allergies occur when the body's immune system produces antibodies. This is in response to the body's repeated exposure to a substance or antigen that is normally harmless.

Wherever the defense reaction is more noticed in the body is where disruptive and uncomfortable symptoms will be most intense. For example, extreme mucus congestion and breathing difficulties arise if the reaction is in the nose, sinuses, or lungs.

In the prostate, an allergic immune reaction could lead to an enlarged prostate. For women, a similar immune response may cause ovarian cysts.

Imagine if you have a toxic diet and suffer from constipation. This allows a lot of time for toxic absorption across the thin rectal wall into the prostate. Every time you pee, toxins pass right through your prostate. What you eat counts big time! You can pretend otherwise if you haven't developed symptoms yet, but most Western men eventually develop prostate problems.

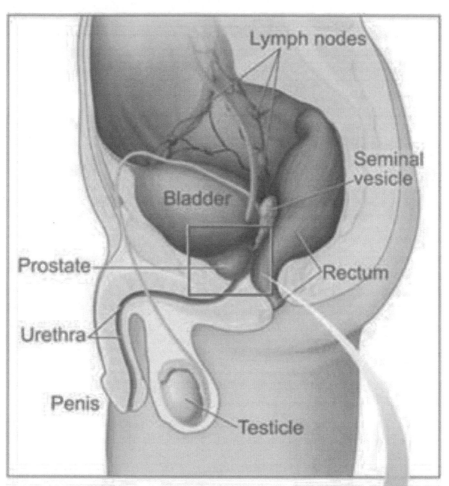

This shows the prostate and nearby organs.

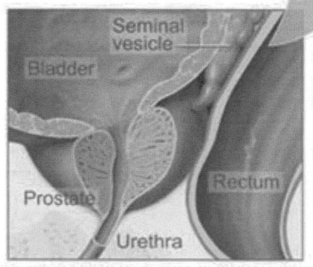

This shows the inside of the prostate, urethra, rectum, and bladder.

The answer is clear: you are what you eat. Food can be your medicine or your poison. We have come so far from a natural healthy food diet. Highly processed food has become the norm. We are sadly way off base if real men's health is the goal. Just as poor quality non-foods cause disease, so too can healthy food be a medicine to create a vital body and prostate.

The Bad and the Good about Red Meat and Dairy

Let's take a closer look at meat. Meat today is so far removed from our natural meats of yesteryear that they have become killer foods. The fat changes from being healthy—with the perfect balance of omega fats—to an unbalanced form filled with hormones (to increase meat and dairy production) and antibiotics (to deal with rampant animal disease). The feed for these animals is toxic and the animal living conditions are horrid. Meat becomes a killer, and burgers are a toxic time bomb!

It is no mystery that we have heart disease, cancers, diabetes and chronic health conditions, such as the aforementioned allergies. We eat poison! We have let our governments and industries deliver to us the lowest grade cheapest food possible without real concern for health, and all of that unhealthy food is certified as Grade A ("A" should be for "awful")! What we have done to our food supply is a travesty. Hey, your nose never lies. Have you ever driven by a factory cow or pig farm? The stench is unbearable! Think that food is healthy? Yum bring it on!

Changes in hormonal balance are perhaps the key to why Western prostate conditions, including prostate cancer, have risen drastically. So what causes this hormonal change? Doctors say it is a natural consequence of aging. Alternative practitioners often blame high fat, high dairy, high meat diets as the culprits that affect our hormonal balance.

I contend that it is none of the above and that health professionals are confusing observations with cause. Yes, there is some truth to this, as high protein is a factor in many chronic diseases, but it is not the protein or the meat itself, rather it is the changed nature of the meat resulting from feeding animals the wrong food (grains not grasses) and the added chemicals, antibiotics, and growth hormones that alter once-healthy animal meat into toxic food for humans.

The real cause is that hormonal balance changes as a result of the degeneration of the quality of our food and the toxic overload of estrogen-mimicking chemicals now so all pervasive in our food and water supplies. The effect alters our hormone balance and leads to prostate problems. Men now have extremely high levels of estrogen, causing changes in men's testosterone levels, and we get all forms of prostate troubles as a consequence.

Men are almost guaranteed to have some form of prostate disease as they age unless they stop the prime causes, as I have outlined in this book. This includes prostate cancer. One piece of good news about prostate cancer is the fact that it is so slow growing, so the best course of action is to avoid cancer treatments (none of the conventional treatments improve the chances of survival, as I discussed in the "Prostate Cancer" section of Chapter 3), and some doctors admit as much. As shown by many of the latest studies, watchful waiting is now the recommended course of action.

You can go further than simply waiting and doing nothing! You can implement changes that minimize the inputs of toxicity and maximize cleansing and high quality food inputs. You can reverse the damages done over the decades or at least delay the slow growth of the cancer.

Today hormone-disrupting chemicals are impacting our health and our prostates in an unprecedented way. Known as "xenoestrogens," these hormones have invaded our lives and prostates.

Pesticides, insecticides, processed foods, household cleaning products, fireproofed mattresses, synthetic clothing, and some plastics used in food containers and plastic bottles contain these xenoestrogens. When absorbed by our bodies, these hormones mimic estrogen and create a host of toxic conditions. In men xenoestrogens create hormone imbalances raising the ratio of estrogens to testosterone, impacting our prostates with disease and cancers, growing male breasts, creating erectile difficulties, and lowering sperm count, never mind the increase in obesity.

Estrogen is also fed to cows to fatten them up and increase milk production. So we are overloaded with estrogen when we eat conventional dairy and meat products. The result is a very unhappy body riddled with growing toxins and a sad, mad prostate!

Let's take a look at these lists to see the differences in food choices. Where do you rank on this scale?

Meat

Meat can be an emotional issue for many people, especially vegans and vegetarians. I know because I was one for decades!

I went trekking in Nepal with my daughter in the Mt Everest region. When we got to the Sherpa mountain village of Namchi Bazar, after which she was named (I liked the name!), we celebrated the first part of our journey by going to a bakery. She had a cookie. I had chocolate cake. There was something in it that was no good and by nightfall I was very sick with extreme diarrhea and fever. It lasted 4 days. In the cold of the high mountains at 11,300 feet, I was severely weakened.

I finally felt better and much to the surprise of our guide, I wanted to head higher up towards Mt Everest. He was surprised because in his experience when Westerners got as sick as I was, they would go down not up as I wanted!

Two days later around noon we came upon a very isolated tea house/home at over 14,000 feet where we stopped for lunch. The owner had just slaughtered a Yak (the high mountain animal that survives only in the high terrains). The meat was drying in strips outside in the wind and sun.

I knew immediately that I had to have some! I ordered two big portions that he fried up. I ate that with such relish after being a vegetarian for so long! It was so nutritious

If you are going to eat meat here are some guidelines:

1. Eat only meat from grass-fed, free-roaming, pastured animals—animals like they were meant to be. New Zealand lamb by law must only be pasture raised. It is quite widely available.

2.
   Avoid commercial toxic meat completely—it is deadly because of the feeds used and toxins and estrogens accumulated in the meat.

   Grain-fed organic beef, while much better than commercial meat products, still have an improper ratio of omega 3s to omega 6s, which is caused by the cattle being fed grain, a completely unnatural food source, even if organic!

   Grass-fed meat is best. Grass-fed cattle produce meat with much higher levels of the beneficial omega-3 fatty acids and lower levels of omega-6 fatty acids than grain-fed cattle. Grass-fed beef is also higher in beta-carotene, calcium, magnesium vitamin E, potassium, some B vitamins, and is also higher in beneficial conjugated linoleic acid (CLA), which is known to have anti-cancer properties.

2. Eat meat with saturated fats—not lean meats. Saturated fat is good for you! This takes a shift from decades of brainwashing as to its supposed harm. It is not the protein that we need in high amounts, rather it is protein combined with the saturated fat! I know this is hard to grasp as we have been brainwashed so thoroughly that protein is good and saturated fat is bad. But read the literature at Weston A. Price Foundation [http://bit.ly/qfzk3u] and see for yourself. You decide and you can easily personal test (something I teach later in Chapter 11) to see what your body prefers. I discuss this more later on.

3. Eat smaller portions of meat (a good portion size is the size of the palm of your hand, about the thickness of your middle finger).

4. Eat organ meats like liver from time to time.

5. Avoid high temperature cooking. Stews, slow roasted meats, lightly sautéed food, and soups are ideal.

6. Avoid BBQ meats as much as possible. The charring creates carcinogens, which is not good for a prostate! More on this later.

7.
For an in-depth review of traditional and primitive diets from around the world and the conclusions on saturated fats, meat, a balanced whole foods diet and more, please read this wonderful and educational article [http://bit.ly/o9l289]:

For an in-depth look at meat, read this book:

Why Grass Fed Is Best!: The Surprising Benefits of Grass Fed Meats, Eggs, and Dairy Products [http://amzn.to/p10G7C]

Milk and Dairy

Most milk today is ultra-pasteurized, even organic milk. Ultra-pasteurization is the process of heating milk to a temperature of at least 280°F, well above the 212°F boiling point, for a few seconds. This is done to give milk a longer shelf life. What is less known is the effect that the ultra-pasteurization process has on the natural enzymes in the milk and consequently the effects this has on the human body. The Weston A. Price Foundation [http://bit.ly/qfzk3u] states:

> *"Rapid heat treatments like pasteurization, and especially ultra-pasteurization, actually flatten the molecules so the enzymes cannot do their work. If such proteins pass into the bloodstream (a frequent occurrence in those suffering from 'leaky gut,' a condition that can be brought on by drinking processed commercial milk), the body perceives them as foreign proteins and mounts an immune response. That means a chronically overstressed immune system and much less energy available for growth and repair."*

Not to mention the ill effects of milk packaging! Read from the same website about the dangers of this health destroying process and the risks of the plastic containers that are common today.

> *"While the processing of [ultra high temperature processed] milk creates palatability problems and possible health risks, so does its packaging—both the aseptic boxes and plastic containers. For example, phthalates and other endocrine disrupting compounds (EDC) can leach into the milk."*
>
> Forristal, L.J. 23 May 2004, "Ultra-Pasteurized Milk". www.westonaprice.org/modern-foods/ultra-pasteurized-milk [http://bit.ly/pOvUsd] (Accessed 29 March, 2011)

The normal pasteurization process heats milk up to around 250°F and uses pressure as well. Perhaps it is a bit better than the ultra-pasteurized type, but still is not a healthy or whole food.

Andreas Moritz in *Timeless Secrets of Health and Rejuvenation* [http://amzn.to/nmUh4Y] also describes the problems with milk pasteurization:

> *"Once milk is pasteurized, or ultra heat-treated, its natural enzyme population is destroyed. Yet the enzymes are needed to make the milk nutrients available to the body cells. <u>Newly born calves die within six months when fed with pasteurized cow's milk.</u> One can only imagine the turmoil that must be going on in the tiny intestinal tract of a baby who is fed with pasteurized milk or sterilized milk formula. As mentioned before, such babies usually develop colic, bloated and chubby, discharge mucus, catch colds frequently, are restless, and cry a lot."*

My conclusion is to find a source of raw milk if you are going to drink milk or milk products. I finally found some and was able to personally test it. Commercial milk and the best organic pasteurized milk I can find, including yogurts of most brands, have a test result of NO for me but the raw milk and the raw milk yogurt made at 180°F have a YES test result. In addition, when I consume raw milk my tongue does not have a white coating in the morning, which is a sign of poor digestion.

I was also able to find some delicious raw milk cheeses at the health food store, so look for those and perhaps at extensive cheese counters in upscale supermarkets, as they may have some as well (especially Quebec or French ones). I also tested YES for raw milk cheese while other pasteurized cheeses, including organic ones, are NOs for me.

In *Timeless Secrets of Health and Rejuvenation* [http://amzn.to/nmUh4Y], Moritz goes on to describe how boiling milk can be beneficial. To differentiate, slowly boiling at a lower temperature or about 180 to 220°F, rather than a rapid heating under pressure to temperatures between 250 and 280°F for pasteurization are two completely different processes. The slow boiling at a lower temperature is something that traditional cultures have done for a long time…

> *"Boiling fresh, non-pasteurized milk before consumption seems to have a beneficial effect. Milk protein begins to break down into amino acids during boiling, which makes it easier to digest and absorb. This may be one of the reasons why East Indians always boil their milk before use. They also know that milk has adverse effects when its fat is removed…"*

And just a note on digestibility and milk temperatures, Moritz lets us in on the life of enzymes and the ideal environment required for maximum digestion:

> *"Cold milk is very difficult to digest. As the cold milk touches the warm stomach lining, the nerve endings of the stomach become 'numb' or insensitive, and its cells tighten or shrink. This inhibits the secretion of gastric juices, which is required to digest milk protein. The cold condition of the milk may even be responsible for leaving those proteins undigested that are known to cause allergic reactions. Enzymes require a specific temperature to be able to act on the food; if the temperature is too low the proteins will not be broken down properly, hence the intense irritation of the mucus lining."*

Fats

There is more and more research pointing its finger at our Western diets, in particular at our over consumption of meats and fats. It is definitely true that rural Asian men have a tiny fraction of the prostate diseases than we have in the U.S. Their diets have a lot more fiber, vegetables, legumes, and fish and much less red meat, dairy, and fats.

The table below contains World Health Organization data, providing age-standardized rates of incidence and mortality in males (per 100,000) in 2002:

Country	Incidence of Prostate Cancer (per 100,000)	Mortality (per 100,000)
China	1.7	1.0
Thailand	4.5	2.9
Korea (South)	7.6	2.8
Japan	12.6	5.7
New Zealand	100.9	20.3
Australia	76.0	17.7
Canada	78.2	16.6
UK	52.2	17.9
USA	124.8	15.8

The information in this table is overwhelming—American men have a huge risk of prostate cancer compared to Asian men.

After examining this table, it certainly makes sense to eat more vegetables and increase the right kind of fiber. I believe that it is mostly the transformation of our once-healthy grass-fed meat and unpasteurized milk into toxic meats and dairy that we consume today that contributes greatly to our inflated rates of prostate disease as well as the addition of highly processed vegetable fats like margarine and trans fats.

We need to eat meat and dairy as they were produced for thousands of years, not the way they are adulterated and poisoned today.

When looking at fat, it seems that the culprit is always saturated fats and trans fats. Clearly trans fats are highly processed dangerous fats to consume, but we have to be very careful about the argument that saturated animal fat is bad for us. What is certainly bad for us is what is found in the saturated fat of today's animals.

Read this article that exposes the myths that cholesterol from saturated fat is the major harbinger of heart disease and death:
"You Have Been Lied To About Cholesterol And Fats" [http://bit.ly/rps3Af]

I have explained that the meat and dairy we consume today are bad for us because of the toxicity from the animals being fed grains, hormones, and antibiotics, and being crammed into small stalls—this problem is even worse for the fat. The toxins, hormones, and antibiotics concentrate even more in the fatty tissues of these animals and in the fats in dairy. So the more we consume these toxic foods, the more our disease rates explode. But is it the fat or what we have allowed to take residence in the fat?

I believe the evidence is clear—toxins are the culprit. How in the world could the human race have survived if animal fat itself were toxic? The fat and the animal organs were the prized parts of animals and provided many health benefits (more on this later). Read this article called "The Skinny on Fats" [http://bit.ly/rc1KCz] if you want more info.

Another thing to consider is the omega-6 to omega-3 ratio. It is the omega-3s that we are deficient in. The omega-6/omega-3 fat ratio has become too extreme and we are eating way too much omega-6s. This crops up in areas of our diet that we don't even think about, like regular store or restaurant meats

For example, grass-fed beef contains omega-6 and omega-3 fatty acids in close to the healthy 2:1 ratio. But grain-fattened commercial beef, which most people eat, contains fat in an imbalanced ratio that parallels the ratios found in the grains used to fatten them, which are 20:1, 30:1, and even 50:1 in favor of omega-6!

Omega-6 polyunsaturated fatty acids have a tumor-promoting effect while omega-3 acids have a protective effect.

Jon Barron's article, "Fats and Oils Made Simple" [http://bit.ly/qCEN4J]

After writing this, I went downstairs for lunch. The plan was to have cold adzuki beans on toast that I had cooked last night after reducing the phytic acid content by soaking the beans for 24 hours and by cooking with kombu seaweed (a trick the Japanese use to reduce the phytic acid as well as to reduce flatulence). The beans certainly tested positive when I personally tested it after cooking.

I tested the food again, just to double check. I then had the idea to see what my body would prefer. I had some grass-fed bacon full of fat in the fridge. I have been slowly adding grass-fed meat to my diet after decades of being mostly vegetarian and vegan.

So I have been going slowly in this change to meat eating. What would my body prefer? So I did the personal test for the beans, got a yes and the same for the bacon. Now I did the test to see which one would be better for me—the bacon won!

The "STOP" Lists

This section summarizes what to stop eating. Most items have been covered earlier. For many people, it is not obvious that food is medicine and crucial to ensuring good health. We become victims of our daily habits. Many of the bad foods we eat are addictive. The toxic assault these foods provide to the body result in weight gain as the toxins are forced out to exterior tissues because they cannot all be eliminated by the overburdened system of elimination.

Our guts become a toxic wasteland. Our prostates bear a huge burden. Eliminating toxic foods is essential to give your body a chance at natural healing. Review this list and see if it makes sense to you.

Stop Consuming the Following "Non-Food" Products:

- Stop eating commercial manufactured food. This includes: cookies, candies, muffins, cakes, breads, crackers, frozen dinners, soft drinks whether of the sugar kind or artificial sweeteners, sauces, oils, white flour products, white rice, and spaghetti-like foods. Basically, avoid most of what you find in today's supermarkets.

- Stop eating most commercial, conventionally-grown, pesticide-contaminated fruits and vegetables.

- Stop using refined sweeteners such as sugar, dextrose, glucose, high fructose corn syrup (recently found to contain mercury in over 40% of products tested by the FDA); bottled fruit juices (they have as much sugar as a Coke), "energy drinks", etc.

- Stop using all sugar substitutes like Aspartame and Splenda brands, etc.

- Stop eating all hydrogenated or partially hydrogenated fats, trans fats and oils no matter how "healthy" the marketing departments make them appear. This includes canola oil (the first GMO food made from toxic rapeseed oil), corn oil, soy oil, margarines, safflower oil, cottonseed oil. Replace with butter, ghee, lard, extra virgin coconut, olive, and avocado oils. Learn more here "Know Your Fats" [http://amzn.to/oTm9XB] and here "Canola Oil is Another Victory of Food Technology over Common Sense" [http://bit.ly/ojo2E5].

- Stop consuming commercial pasteurized and homogenized milk and dairy products. Replace with raw milk ones (ideal) or organic versions (not as beneficial as raw). Learn more here: www.realmilk.com/why.html [http://bit.ly/ntX38m]

- Stop eating commercial factory eggs, fowl, meat, and processed meats of all kinds. Replace with organic or grass-fed, free range products (ideal).

- Stop using commercial salt. Use sea salt instead.

- Beware of health food store products that contain many of the above restrictions. Many health food store foods are unhealthy.

- Stop consuming Genetically Modified (GMO) or Genetically Engineered (GE) and irradiated foods. The American Academy of Environmental Medicine has issued a warning urging the public to avoid genetically modified foods: www.aaemonline.org/gmopost.html [http://bit.ly/nz8Anm]

- Stop eating commercially farmed salmon and fish unless organic—these fish are fed toxic feeds and antibiotics.

- Stop eating fish that are very high in mercury, like king mackerel, swordfish, tilefish, grouper, marlin, orange roughy, walleye, and tuna. Eat these fish instead: catfish, clams, flounder, haddock (Atlantic), herring, mackerel (North Atlantic, chub), mullet, oysters, perch (ocean), plaice, pollock, salmon, sardine, scallop, shrimp, sole (pacific), squid (calamari), tilapia, trout (freshwater), and whitefish. See this consumer guide for a complete list of the best and worst fish: "Consumer Guide to Mercury in Fish" [http://bit.ly/oIznaR]

- Stop consuming canned foods. Not only are the can linings toxic (coated with BPA), but also the food is devitalized and nutrient poor.

- Stop drinking caffeinated commercial products and drinks.

  Stop taking powdered protein concoctions and mixes.

- Stop eating commercial cereals, grains, nuts, and seeds and granolas that contain phytic acid (phytates), as these deplete the body of vital minerals. These foods, including organic grains, nuts, and seeds, must be soaked first to reduce this irritant. The worst foods in this category are extruded ones like puffed cereals and flakes (often coated with oils and sugars), rice cakes, shredded cereals. (More on this later.)

- Stop consuming soy products like soymilk, tofu, frozen soy desserts, etc., as they contain very high levels of phytic acid as well as cause many problems, especially related to hormones. Miso, tamari and tempeh are the okay soy foods as they have been fermented. Avoid all others. Buy organic versions of miso, tamari, and tempeh, as most soy products are now genetically modified. See this article called "Soy Alert" [http://bit.ly/pA2fY1] for more info, and this article called "The Truth About Unfermented Soy and Its Harmful Effects" [http://bit.ly/pRd9SE].

- Stop fluoridated water. It depletes iodine from the body causing hypothyrodroidism and immune deficiency as well as weight gain and heart disease. See this article "Flouridation: The Scam of the Century" [http://bit.ly/mQLGxp] and this article "Flouride Depletes Iodine in the Body, Causing Hypothyroidism and Immune Deficiency" [http://bit.ly/rtDwTY]

- Stop drinking chlorinated water. Chlorine is highly toxic and can mix easily with other trace contaminants in the water to make highly carcinogenic chemicals. Remove chlorine and other toxins from your water.

- Stop eating BBQ'd meats with flames burning the fats causing carcinogens (polycyclic aromatic hydrocarbons). Slow cook your meat instead.

- Stop eating commercial foods containing Monosodium Glutamate (MSG) and other food enhancers like vegetable protein, hydrolyzed protein, hydrolyzed plant protein, plant protein extract, sodium caseinate, calcium caseinate, yeast extract, textured protein, autolyzed yeast, and hydrolyzed oat flour.

- Stop eating at fast food outlets whose foods contain massive amounts of Food STOP List products.

- Stop using aluminum cookware and non-stick cookware. Use stainless steel, cast iron, stoneware or glass and ceramic pots and pans instead.

- Stop smoking and stop drinking distilled alcohol. Drink red wine and small brewery organic beers in moderation instead.

- Stop as many pharmaceuticals as possible and choose natural medicines instead.

- Stop getting vaccines. For more info, read this article on the dangers of vaccines and the impact on your immune system: "Vaccine Epidemic: How Corporate Greed, Biased Science, and Coercive Government Threaten Our Human Rights, Our Health, and Our Children" [http://amzn.to/ouZdBA]

- Stop using your microwave. It kills your food. (Read the next section on microwaved food for more info.)

- Stop using disposable coffee cups and foam take-out containers. These contain formaldehyde preservatives as well as styrene (another chemical additive), which have both been added to the federal government's list of known or suspected carcinogens [http://nydn.us/oTuO0a].

Stop Eating Microwaved Food

The Russians did a lot of research on microwaves. Microwave cooking destroys the B complex, C, and E vitamins that are linked with the prevention of cancer and heart disease, and it also destroys trace minerals in your food. Microwave-cooked food is nutritionally useless. Increased rates of cancer cell formation were found in the blood of people eating microwave-cooked meals as well as increased rates of stomach and intestinal cancers.

See Andreas Moritz's *Timeless Secrets of Health and Rejuvenation* [http://amzn.to/mRERca] page 463:

> *"Reporting for the Forensic Research Document of AREC Research, William P. Kopp now states: "The effects of microwaved food byproducts are long-term, permanent within the human body. Minerals, vitamins, and nutrients of all microwaved food is reduced or altered so that the human body gets little or no benefit, or the human body absorbs altered compounds that cannot be broken down...*
>
> *In a classical experiment 2,000 cats were given only food and water that were previously placed in the microwave oven, even for just one minute. The foods selected were the most nutritious and natural ones available. Within six weeks, <u>all cats mysteriously died</u>. While investigating the surprising result of the test, it was discovered that, although the cats looked well fed, the cells in their bodies virtually contained no trace of nutrient-components. The cats literally starved to death, despite all the nutritious foods. Microwaves turned their food into deadly poison."*

Yes, I know it's fast and convenient, but microwaved water kills plants dead, fast! If you would like to read more about the dangers of microwaved food, this article describes the deadly effects of microwaved water: www.eutimes.net/2011/03/experiment-microwaved-water-kills-plants [http://bit.ly/ojQCTr]

To read more about the dangers of microwave ovens, click on this link: "Ninety Percent of Homes Contain This Health Risk" [http://bit.ly/qlxcjb]

To read more about how microwave-food causes cancer, click on this link: "Why and How Microwave Cooking Causes Cancer" [http://bit.ly/ngtASv]

Now imagine what microwaved food is doing to you and your prostate!

Stop Using Toxic Household Products:

Let's go back and revisit the Food STOP List. Above I listed a lot of foods and products to stop consuming if you want to regain your health.

The Food STOP List contains the modern killer foods and the primary cause of epidemic levels of chronic disease and prostate problems today. We are overfed, undernourished, and highly toxic to cannibals!

The good news is that when you replace toxic foods with real, whole foods, you gain back your health and discover how delicious and yummy real foods are! If you start to grow some of your own food then you will be eating fresh food with mouth-watering flavors.

Now let's add some other items to the STOP list. (You thought that list was excessive did you?) Here is the Bodycare and Household Products STOP List:

- Stop using mainstream commercial bodycare, haircare, toothcare and cosmetic products that contain large amounts of toxic ingredients, no matter how inviting they sound. Your skin is your body's largest organ and absorbs the toxins right into the body. None of these synthetic chemical ingredients have been approved as safe for human consumption by the FDA. Be wary of anything that contacts your body. Replace all bodycare products with organic versions that have safe ingredients. For a review of which preservative ingredients are safe, see www.youngagain.org/p12.html [http://bit.ly/pL9LFG]

- Stop using commercial laundry products and fabric softeners. These products get into the air and into your skin when you wear your clothing, as rinsing cannot remove all traces. Replace with organic versions that have safe ingredients.

- Stop using deadly mothballs. These are so toxic that they are banned in Europe. Use natural alternatives instead, like citronella, sandalwood, cloves camphor/eugenin, lavender, or aromatic cedar. See this article for more info: "Get Rid of Moth Balls and Other Harmful Insecticides and Use Natural Alternatives" [http://bit.ly/nmVqMe]

- Stop commercial household chemicals and cleansers of all kinds. Replace with organic versions with safe ingredients. Here is a list of safe and inexpensive alternatives: Household Cleaners and Natural Products [http://bit.ly/nFsX4E]

- Stop using plastic containers for food storage with the numbers 3, 6, and 7 in the recycling codes on the bottom. Code #7 plastics often contain BPA, which mimics estrogen and is very harmful to the prostate. Use glass containers instead.

- Stop using commercial air fresheners and perfumed candles. Replace with essential oil diffusers and beeswax candles.

You may think this list is extreme but the reality is we have compromised our health so drastically that it is time to go back to safe, time-tested products. Give your body a break! Stop the "death by a thousand cuts"! Purge your home and replace the items with safe ones.

We need to step into a time machine and go back a hundred years and have the real vital food our great-grandparents ate. We now have many conveniences to make food prep much faster and easier (except your friendly microwave oven). There are many ways to cook quickly when you take the time to learn how. Make food and your health a top priority and regain your health and vitality.

Stopping the toxic onslaught is the first step to regaining your health and preventing prostate problems from occurring or growing worse.
Remember how close the prostate is to the bladder and rectum. Your prostate can easily absorb toxins from these organs because of its proximity. That is why our diets, in the broad sense of the word, are so crucial to the health of the prostate.

> *"The urinary tract and rectum are organs through which most of the waste products and toxins in our body are eliminated. The higher the level of toxicity in a person's body, the higher the level of toxicity present in their urine and feces. The proximity of the prostate to these organs makes it very susceptible to an accumulation of toxicity – both as urine passes through the prostate, and as toxins leach out of urine stored in the bladder and feces stored in the rectum between bowel movements.*
>
> *The primary cause of most prostate conditions is toxicity in general, and hormone disruptors in particular. Hormone disruptors include pesticides, herbicides and fungicides, plus chemicals that leach into foods and drinks stored or heated in plastic or plastic-lined containers, foods cooked in cookware with non-stick coatings, and chemicals in cleaning and cosmetic products.*
>
> *Additional hormone disruption can arise from the free floating estrogen in our water supply (estrogen is excreted in the urine of women on hormone replacement therapy or oral contraceptives). In fact, all sources of toxicity in our food, water, home and work environments can potentially aggravate prostate inflammation...*
>
> *Other factors that can help prevent or support the treatment of prostate conditions include significantly reducing consumption of foods and liquids stored in plastic or plastic-lined containers; avoiding the use of drip coffee brewers where the water is heated and dripped through plastic (a stainless steel or Pyrex percolator or a Pyrex coffee press are good alternatives); using only natural hygiene and cleaning products (in particular watch out for phthalates, parabens, triclocarbans and dioxanes)."*

Vertolli, Michael. "Prostate Health: Herbs for Treating Inflammation." vitalitymagazine.com/article/prostate-health-herbs-for-treating-inflammation [http://bit.ly/qacxNu] (Accessed 5 May 2011)

Go through your whole house and start to throw out the toxic foods, bodycare, and household products. Replace all of these products with organic and healthful products. Your body will then be able to start to eliminate its toxins.

That's a lot of things to change and stop doing if you want to regain your health, but it is well worth the effort!

In issue #75 of Vista Magazine, an article on chemicals states:

> *"There are 80,000 chemicals that are registered for industrial use by the US Environmental Protection Agency. There are medical tests for only 250 of them. The health agencies have tested samples of people to try to assess the degree of contaminants in the average citizen. They tested for the presence of 210 chemicals and found 167 of them in the people tested. The average number of chemicals in any one person was 91.*
>
> *The obvious conclusion is that we are all toxic to one degree or another. It is no surprise that we are fighting a losing war on cancer, Alzheimer's disease, diabetes, thyroid disease, super bacterial infections and many other chronic degenerative conditions."*
>
> Kuprowsky, Stefan. 4 February 2011. "The Obesity-Toxicity Connection" issuu.com/beaudrystudio/docs/vista_issue75 [http://bit.ly/pTiTZr] (Accessed 5 May 2011)

If you want more information on the dangers of many common household materials, then take a look at this article: "Common Household Materials Contains a Toxic Brew of Dangerous Chemicals" [http://bit.ly/oceN2t]

Yikes! No wonder prostate disease is epidemic in the West!

My purpose is not to scare you but rather to realize why disease can develop based on our inputs. Knowledge is power. You start by making changes where you can, by substituting healthier choices little by little. Over time they will add up and your health will improve.

Using Safe Cookware

Do you want to know more about which cookware is best to use?

> *"There's good reason why glass and ceramic beakers are used in a chemistry lab where it's critical that containers don't taint the experiment. Glass and ceramic are inert or non-reactive...*
>
> *Before making your next kitchen purchase, consider the reactivity of various tools and cookware and, whenever possible, favor inert or non-reactive"*
>
> Wood, Rebecca. "Healthy Cookware" **www.rwood.com/Articles/Healthy_Cookware.htm** [http://bit.ly/pIvC7G] (Accessed 27 March, 2011)

This article provides further evidence of the dangers of non-stick cookware: "Be Informed - Non-Stick Pans Pose Danger" [http://bit.ly/p8STxS]

Here is a list of safe cookware with links to sources:

- Natural Stoneware Bakeware [http://tiny.cc/eqtky]
- Ceramic Cookware [http://tiny.cc/yzlod]
- Glass Cookware [http://tiny.cc/ynahi]
- Cast Iron Cookware [http://tiny.cc/rjaha]
- Stainless Steel Cookware [http://tiny.cc/8dm7f]

Cosmetics and Bodycare Products

I have mentioned that cosmetics, bodycare products, and household products often contain very toxic chemicals. Even ones labeled "natural" are suspect because the word has almost no protection and is not held to any standard or code. The word "natural" is overused and misleading.

The only real way to know if a product is safe is to search here for specific ingredients www.hazard.com/msds and to avoid these specific chemicals:

- Cocoamide DEA, diethanolamine, TEA, triethanolamine, MEA
- Mercury
- Parabens
- Propylene glycol, propylene oxide, polyethylene glycol
- Petrolatum and coal tar
- Phthalates
- Sodium lauryl sulfate, sodium laureth sulfate
- Sodium fluoride

Make sure your toothpaste, soaps, shaving cream, shampoos and conditioners, deodorants, aftershaves, and anything else you use on your body does not add to your toxic load. The skin is the body's largest organ and easily absorbs what you put on it. Then your kidneys and liver have to deal with the chemicals. These toxic chemicals will affect your prostate over time.

Here you can find a product database that rates bodycare and cosmetics products from least to most toxic: www.ewg.org/skindeep

The Environmental Working group has an incredible database of bodycare products from shampoos to cosmetics and sunscreens, all ranked according to toxicity. Now you can easily find safe ones and analyze the ones you are using.

For sunscreens: www.ewg.org/2010sunscreen

For perfume and cologne: www.ewg.org/notsosexy

To avoid prostate problems, avoid using conventional bodycare products. Get smart! Know what you are using. Yes, safe products will cost more in dollars but it will keep you healthy, and that saves a lot of money and unnecessary suffering. Read this article that gives a great perspective on the issue: "Heal Yourself in 15 Days by Cleaning up Your Skin Exposure" [http://bit.ly/nfT24t]

To find excellent sources of bodycare products from small-scale producers visit the: Organic Consumer Association Website [http://bit.ly/nHg3ji]
or here at Amazon: Organic Bodycare Products from Amazon [http://tiny.cc/0ppl4]

My best advise is to find organic bodycare products from a manufacturer that you can trust *and* whose product personally tests positive for you. To be safe, every now and then retest your bodycare products to ensure that minor ingredients do not have a negative reaction over time.

One of my favorite brands that goes a long way for the dollar and is exceptionally high quality and pure is the line of soaps and shampoos made by Dr. Bronner: Dr. Bronner's Bodycare [http://tiny.cc/wpqzs]. Try the almond scent. It's my favorite.

The same story holds for the dangers of household products from laundry detergent to dish liquids, from floor cleaners to air cleaners. Conventional and "natural" versions are highly toxic. If you think the water washes it away, think again. The fumes get into the air you breathe, it seeps through your skin, and the remnants stay in your clothes and also penetrate through your skin.

You don't have to believe me—educate yourself. Read this brief article on the chemicals found in the different rooms and products in your home: Toxic Household Chemicals [http://bit.ly/om7Pp6], and then personally test them to ensure they are okay.

My favorite organic all-purpose super-concentrated household cleanser that you dilute in a spray bottle is called Orange TKO.

> *"Orange TKO is a citrus cleaner/degreaser made from the peel of the orange. It is an emulsifier which contains no synthetic chemicals, petroleum distillates, or detergents. It is also 100% environmentally friendly, biodegradable, and non-toxic. Orange TKO comes as a concentrate which can be diluted with water to handle the toughest industrial cleaning problems, but is safe enough to use in the home, around children and animals. In the home, Orange TKO can be used for all of your cleaning applications."* Orange TKO [http://amzn.to/rgC6Jv]

Two quick tips on how to use this amazing cleaner: always shake the spray bottle before use. And let it sit for 10-30 seconds before wiping. It will then work like a charm! Now you can throw out all your commercial toxic stuff.

Pest Problems?

Here is another safe household item to replace your toxic ones: AlwaysEco Pest Control Products [http://bit.ly/pUvdzT]. These products use completely organic, safe ingredients and at the same time are better than conventional toxic chemicals for your lawn and garden! AlwaysEco Pest Control Products [http://bit.ly/pUvdzT] are also excellent for ridding your home of pests like wasps or bed bugs.

Purge your home! Get rid of all that nasty stuff. Personally test the products you currently have in your home and you will see how many items come back screaming NO! Fill your home with organic household products:
Organic Household Products [http://tiny.cc/qzyg4]

Do not overlook the role of personal and household products on your health. We are so over-exposed daily to toxins. If you want a healthy prostate, then there are no shortcuts. Get smart, and use only safe items in your home and on your body.

Ranking of Food Choices

In this section I rank foods from Poorest to Optimum quality. The food choices shown here are as specific as possible so that you can see the ascending scale of food choices.

Poorest

- Artificial sweeteners of all kinds such as Aspartame (NutraSweet) and Splenda (Sucralose) and their products like diet drinks
- Foods with preservatives, MSG, and other hidden neurotoxic ingredients
- Highly processed manufactured factory foods
- Foods containing growth hormones and antibiotics such as conventional dairy and meat
- Foods sprayed with pesticides
- GM (Genetically Modified) foods that are foreign to the body (90% of soy and its by-products in the US contain GMOs – that is just one item, and it is fed to animals that you eat)
- Food with trans fats
- Artificial foods and food dyes
- Meat from animals fed animal parts and grown in farm factories
- BBQ'd fat flamed food (cancer-causing due to burnt fat)

Most fast food restaurants use many of the above items. How in the world can we be healthy when we feed ourselves non-food products? Of course you don't notice it as you are eating these yucky foods. You may not even be aware what they contain until now. But little by little you are destroying your health, and you will pay a price, either with a major disease or with a slowly deteriorating health for your elder years or an untimely death! Guaranteed.

Poor or Lacking in Vitality

- Refined grains and white flours

- Extruded grain products like puffed cereals and flakes

- Undetected molds in our food

- Unripe sprayed fruit

- Commercial animal fats

- Meat and fowl grown in cramped quarters and stuffed with antibiotics and fed low quality feed

- Ultra-pasteurized and homogenized dairy food and milk

- White and processed sugars and its products

- Desserts with unhealthy fats and sugar

- Canned food

- Table salt

- Microwaved food

- Hydrogenated or partially hydrogenated oils and margarine

- Processed or smoked meats, hot dogs, and deli meats with nitrates and preservatives

- Commercial fast foods

- Highly manufactured packaged food with many ingredients with chemical names you can't pronounce

These items are a bit better than the prior "Poorest" list, but the result will be the same. It just may take a bit longer. By the time you reach your 50s, you are on our way to serious prostate problems. At best, you should only eat these foods very occasionally.

Do you really believe the claims that pesticides and preservatives are not harmful in small quantities? What about the cumulative effects? Could this be why we lose our health over time? Almost all supermarket food is toxic to your health.

It just may take time before you notice prostate problems, and most men will, in due course, have them (at least Western modern men).

Look at our epidemics of disease from diabetes to heart ailments, from cancer to chronic illnesses, from overweight problems to degenerative diseases. Most commercial food and fast foods are highly dangerous to you over time, causing major health problems and diseases.

The highest rates of prostate disease occur in those countries that eat the most animal fat and animal foods (which concentrate toxins up the food chain in a process called bio-accumulation).

Poor food choices rob you of vitality and set the stage for a diseased body. It is just time that is needed for the effects to manifest. Remember the poor frog in the pot that felt nothing until it was too late!

Acceptable but Still Not the Best

- Fresh commercial grade produce
- Home-cooked meals using fresh ingredients
- Free-range fowl and meat
- Frozen seafood
- Non-fast-food quality restaurant food

Good

- Organic produce
- Fresh seasonal local food
- Frozen seafood low on the scale of toxic metals
- Free-range fowl and meat fed with organic grain
- Natural whole foods: grains, beans, seeds, nuts
- Sea salt
- Honey and maple syrup sweeteners

Optimum

- ✓ Homegrown garden fresh organic fruits and vegetables
- ✓ Organic fresh picked berries
- ✓ Super foods (more on this later on)
- ✓ Fresh organic produce from farmers' markets and local farms
- ✓ Organic non-pasteurized grass-fed milk and dairy
- ✓ Organic, pasture-grazed (not grain fed) meat and fowl

✓ Fresh caught seafood and shellfish lowest in toxic metal content

✓ Organic whole foods: grains, beans, seeds, nuts—soaked, fermented or sprouted to reduce harmful enzymes/acids

✓ Fresh wild foods and herbs

✓ Ancient sea salt from salt deposits buried in the earth

✓ Organic unpasteurized raw honey, organic dried date and maple syrup sweeteners and naturally made organic coconut sugar

These lists shout out the differences based on our daily food choices. When people say they eat healthy, think of these lists. Where do you stand?

How much of your food and how much of the time do you eat optimally? Now imagine the cumulative effects of our choices: are they life enhancing or disease promoting? Now you understand one of the main causes of prostate disease.

It is what happens over time that causes our health problems. It can be a challenge to move up the scale, but if you have a prostate disease then this is such a key area to make improvements. In the long run, eating optimally will be the most important decision you can make for your health. Food is the magic key to health or disease based on your choices. Choose wisely.

You don't have to make all the changes right away, unless you are in a severe condition with prostate cancer. Just start to make better and better choices as you go along.

Food can kill or heal. Each choice you make counts.

Tip: STOP your bad food choices now and replace with more "Good" or "Optimum" ones. Better food choices will start you on the way to prostate health and help reverse prostate diseases, and it will also help you drop those unwanted pounds!

I remember a headline in the British Press that read: "He was bright orange when he died!"...

A man had become obsessed with drinking carrot juice because he had heard how healthy it was. I call that an excessive personality!

This man proved the saying: "Too much of a good thing can be bad for you."

Eat a broad range of foods and in moderation.

SAD—The Standard American Diet

It is SAD. Many natural health advocates beat up on the Standard American Diet, abbreviated as SAD. The health advocates claim that the Standard American Diet is the cause of our rampant chronic diseases.

The reality is that we have allowed ourselves to become duped, thinking that the cheapest, fastest food is okay to eat, and that there are no consequences for living this lifestyle. It is not necessarily the food per se but rather what has become of a once life-sustaining healthy diet of homegrown natural foods.

We indulge in denatured, devitalized foods like the Whiteys: white flour products and white sugar (breads, donuts, cakes, cookies, cereals and much more) or their artificial substitutes, combined with oils that are unfit for human consumption. We treat our animals with the opposite of respect, caging them in prisons, feeding them atrocious foods including animal parts, injecting them with massive amounts of hormones and antibiotics, and killing them without the least amount of dignity for an animal that has given its life to nurture us.

Compare that to the dignity expressed by our ancestors and farmers who treated animals with the respect and care that allowed an animal to live a life that ended with kindness and appreciation. Merciless killing of animals changes the chemical composition of the meat as fear-based hormones are released when the animal is frightened in the killing cages of today, rendering these foods even further more acidic and toxic and even more unfit for human consumption.

We have poisoned our fields with toxic fertilizers that rob the soil of its nutrients and use seeds that are so modified that they have become a source of future contamination of our whole food supply. We have sprayed toxins of all kinds on our fruits vegetables and grains that result in massive amounts of toxic wastes and chemicals amassing in our bodies.

Men's sperm counts have dropped dangerously, our infants all start life with inherited chemicals, and breastmilk is unsafe for our babies' consumption because toxins are all pervasive. Our government agencies do not protect us. They have become a conduit for special interest groups that put the financial health of corporations ahead of human safety and real health.

We have played along as consumers, believing the commercials, the agencies, and the businesses that all is well with our food. We shirk our responsibilities to our own health by ignoring what is obvious all around us, eating massively processed foods whether from the supermarkets or fast food outlets, that use concoctions of ingredients designed solely to gratify our habits with no sense of health and even the so called healthy choices are a lie when you really examine what is in them.

We are <u>all</u> guilty of letting our health degenerate to a level that is killing us and robbing our nation to pay for chronic diseases that could be avoided with conscious choices and changes to make a safe food world.

Sadly our Standard American Diet has become the Sick American Diet, and that is why we have unprecedented rates of chronic disease. The solution is not more research, new pills, or new techniques to allow the same old damaging patterns to continue.

The only realistic solution is to change our Sick American Diet and get at the very root of the problem, not to treat the massive symptoms we see all around us. Sure you can take poison pills, be irradiated, or sliced and diced and call that a "cure," but that is a joke. A cure must get to the root causes of the problem, otherwise we are living with our heads in the sand, whether you are the patient or the healthcare provider.

Prostate disease along with all the other chronic health problems is a disease of our ignorance. Sadly again, there is no bliss in this but rather the misery of a life of more and more loss of vibrancy instead of vitality and quality—a pain-free, fully-functioning life until an old age.

It is time to put our SAD to an end. We must start with ourselves by making changes day by day, bit by bit to STOP, CLEANSE, and REVITALIZE by choosing the healthiest foods and products that we can. Each of us needs to become aware of our choices and become our own caregiver. That is how we overcome prostate disease. That is how we regain our lost paradise of health.

The diet suggestions are laid out for you to embrace those changes with the promise of a renewed and healthy you with a zap in your sex life and a pee that flows strong and long!

Electric stoves in the Sherpa village of Namchi Bazar, Nepal, at 11,300 feet above sea level.

We traveled there, father and daughter, as described earlier. The people of this high mountain village were the beneficiaries of a Swiss mini hydroelectric project that brought electricity from 5 km away from a mini dam turbine. Never before had there been electricity in this village.

The villagers were ecstatic about having lights for the night but were much less so about using electric cooking stoves. This is what so many of them told us: the food cooked on the electric stoves had lost the vitality of foods cooked in their traditional way on fires. They said they never felt properly nourished by the food and they blamed the new electric stoves even though they were big energy savers. Many of them still used the old ways and cooked the food for the Western tourists on the electric ones!

Remember the cat experiment with the microwave ovens that killed them all.

Perhaps natural gas stoves are an even better choice than electric versions if you have a choice! At a minimum, stop irradiating your foods with a microwave!

Stress and How it Affects the Prostate

Stress plays such an important role in men's prostate health. Research has proven that stress is one of the major causes of all diseases not just men's prostate diseases. Men are susceptible to poor stress management because of our more aggressive makeup and activities.

If you have prostate problems or prostate cancer, then make managing stress symptoms a key area to master. This is crucial to your well being!
Let me explain why this is so important to your prostate health. I'll tell you a story, and it's true.

In my third year of my enlarged prostate condition, I got a call that Canada Revenue Agency (the Canadian equivalent of the IRS) wanted to come see me for an audit of my personal and business affairs. I knew I had nothing to hide, yet I could see why they had chosen me.

My personal income was very low while I was involved in a new start-up. It was the old bootstrap entrepreneur story. I knew all I had to do was show them my credit cards and they could see how I was living and financing the business. So, I told myself to relax and that I had nothing to worry about.

I live on a remote island and two auditors came to see me—a day's journey each way from their office! When they came, I thought that I was relaxed enough and ready. I guess I felt a bit intimidated by all the questions they asked and the documents they wanted to see. It was quite invasive.

As time progressed, I found myself shutting down. My already enlarged prostate enlarged significantly more during the three-hour meeting, and I urgently had to go and pee often.

While trying to pee, a few drops came out and then during the last hour or so of the audit nothing would come out! Every 5-10 minutes I had to go try again, but still no luck and the pain was getting unbearable. I had a complete prostate attack! Total shut down caused by stress!

By the time they left, I rushed upstairs grabbed my catheter and was able to release the urine! I learned then that stress plays a *major* role in prostate disease.

Sperm Count and Prostate Cancer

The findings of a study that examined 20,000 men suggested that prostate cancer and flaws in sperm production have a common origin. This study looked at men who had problems with sperm count in their younger adult years. It suggests that later on these men are much more likely to get severe prostate cancer. Here is a summary:

> *"Men who struggle to father a child while young are more than twice as likely to develop the most deadly form of prostate cancer when they age, research shows.*
>
> *A study of more than 20,000 men revealed those classed as infertile by [in vitro fertilization] doctors were up to 2.6 times more likely to go on to be diagnosed with the fast growing and spreading, hard-to-treat form of the disease as other men."*

> Macrae, Fiona. 22 March 2010. "Young infertile men are '50% more likely to develop aggressive prostate cancer'" www.dailymail.co.uk/health/article-1259714/Young-infertile-men-50-likely-develop-aggressive-prostate-cancer.html [http://bit.ly/nPLMn6] (Accessed 12

April 2011)

To me the decline in sperm count correlates well with the decline in our food quality and the increase use of toxic chemicals. The drastic decline in the sperm count over the past 50 years, with the higher rates of prostate cancer in those men later on, suggests to me that with the extra time those toxins are doing their job well: weakening and poisoning men's prostates. The lowered sperm count is a shot over the bow for younger men, especially those with infertility problems, to get with it! Smarten up and make the diet changes outlined in this book now!

I talk more about electromagnetic fields in a later section, but I'll introduce the idea here, as this quote relates to sperm count:

> *"Men who use mobile phones for long periods at a time may be at risk of damaging their sperm…*
>
> *Dr Agarwal said mobile phone radiation may harm sperm by damaging DNA, disrupting cells that produce testosterone in the testes, or shrinking the tubules where sperm are created."*
>
> Sample, Ian. 24 October 2006. The Guardian. "Warning to male mobile phone users: chatting too long may cut sperm count" www.guardian.co.uk/uk/2006/oct/24/mobilephones.science [http://bit.ly/qP4s6v] (Accessed 7 May, 2011)
>
> *"A recent study out of the University Hospital San Cecilio, Granda, Spain, found that common pesticides used on food crops lead to poor quality and lowered sperm counts …"*
>
> Benson, Jonathan. 11 April 2011. "Sperm counts continue to plummet, say researchers." www.naturalnews.com/032031_sperm_counts_radiation.html [http://bit.ly/pc9gcT] **(Accessed** 5 May 2011)

Another article by BBC News makes reference to a Finnish study carried out at the University of Turku. It concluded that in recent years there has been a significant deterioration in sperm quality, while at the same time testicular cancers increased. There is definitely a correlation here.

You can read the study in International Journal of Andrology [http://bit.ly/qrsvEb]. The subjects were men born between 1979 and 1987. These are young guys! The study suggests that environmental reasons, in particular exposure to industrial chemicals, could be responsible for both observations, as the title of the BBC article suggests.

BBC. 4 March 2011. "Cancer Rise and Sperm Quality Fall 'Due to Chemicals'" www.bbc.co.uk/news/health-12634109 [http://bbc.in/naIJTC] (Accessed 5 May 2011)

Mercury Fillings

Some natural health practitioners claim that mercury amalgam teeth fillings pose a risk to your health. Some practitioners will advocate the removal of mercury fillings and replacement with enamels. Their rationale is that the mercury is toxic and has been banned in many countries for use in fillings as mercury fillings leak and cause many health problems. Yes, never get a new filling with mercury. The question is should you remove the old ones? Here is how I would approach that question:

1. Are your fillings stable? Your dentist can verify their status. If your mercury fillings are cracked or damaged then replacement may be warranted because of the dangers of leakage. While some alternative dentists will say that any fillings are harmful, my question is this: where is the evidence?

2. I would be wary of replacing all your fillings. I know many people who thought that mercury fillings were the cause of their health problem and had their fillings replaced, but it did not solve their health issue—many thousands of dollars later!

3. If you suspect a problem, a blood test for mercury and heavy metals is ideal, not a saliva test, urine test, or hair analysis. Do not let someone muscle test you to see if you have a problem with mercury fillings (especially a practitioner with a vested interest in selling you their products or services). I did a blood test and the results came back at the low end of normal results.

The Personal Heavy Metal Screen Test is a new test that can be a starting point for further tests if your blood test shows toxicity or to give you an idea of your general toxicity. It is a simple, inexpensive, and fast way to test for heavy metal toxicity right at home. You can read a lot more at the website on the background of the test:

> *"The Heavy Metal Screen Test gives you a quick, reliable method for determining if heavy metal ions are present at a high, medium, or low concentration, or not at all."*

> www.nissenmedica.com/pages/products/heavy_metal/ [http://bit.ly/oPBJWU]

It doesn't seem like you can order it on their site but you can at Amazon: Heavy Metal Test [http://tiny.cc/gekdl] or through LifetimeHealth here: www.lifetimehealth.ca/category_s/2.htm [http://bit.ly/qaFcjx]

If you test positive for heavy metals, you can get heavy metal cleansing kits here: LL's Magnetic Clay Bath from LifetimeHealth [http://bit.ly/ooQYzP] or here: LL's Magnetic Clay Baths [http://bit.ly/qBYtQe]

Clay has been used for thousands of years to heal the body. It has uses both externally as a poultice or as a mineral bath and internally to bind with toxins and expel them from the body. I often take Swanson's French Green Clay [http://bit.ly/q4zcS6] capsules for this purpose.

4. You can also personally test with a pendulum by putting the pad of a finger on each tooth and test to see what you get. When I do that, all my teeth come back YES (meaning they're okay), whether they have a filling or not. (You will learn about Personal Testing further on.)

5. Replace your fillings with enamels only as needed—when they need to be replaced or other work is happening on the tooth.

6. If you do decide to replace your fillings, then use a holistic dentist who practices safe procedures for removing mercury.

EMF Radiation and Prostate Health

Electromagnetic Field (EMF) radiation is generated by electrical devices, power lines, WiFi stations, cell phones, handheld phones, computers, airport scanners, hospital testing machines, and more. Electromagnetic fields are created from electric current flows, such as when using a portable phone, microwave, computer, or a cell phone. It is also known as Electromagnetic Radiation (EMR).

There is a growing body of concern that our unprecedented exposure to EMFs may have a serious yet hidden ill-health consequence for many people, particularly the very young, individuals with weakened immune systems, or with others who are more sensitive and actually feel a response to EMFs.

EMFs are a sleeper health issue, invisible, and very slow to manifest in chronic health conditions. EMF radiation is a controversial subject because conclusive evidence could devastate many modern electronic device industries until they could find a way to produce items that minimize the risks. Industry-funded research shows no harmful effect and supposedly neutral organizations may still have industry support or affiliations.

For more precise information, read this report: "Cellphones and Brain Tumors: 15 Reasons For Concern" [http://bit.ly/o5FgNZ]. It explains the risks of brain cancer, the higher risks for children, and the real dangers of testicular cancer and lowered sperm counts in boys and men who wear their phones in their pants pocket.

You can also watch a short YouTube video here: EMF Radiation Research Trust [http://bit.ly/piSruz]

An ever-increasing number of independent doctors and groups are warning about the dangers. If you think about the issue, you'll realize that in any city we are now bombarded by exposures from all directions around us, crisscrossing us with invisible EMF fields. As an example, my WiFi picks up over 25 signals while I am typing this in Vancouver and that is only EMFs from WiFi. Cell phone tower signals are everywhere, as are portable and cell phones.

I am no expert on this area, but I will provide links for you to make your own informed decision. I certainly err on the side of caution and try to limit my exposures by using wire connections whenever I can for the computer or phone. I minimize my cell use, hold the phone away from my head as much as possible and use the speaker phone of my portable instead of holding it next to my ear.

Read these articles for more information about this issue: "Electro Magnetic Field (EMF) - Hazardous to Our Health?" [http://bit.ly/qzzBr8] If you have a prostate problem, especially cancer, then use caution.

The EM Watch website [http://bit.ly/oYYOjD] has lots of good information, so spend time there exploring and reading more about EMFs. This site offers great advice on how to minimize exposures.

Devra Davis' book explains a lot more about cell phone dangers, including why Lloyds of London refuses to insure cell phone manufacturers against health-related claims: *Disconnect: The Truth About Cell Phone Radiation, What the Industry Has Done to Hide It, and How to Protect Your Family* [http://amzn.to/ok6ILa].

Here is an excerpt from an article that discusses the dangers of EMFs:

> *"Studies show that myriad wildlife abandons terrain when cell towers are installed. Cows have increased cancers, lower milk production, agitation, immune system disorders, more mastitis (breast infection), miscarriages, and birth defects in offspring near cell towers. Birds with nests near antennas display lower reproductive rates, and chicks are born with birth defects. In simulations of whole colony collapse disorder, bees have disappeared entirely when transmitting cell phones were placed next to their hives. It is thought that RF interferes with their navigational abilities by coupling with a natural magnetic material called magnetite in bee abdomens.*
>
> *Meanwhile, hundreds of studies done with laboratory animals found numerous cancers, immune disorders, and increased mortality from chronic, low-level exposures. This body of work should make us ponder the accuracy of the data— and humaneness - when biologists attach RF transmitters to elk, marine mammals, big cats, and other species to study them."*

Levitt, B. Blake and Glendinning, Chellis. 22 March 2011. "The Problems With Smart Grids: Dumb and Dangerous" www.culturechange.org/cms/content/view/714/63/ [http://bit.ly/r6ZlLL] (Accessed 29 March 2011)

Trees also die-back near towers. Whole forests near broadcast antennas in Europe have suffered. This same article discusses the dangers of smart metering, which emit EMFs non-stop:

> *"The problem: smart metering will turn every single appliance into the equivalent of a transmitting cell phone, and this at a time when public concern about the safety of exposure to the radio frequency radiation (RF) of wireless technologies is on the rise. Heads up: that's every dishwasher, microwave oven, stove, washing machine, clothes dryer, air conditioner, furnace, refrigerator, freezer, coffee maker, TV, computer, printer, and fax machine...*
>
> *And that's just the indoor part. All transmitters inside your home or office will communicate with a Smart Meter attached to the outside of each building. That meter, in turn, will transmit at an even higher frequency to a central hub installed in local neighborhoods. In what are called "mesh networks," signals can also be bounced from house-meter to house-meter before reaching the final*

hub. So exposures will not just be from your own meter, but accumulating from possibly 100-to-500 of your neighbors' as well. That's a hefty barrage of radiation.

Levitt, B. Blake and Glendinning, Chellis. 22 March 2011. "The Problems With Smart Grids: Dumb and Dangerous" www.culturechange.org/cms/content/view/714/63/ [http://bit.ly/r6ZlLL] (Accessed 29 March 2011)

EMFs and Hormones

This article on breast cancer and EMFs also talks about the effects on hormones including men's testosterone and prostate cancer.

*"Experimental physiologist Dr. Charles Graham's research found that magnetic fields had an effect on two other hormones. Overnight exposure of women to elevated levels of EMR in the laboratory significantly increased estrogen levels which is a known risk factor for breast cancer. **In men, EMR exposure reduced levels of testosterone—a hormone drop that has been linked to testicular and prostate cancers.**"*

Sellman, Sherrill. November 2007. "Effects of Electropollution On Hormones and Breast Cancer" www.vitalitymagazine.com/article/effects-of-electropollution-on-hormones-and-breast-cancer/ [http://bit.ly/mTpD2h] (Accessed 10 March 2011)

Still not convinced? As of May 31, 2011, The World Health Organization's International Agency for Research on Cancer "IARC Classifies Radiofrequency Electromagnetic Fields as Possibly Carcinogenic to Humans" [http://bit.ly/n0q9HI]

Dear reader, this is a conservative organization that is making this statement. I would pay attention and use the suggestions I have listed on how to limit your exposures. Remember how long it took for the powers that be to finally agree that asbestos, DDT, cigarettes, and lead in gasoline were hazardous to health and enacted legislation? When billions of dollars are at stake, it takes a long time for change at the regulatory level. But you can adapt any time you choose. Play it safe with exposures to EMFs, or play and pay with your health. Your choice.

A report issued by the Council of Europe's Parliamentary Assembly calls for a school ban on cell phones: "The potential dangers of electromagnetic fields and their effect on the environment" [http://bit.ly/qDYRVW]

Protect Yourself Against EMF Radiation

If you do searches, you will no doubt encounter supposed protective devices that you can attach to your electronic devices like cell phones or laptops to "protect" you from EMFs. In addition there are devices that you can wear that also supposedly protect you.

Although these devices sound good in theory, I would take most of these claims with a big grain of salt no matter how much "science" there is around them. The reason is that they work by switching the energy from one part of the body to another. You may feel temporarily better but then find health problems manifest in other parts of the body later.

I had such an experience where an alternative health practitioner sold me a device to wear even while I slept. During the second night I awoke and almost blocked completely. I traced the reaction back to the device and got rid of it.

I advise you to be careful with any of these devices. The devices work by hyper-stimulating your nervous system so you initially feel much better - while new problems start developing - shifting the sensitivity to EMFs from one area of the body to another. You feel good for a while but then other symptoms develop. Do not trust the "scientific" claims. The best solution is to practice safe EMFs! For some excellent tips read this article: EMF Protection and Safety [http://bit.ly/oYYOjD]

DLan plugs are a simple way to wire your house for computers without a wireless WiFi network. It works by using the dLan plug to connect your router through the electrical system. You just plug into another room's electrical socket and you have Internet connection without any WiFi EMFs: [www.devolo.com]

Another EMF risk comes from the compact fluorescent lights that emit EMF radiation (because that is how the technology works) and are an environmental nightmare because they contain mercury and are hazardous to get rid of. How many light bulbs have you broken in your life? Now you have to deal with spilt mercury, which is a serious toxin:

> *"The voltage reduction technology in CFL bulbs causes high amounts of EMF pollution to be emitted. Similar to the kind released from mobile phone antennas and food irradiation machinery, EMF [http://bit.ly/qqGX2s] radiation poses serious health threats to humans who are exposed to excessive amounts of it. CFL bulbs have been found to greatly increase EMF exposure as they are often the most significant EMF polluters in homes that use them."*

> Huff, E. 27 January 2010. "Compact Fluorescent Lights Dumping Mercury Directly into Landfills"
> www.naturalnews.com/028034_mercury_compact_fluorescent_lights.html [http://bit.ly/p5glpU] (Accessed 25 April 2011)

You can read more on CFLs here: Compact fluorescent bulbs release cancer-causing chemicals when turned on, says new research [http://bit.ly/pf1w3w]

Germany just banned fluorescent light bulbs because they cause cancer in mice and contain unacceptable amounts of mercury. Germany is also calling for a drastic reduction of CT scans, because of the increase in cancer incidence from radiation.

How to Minimize EMR Exposure

- Minimize usage of wireless communication: cell phones, cordless phones, and WiFi devices.

- Turn your cell phone off when it is not in use.

- Do not use your cell phone to play games, as you are unnecessarily increasing your exposure.

- Keep the cell phone at least 6-7 inches away from your body while talking, texting, and downloading.

- Use air tube headsets or speaker mode when talking. Keep in mind that wireless and wired headsets still conduct radiation.

- Never keep the cell phone in your pocket, purse, back pocket, or on your hip all day. Your hips produce 80% of the body's red blood cells and are especially vulnerable to EMR damage. Close proximity may also affect fertility.

- Do not talk on a cell or cordless phone when pregnant or with a baby or small child in your arms.

- Children under age 16 are very vulnerable and should minimize their exposure.

- Do not talk while in a vehicle (car, train, plane, subway). Radiation gets trapped and is higher in these closed metal zones!

- Replace all cordless and WiFi items with wired, corded lines (phones, Internet, games, appliances, devices, etc.). The cordless phone base emits high levels of EMR, even when no one is making a call.

- Keep laptops off of the body and away from metal surfaces.

   Strachan, Tim. Health and EMR – What you can do
   www.geopathic-stress.info/index_files/health_emr.htm
   [http://bit.ly/qXw01X] (Accessed 8 May 2011)

The Environmental Working Group has created a list of Best and Worst Phones [http://bit.ly/oRsoK2].

Conclusion

Take a precautionary approach to EMFs. If you are having a prostate problem, then reducing these possible irritants just makes sense.

This is not going to be easy to do, but start making efforts where you can. This is a long-term exposure problem with no immediate observable benefits. The symptoms occur down the road. Let's hope it is not an early dead end.

Chapter 6: Diets, Diets Everywhere!

We Are All Unique

I spent quite a bit of time writing about food and diets. Why? Because it is central to good health and there is so much competing misinformation, so I decided to cover all the bases. If you want a healthy prostate then it would be useful to know what you should eat that works for you (not someone else). You need to know for sure that what you are eating is best for you!

The perfect diet for <u>you</u> is **not** for everyone!

I will give an example. I grow kale in my garden, and last spring a whole lot started growing all over from seeds that had fallen and spread in the fall. I like kale a lot and, when young, it's really delicious both raw and cooked. So I ate some every day, and some days had big portions. We all know the claims of how good kale is for you! "Kale is widely regarded as one of the world's most powerful superfoods." "Discover the Superfood Power of Kale" [http://bit.ly/qNRu4u]

One night my prostate blocked, and I couldn't pee and had to use a catheter. In the morning I traced back everything I had eaten and tested them with personal testing to see what the culprit could be. Everything was fine. The only thing I hadn't yet tested was the kale. I just assumed that something so nutritious and described by many as being very beneficial to the prostate (part of the cruciferous family) that it was fine. At this point I was at a loss as to what had triggered the prostate attack. I decided to test the kale and lo and behold I got a NO for kale! I had surpassed my limit on this healthy food and it was now toxic for me!

It doesn't matter how many beneficial vitamins and minerals a food has or other merits claimed by food pundits. It was no longer good for me and caused a severe reaction. I guess the old saying is true—"Too much of a good thing is no good!" Like the carrot guy!

We are all so unique. No prescribed diet can be good for everyone, everywhere, all of the time. To believe so is just faulty thinking. That's the problem with the diet gurus who claim their way is <u>the best way</u>.

You are the master when it comes to knowing what is best for you to eat, but "knowing" requires learning and tuning inwards, listening to what your body needs. I will provide you with a tool that will help you do that. It is called personal testing (see Chapter 11 for more information).

Diet is a very important topic. There is much to learn. When it comes to food it is easier to say what is best not to eat. So let us start there.

I do believe that my Food STOP list (see Chapter 5) should be followed as much as possible because these foods have become toxic, denourished, or altered and processed so much to become almost alien to our bodies. Once you know how to personally test foods, you can test these non-foods for yourself to see if they are good or bad for you to eat.

A crucial step to take is to stop eating the foods that are identified as most harmful. The next step is to replace those harmful foods with healthy alternatives.

When it comes to what you should eat, you will find many diets with compelling reasons to follow the proponents' ways. The problem is that there may be foods the diet says you should eat that may actually be harmful for you, and there may be foods that the diet says you should never touch that may be exactly what your body needs right now.

In this section, look at the many diets and try to assess what makes sense in them and what doesn't. Then apply that to you and your unique constitution and condition right now. Since we are constantly changing and in need of different things from our food, what may well be ideal for you today may change and become less so or even harmful. This can be true for even the healthiest of foods.

We are all unique. There is no one diet that is perfect for everyone, and what is perfect for you today may not be perfect tomorrow. This is contrary to virtually all health practitioners who claim that their way is the best way and all others should take the highway!

The reality is that we are all so very different from each other. I hate olives and can't stand even the sight of them! Others would die for them! You see this all the time. What one loves, another hates!

The only way to know what is healthy for you at this time is to personally test to see and to retest over time to ensure that what you are eating is still good for you. Keep in mind that the foods that once tested as NO may change and become okay for you to eat again later.

In Chapter 11 I teach you how to personal test to know what is good and what is bad for you at this moment. It is a simple and invaluable tool.

Remember too that something that is wonderful for you may be the opposite for someone else. That is why all recommendations no matter how great the source and science behind it need to be critically examined with personal testing.

Popular Diets

What follows is my take on the recommendations of many other diets. Use the lists in this section to test what would be best for you. This will help you create a great list of potential foods to eat. We will do the same with supplements and herbs in a later chapter.

Raw Food Diet

This diet is all about eating foods in their natural state without cooking, but allows for processing at low temperatures to dehydrate some foods.

The theory is that raw foods contain many more enzymes than cooked foods and are, therefore, best eaten raw for optimum health.

This may be true to a point, but what I believe is missed here is that the key is what the body is <u>able to absorb</u>. Cooking makes many foods much more absorbable, so the question becomes, which has the most net gain, cooked or raw?

Why is it that virtually all primitive cultures cooked their food? The reason is to make the food more digestible and to remove harmful anti-nutrients sometimes found in raw food. Andreas Moritz in *Timeless Secrets of Health and Rejuvenation* [http://amzn.to/n71lG7] does a great job in critiquing this diet. He explains why it seems to work for a while but describes some of the very real risks in this way of eating.

That said, for some people coming off a toxic diet, the best choice may be raw food for a while, as it can help detox the body. However, a raw food diet may not be a healthy long-term choice. Perhaps mixed with some cooked food, it would be more balanced. Most raw foodists are also vegans, which has other risks added to the mix.

Raw foodists also eat sprouted foods. Sprouting does make foods more digestible but not as much as soaking and cooking. People who only eat raw foods also like eating "greens" in the form of sprouts like wheat grass or in dried powdered forms. Watch out—these types of foods can be a real irritant. I have had complete shutdowns taking supposed super healthy greens!

This diet seems to be best suited to certain geographic climates. Eating raw in more northerly climates in the winter will be a challenge, as you must rely on foods being brought in from far away. Eating food "in season" is also something to take into consideration. Eating watermelons in Alaska in January may not be the perfect food! Personally test seasonal items from far away and you may be surprised to get a NO.

Another raw food diet weakness for many is that a lot of the foods are juiced. Many claim that eating a whole food is better than drinking a juiced food, because you absorb more nutrients from the whole food.

Eating foods like sauerkraut can accomplish what the raw food diet tries to do—maximizing enzymes. Most foods aren't great sources of enzymes, which help digestion in the upper stomach where digestive fluids are lacking.

Lacto-fermentation (a fermentation process) improves the amount of enzymes and when eaten with cooked food compensates for the loss of enzymes in the cooked food. This fermentation process also provides lactic acid and good bacteria that survive the digestion process and make it into the intestines. Lacto fermented foods can be considered "super-raw."

Miscellaneous Food Questions [http://bit.ly/qLejwh]

My take on this is to try eating only raw foods if it appeals to you, but do not do this obsessively and personally test everything. That way you will know if it is good for you and how much to have. Most of us need to eat a lot more raw foods mixed in our diets in the form of salads and vegetables. Be careful of having too many fruit juices, which can deliver too much sugar to your body. Read the links in the next section on "Vegetarian Diet" for more information.

Vegetarian Diet

The Vegetarian Diet is a very popular diet with many variations and is claimed to be superior by many. However, many weaknesses have been found in this diet. For example, eating the wrong kind of dairy (i.e., pasteurized) will be harmful over time. Many vegetarians consume too many sweets and can become quite unhealthy. The difference in life expectancy between vegetarian peoples of southern India and the wider-eating peoples of northern India (who also eat animal foods) is significant.

Vegetarians are often deficient in vitamin B12 because it is not found in plant-based foods. You can read more on this here:

Fallon, Sally and Enig, Mary G. 27 July 2005. "Vitamin B12: Vital Nutrient for Good Health"
http://www.westonaprice.org/vitamins-and-minerals/vitamin-b12
[http://bit.ly/mSMWIc] (Accessed 24 August 2011)

You can easily test non-vegetarian foods like eggs, fish, fowl, and red meat to see if these foods test positive for you. If so then you may well need them in your diet! If you need meat, eat high-quality, grass-fed organic meat products.

To read more about the dangers of the vegetarian diet, read these articles:
- "Twenty-Two Reasons to Not Go Vegetarian" [http://bit.ly/oQ7Gfl]
- "The Vegetarian Myth" by Lierre Keith [http://bit.ly/qSvwqj]
- "Vegetarianism and Nutrient Deficiencies" [http://bit.ly/qfnaWW]

Hey, I was mostly vegan/vegetarian for years and I paid the price—I developed a prostate problem! So if you are vegetarian, you may want to consider the impossible: some animal foods of the right kind may be very beneficial for you!

Vegan Diet

This is essentially a vegetarian diet, but with no animal products like dairy or eggs, that vegetarians often eat. This diet often includes a large raw food component. Please see the above "Vegetarian Diet" section for information on vitamin and nutrient deficiencies.

Macrobiotic Diet

This diet is a variation of the vegan diet with some fish allowed and lots of grains, beans, nuts, seeds, sea vegetables, and vegetables. Basically, it's a high complex carbohydrate, low fat diet.

I know now that many of these recommended foods contain phytic acid or phytates that are so harmful over time if not removed by traditional methods of soaking and fermenting. I only discovered this recently, and I believe it has been the major factor in causing my enlarged prostate.

Phytic acid has a strong binding affinity to important minerals such as calcium, magnesium, iron, and zinc. When a mineral binds to phytic acid, it becomes insoluble, precipitates and will be non-absorbable in the intestines. This process can, therefore, contribute to mineral deficiencies in people whose diets rely on these foods for their mineral intake. See Wikipedia's webpage for more info on Phytic Acid: en.wikipedia.org/wiki/Phytic_acid [http://bit.ly/oAF2Wc]

Please note that the Macrobiotic Diet removes zinc from the body. Zinc is a crucial mineral for the prostate. Please read the links in the "Vegetarian Diet" section of this chapter for more info.

I wish I had known how to personally test foods many years ago (which I explain in detail in Chapter 11). I had been mostly macrobiotic for well over 30 years, never knowing the dangers I know now, which I could have avoided had I been able to test those foods for phytates.

Alkaline Diet

Also known as Acid/Alkaline or pH Diet, this diet is growing in popularity. It looks at food from the point of view of how alkaline or acid-forming the food is in the body.

The goal of this diet is to eat foods so that the body maintains an alkaline state. The reason claimed is that an acidic state is the cause of many of our modern diseases. Most of the foods on my Food STOP list (see Chapter 5) are too acidic.

The ideal diet here is one that is largely vegetarian or vegan and often raw with at most small portions of animal foods. It also minimizes most grain and bean products because most are too acidic.

The goal is to eat approximately 75% of foods from the alkaline list and only 25% from the acidic list. Many claim success healing many diseases and cancer with this diet.

You will find variations from different pundits on what constitutes the degree of acid/alkaline of a particular food, but the bulk of foods seem to agree with each other's assessment.

Go here for more information:
- *Acid/AlkalineDiet* [http://bit.ly/qsjhwT]
- *TheAlkalineDiet* [http://bit.ly/mUfd0x]

This diet may be beneficial for a short period, especially after a long-term diet of foods found on my Food STOP list but, in my opinion, this diet is harmful in the long term. The key to health is not low acidity but in taking nutrient-rich foods. Eating an Alkaline Diet for a while will provide many more nutrients, but the restrictions on saturated fat may become costly over time.

It's what we absorb and what minerals are maintained by the body that is the essential key to health, not the acid content of foods even though it appears that way. Perhaps the reason many benefit from this diet is that they are eating real food instead of manufactured foods, which they may have been eating for a long time. Thus immediate benefits are felt, but in the long term people on an Alkaline Diet may suffer, as do vegans and vegetarians.

Look at this conclusion from an amazing researcher, Dr. Weston Price, who in a published paper called "Acid-Base Balance of Diets Which Produce Immunity to Dental Caries Among the South Sea Islanders and Other Primitive Races." Dr. Price compares the amount of acid ash and alkaline ash minerals in the diets of primitive Swiss, Gaelic, Eskimo, Native American, and South Sea Islanders.

> *"In all but the South Sea diet, acid ash foods predominated. But the important point is that the overall mineral content in every primitive diet was at least four times, and sometimes more than ten times, higher than the mineral content in the modernized diet." (A. Price, Dental Cosmos, September 1935)*

> www.westonaprice.org/basics/the-right-price [http://bit.ly/reBm89]

Note the date of that article... 1935. Imagine today how much more the modern diet would be depleted of minerals! My best advice is to use this alkaline diet as a transition, and personally test all the foods. One can easily become too alkaline, like I did with my kale episode!

Ayurvedic Diet

This is a time-tested and traditional diet based on Ayurvedic (ancient tradition) principles from India. It describes three basic body types and shows which foods are best for each body type and why. Many valid and insightful teachings can be found here, including daily practices that promote health, like tongue scraping in the morning after teeth brushing (I highly recommend this practice because scraping removes toxins on your tongue after sleeping that no amount of brushing can do.

Take a look at these: Tongue Scrapers and Cleaners [http://tiny.cc/kvv54] (I recommend that you try the Pureline ones, that's served me well for years).

Here are two books about this diet:
- *Ayurvedic Healing, 2nd Revised and Enlarged Edition: A Comprehensive Guide* [http://amzn.to/okRlD4]
- *Ageless Body, Timeless Mind: The Quantum Alternative to Growing Old* [http://amzn.to/nkEzy0]

The Ayurvedic Diet may be largely vegetarian in its recommendations, so please do personally test foods to confirm the suggestions, otherwise with time it could be too restrictive. I could not follow that diet today without reactions, especially since many phytate foods are recommended. Make sure you read the information on phytic acid (found in Chapter 8) to learn how to minimize this substance in this diet regime.

Low Glycemic Diet/South Beach Diet

This diet uses what proponents believe is the perfect guide: the glycemic index of foods. The Glycemic Index (GI) is a numerical scale used to indicate how fast and how high a particular food can raise your blood glucose (blood sugar) level. Supposedly the lower the GI the better. You can read more here: Glycemic Index on Wikipedia [http://bit.ly/pnYcin]

To me the whole concept of GI is flawed because it classifies whole grains, such as rye bread, as being identical to jelly beans! Something is off base here!

Diets based on low glycemic index foods ignore one important fact: fats lower the glycemic index as can cooking time! Put butter on your rice or bread and the glycemic index of these foods comes down, which means that these foods are absorbed slowly into the bloodstream rather than in one quick burst, which is what happens supposedly with high-GI foods.

High-Carb-Low-Fat Diet or Low-Protein Diet; the Hunter-Gatherer Diet, Primitive Diet, or Paleo Diet; and the Low-Carb-High-Protein Diet

I am grouping these diets together because the questions of fat, protein, and carbohydrates are common to all.

Weston Price, the researcher who was quoted above, says the high carb-low-fat diet is risky. People who live in industrialized societies, as we do today, consume non-fermented carbohydrates, avoid nutrient-dense foods, and have a difficult time avoiding refined and devitalized food because these foods are everywhere. These diets are completely out of balance. Dr. Price added:

> *"Higher levels of animal foods in conjunction with quality animal fats supplying ample amounts of vitamins A and D, provide an extra measure of protection in Western diets."*

> www.westonaprice.org/basics/adventures-in-macro-nutrient-land [http://bit.ly/pX9vdY] (Accessed 5 May 2011)

The Paleo Diet says that we should eat what our ancestors ate before the advent of agriculture about 10,000 years ago. Paleo diet enthusiasts claim that it was low in carbs and high in protein from meat and fish. The modern version often recommends lean cuts of meats. The result is, in fact, a diet very different from what our ancestors ate because it contains too little fat and too much protein, resulting in deficiencies.

The problem is similar to the Low-Carb-High-Protein diets:

> *"Dieters often add protein powders to up the protein content without adding too many calories at the same time. The result can be a diet unnaturally high in protein, something that all primitive peoples avoided. Protein requires vitamin A for its metabolism and a diet too high in protein without adequate fat rapidly depletes vitamin A stores, leading to serious consequences—heart arrhythmias, kidney problems, autoimmune disease and thyroid disorders. Diets too high in protein also cause a negative calcium balance, where more calcium is lost compared to the amount taken in, a condition that can lead to bone loss and nervous system disorders."*

> www.westonaprice.org/basics/adventures-in-macro-nutrient-land [http://bit.ly/pX9vdY] (Accessed 5 May 2011)

The bottom line on these diets is that they are better than eating the way most Americans currently eat, which is mainly consuming foods that are on the Food STOP list (see Chapter 5). But are these diets ideal for you? The only way to know is to personally test the foods.

The other major problem with these diets is that they either recommend low-fat foods or vegetable fats instead of saturated fats. The vegetable fats have too high a ratio of omega-6 fats and if these fats are from the Food STOP list they can be very harmful. We will discuss the dangers of a low-fat diet later. For more insights on low fat diets, read this article: "Low Fat Diet Missing Essential Brain Nutrients and Leads to Cognitive Decline" [http://bit.ly/pDRn6s]

The Weston A. Price Foundation's "Health Topics" web page is the most comprehensive site I've found in 8 years of research into what foods are best to eat: www.westonaprice.org/abcs-of-nutrition/health-topics [http://bit.ly/qMcyor]

The Weston A. Price Foundation does an amazing job in describing the "what" and "why" of foods. It is well worth spending time reviewing and searching the site. I guarantee that you will learn a lot.

www.westonaprice.org/basics/adventures-in-macro-nutrient-land
[http://bit.ly/pX9vdY]

Again, I want to remind you that when you are researching online, no matter what great research and insights you find, the final test is to check and see what foods work for you right now. The only way to know is to personally test foods before eating them.

Chapter 7: The Happy Zappy Prostate Diet

Well - finally we come to what I feel is the most important part of the book: the healthy prostate diet! I call it the Happy Zappy Prostate Diet for a good reason—if your diet makes your prostate happy, then you will be in great shape with lots of get up (pun intended) and go!

I say this because what we eat is the secret to our health and wellness, or our sickness and misery. Food, in its broadest definition of your daily inputs, is the single most important determinant of your prostate's happiness.

If you ask someone how well or how healthy they eat, most will say that they eat pretty well. Unfortunately, most people's knowledge of what is healthy to eat is not very accurate. Generally, knowledge comes slowly with the understanding of the consequences of wrong food choices and with the awareness of the full range of what is available to choose from, as well as other things like learning how our food is grown and how it needs to be prepared, such as in phytate-reducing ways.

If your prostate is happy then the well-head of your manhood can allow you a life of vitality, but if it gets sick, then your life will change dramatically as the symptoms start to limit your life and restrict your health and day-to-day living.

Food is so fundamental because it is our daily actions that little by little cause us to sink or rise in health. In this chapter, I explain what to eat, how to know what is the optimum food for you and no one else, and what supplements and healing herbs would be good for you and your prostate. This discourse will go beyond anything you have read elsewhere because in all my studies I have never fully encountered the depth of what I offer here to you: the perfect diet for you and your prostate!

The Happy Zappy Prostate Diet is not a one-size fits all diet. This diet puts the focus on you and your specific needs. I will show you how to learn and discover what works for you!

It is important to realize that there is diet theory and then there is reality. I have followed expert advice and it often made my health condition worse. Your body already knows what it needs and what it is lacking. You just have to learn how to know what it is your body needs. I will teach you.

Every book I have read on health and diet, and every practitioner I have met, all seem to have very specific ideas about what constitutes the ideal diet. I have followed recommendations to a tee, yet health improvements eluded me. My prostate only seemed to get worse! There certainly were good elements in their diet plans, so why in the world did I get worse instead of better?

I was fortunate enough to live on an island where the quality of air, water, and food was excellent. Because I worked from home, I could easily implement health regimes without having to compromise. You could say I was the perfect candidate to test the various diets. I started to learn that deviations or indulgences (which were very rare let me tell you!) could be very costly to me, so I avoided them as much as I could.

Once I had a homemade cookie and I ended up having my prostate shut down the pee tube and had to use a catheter. It was no fun! So I stayed on the recommended path, but better health still eluded me. Sometimes out of the blue I would have a sudden shut down strike me in the middle of the night.

I then learned two things that provided a huge breakthrough:

1. How to personally test to know if something I was going to eat would be good for me or not (see Chapter 11 for info on personal testing), and

2. How to avoid or prepare many common foods to minimize a relatively unknown harmful anti-nutrient that was weakening me and causing an almost allergic reaction (see Chapter 8 for info on phytic acid).

These new breakthroughs were so profound that they started a shift in my health, and at long last I began to recover.

It's easy to get stuck thinking that the foods you eat or the diet you are on is the best. You've studied it, adopted it, and have a lot invested in your choice and opinion.

Hey, I know! I did that for 35 years! I just knew mine was the best! And I made my diet even stricter when my condition developed. Still nothing worked, and my health got worse even though I was on supposedly the healthiest diet advocated by experts.

Sometimes we just need to let go and allow something new to take its place. The Happy Zappy Prostate Diet is your perfect diet, customized for you by you, dynamically evolving in real-time and based on key principles that will make complete sense to you.

For most of us change is not easy, because we get comfortable in our ways. But in the case of your prostate condition, the benefits of being pain free and healthy are well worth the effort to change.

Look at some of the potential rewards of a healthy prostate diet:

✓ Avoid the risk of some serious side effects from conventional medical options like incontinence and impotence. I don't know about you but these two alone were enough to motivate me!

✓ Improve your overall health and well being, which can add years to your life and life to your years with fewer "what ails ya?" as you age.

✓ Feel and look younger.

✓ Lose weight and feel great!

✓ Save money, if you have to pay for conventional healthcare. Avoiding costly procedures can be a significant saving in both money and time.

I am now going to share what I believe will be the answer to set you on the road to health.

We start with diet to change the conditions, move to cleanses to remove past toxins, and add healing herbs and supplements to give a boost, followed by specific prostate treatments to accelerate the healing.

You Are The Cause!

First, let us recap that a prostate problem in your life means that you are doing something harmful to your body. Disease does not mysteriously arise without causes. This insight should be the basis of all medical practice but sadly it is not. Western conventional medical practice only sees the condition or symptom and fails to truly find the causes in order to change them and allow healing to happen.

For me this is so fundamental. It was what gave me the courage to go on when it seemed dark days surrounded me. I just knew the answers were there, but I hadn't yet discovered them! So embrace the notion that finding the causes and making changes is the foundation of your healing.

In our modern lifestyle we have moved so far away from natural eating wisdom, it is no wonder we suffer so much chronic disease. Our supermarkets and fast food outlets are filled with tantalizing choices of so many food items that we have let ourselves indulge without knowing the price we would have to pay down the road. Kind of like the government printing money and growing the debt. Looks good today but look what's coming down the pike!

We evolved over thousands of years based on eating real food, not artificial manufactured food that dominates our diets today. We thrived unless adequate food and sanitation were unavailable, and then disease would develop. When manufacturing began, we suffered from unknown pollutants like lead pipes and cups and the air became toxic, as in London during the industrial revolution. But traditional societies or groups continued to do very well when adequate healthy food was to be had.

Is it possible for today's foods to be healthy when they contain chemical ingredients that we cannot even pronounce? Can foods grown in soil containing artificial fertilizers and doused with pesticides and herbicides really be health enhancing? The fast foods we eat that are grown in such a toxic environment and then modified to contain high fructose corn syrup, trans fats or even high omega-6 poly-fats, or meats from animals fed toxic foods, hormones and antibiotics—can these foods really nourish and sustain us in a health enhancing way?

You know the answers! You have let down your guard out of ignorance and youthful exuberance, saying, "I don't feel anything, so it must be okay." Or perhaps you let your guard down because these unhealthy foods taste good due to the excessive sugars and unhealthy fats and commercial salt added, and you simply weren't aware of the price tag down the road. Some of us are addicted and might have just pushed it out of our minds for the instant convenience and gratification we get when we eat these foods.

We eat massive amounts of sugar and fats that are toxic to our health. We consume so many foods laced with chemicals that our bodies are fighting to survive. Chronic disease is the outcome of the body's last-ditch effort to isolate the toxins to protect itself to survive the onslaught.

As a result, prostate disease is now epidemic in the West, where our indulgences are finally catching up with us. The prostate is vulnerable because it is an easy place to store toxins in the body, away from more vulnerable organs and because of its proximity directly opposite the colon, so toxins can easily migrate into it, or from the pee tube that passes through it.

You know that the first step is to stop eating toxic food. The next step is to start eating healthy foods.

Eat Real Food!

When people eat real food, they are healthy and long-lived, as is evidenced by the isolated peoples found today in more remote places and mountains who practice these time-proven habits:

- ✓ Eat meat from grass-fed, free-roaming, pastured animals and eat fowl that are free roaming and feed on scraps and insects.

- ✓ Eat eggs from birds that are free range and feed on scraps and insects; these eggs will be rich and healthy with deep yellow yokes.

- ✓ Eat vegetables and fruits grown in healthy soils, with no sprays and toxins added.

- ✓ Eat healthy fats and oils.

- ✓ Eat grains, beans, pulses, and nuts and seeds prepared in the traditional manner (more on this crucial step later).

- ✓ Eat wild foods when they are in season (e.g., berries, mushrooms, nettles, etc).

- ✓ Use real sea salt and eat some sea vegetables filled with trace elements and minerals.

- ✓ Use natural, minimally processed sweeteners from plants, bees, and trees.

- ✓ Use spices and herbs and drink teas grown in home gardens or harvested locally.

- ✓ Drink clear, uncontaminated water.

- ✓ Breathe fresh unpolluted air filled with oxygen.

- ✓ Increase your exposure to natural sunlight.

When it comes to meat, poultry, and eggs, commercial varieties are just too toxic to eat. The best meats are grass-fed, free range, and are never fattened with grains. The next best is organic, but even organic producers will often use grain for fattening in the last month or two. The best dairy is raw grass-fed and non-pasteurized. Pasteurization and homogenization destroy the crucial enzymes needed to digest them.

Modern agriculture robs our food of nutrients. Food processing, pasteurization, and the widespread use of preservatives, artificial flavoring and coloring, stabilizers, genetically-modified (GMO) foods deplete life-giving enzymes, natural healthy bacteria, and nutritional content. Our food is stripped bare and the result is "no-food" or "junk food," which in reality is "poison food".

We have become a toxic species! Food is no longer health giving and enhancing but health destroying. When food does not nurture you, it taxes your system putting a heavy strain on the digestive system. Once vital foods that nourished us are now reversing that role and are harming us.

Your prostate is your barometer of how healthy you are. Pay attention to its message and learn how to feed yourself for health and well being.Here is a food guide that is not bad except for not revealing the difference between healthy grass-fed dairy, fats, and meat. Ignore the soy recommendations:
See the Honest Food Guide [http://www.honestfoodguide.org]

Food is your medicine; a supplement cannot make up for what the complex structures of nutrients that real food provide the body. Yes, there are some excellent products that can help you, but remember that food is the foundation of your health. Compromise on this at your peril. **Eat real food!**

The Whole Wide World of Food and What Should You Eat

Talk about a challenge to simplify all the conflicting information one finds from a multitude of health sources and well-meaning practitioners, let alone how personal food is for each of us with our likes and dislikes—you have a mighty task for yourself!

Well my approach is different from others in that the first rule is to eliminate all the well-known harmful foods first, then analyze the data on what foods are "best" for our health, and then to give you a tool that you can use to KNOW what is best for you. KNOWING is the final key that will set you on your road to health.

How can you know? By doing a Personal Test—this skill is so important for you to learn. It is perhaps the most important personal tool you can have in your quest for real health and vitality. You can jump ahead to Chapter 11 to read about personal testing, or you can continue here, get the foundation, and then you try the personal testing after.

So let us begin with **the Happy Zappy Prostate Diet!**

In this section, we will look at major food groups and then look at some very specific foods to see what makes sense.

Let's simplify and see if we can agree on some principles.

1. Food is powerful medicine, which can both heal and harm. Because food is our daily input that renews our cells, the quality of the food we consume has a direct impact on our health.

2. Food effects can take time to be noticed or no time at all. Some people can eat horrible nutrient-poor, toxic food and not appear to suffer any consequences for years or decades, while others are so sensitive they can react right away to an improper food. Our food will help or harm us as we make our day-to-day choices. Some will find those impacts can take decades to be realized, and when they do surface the severity of disease can be extreme.

3. We are all so unique and different that every diet must be customized for each one of us. What is beneficial to me is harmful for you. It doesn't matter how wonderful the research or popularity is on a particular food, herb, or supplement. We are the master and must learn for ourselves what works for us, starting with broad guidelines and personal testing to verify them as helpful or harmful.

4. Everything changes including ourselves—our bodies change and require different inputs day by day. A food that is not good for you today may in fact be ideal on another day or year.

5. What we consume is more than food; it also includes inputs to our bodies as liquids like water, what passes through the skin, and the air we breathe.

Fats

Fats are a complex category because there are so many viewpoints. Fats are probably the most important food because of their potential to harm or heal us. Fats also have the highest calorie content of all food groups. I have already discussed some aspects of fat earlier but I will expand on that information here.

Today even mainstream medical organizations, not just holistic health sites, say that to improve prostate health people should reduce their fat consumption, especially the deadly saturated fats.

Some assume that all fats are harmful and that all fats should be reduced (e.g., low fat diets). Could it be what's in the fat or the type of fat that is harmful rather than the amount of fat? To me this is the essential question to decide what type of fats and how much to eat for optimum prostate health.

For information on the dangers of low-fat diets read this article: "Low Fat Diet Missing Essential Brain Nutrients and Leads to Cognitive Decline" [http://bit.ly/pDRn6s]

In traditional cultures over the millennia, fat (mostly saturated fats) was revered for its health benefits, as were the internal organs of an animal.

Take a look at this major study: In October 2010, the American Journal of Clinical Nutrition reported that saturated fats are NOT associated with an increased risk of coronary heart disease (CHD) including stroke or cardiovascular disease (CVD)!

> **"Conclusions:** *A meta-analysis of prospective epidemiologic studies showed that there is no significant evidence for concluding that dietary saturated fat is associated with an increased risk of CHD [coronary heart disease] or CVD. [cardiovascular disease]"*
>
> Siri-Tarino, Patty W.; Sun, Qi; Hu, Frank B.; and Krauss, Ronald M. 13 January *2010*. "Meta-analysis of prospective cohort studies evaluating the association of saturated fat with cardiovascular disease" www.ajcn.org/content/early/2010/01/13/ajcn.2009.27725.abstract [http://bit.ly/osfTgn] (Accessed 6 May 2011)

This conclusion destroys the myths of the supposed dangers of saturated fats. Taking this study's conclusions one step further, I believe that the rise of heart disease (and many chronic conditions like prostate disease) in modern societies should be attributed to:

1. the harmful, highly refined vegetable oils manufactured today and encouraged by virtually all government bodies and organizations like the American Cancer Society and the American Heart Association, which are anti-saturated fats; and

2. the changed nature of commercial saturated fats from modern agri-biz methods with all its toxins and omega fat imbalances, as discussed in earlier chapters.

Good Fats to Eat

Eat nutrient-rich saturated fats like butter from free-grazing cows and coconut oil. Eat the natural meat fats with your meat rather than lean cuts. Avoid the vegetable oils and commercial meats that contain excessive omega-6s.

Worried about cholesterol? Then read this book that dispels many of its myths being propagated today: *Ignore the Awkward: How the Cholesterol Myths Are Kept Alive* [http://amzn.to/o1jmZs]

After following the advice of natural health pundits and experts for years, reducing all my fat intake and eliminating saturated fat (eating a low-fat diet), my prostate still suffered and was actually getting worse the more diligent I became in sticking to the recommended path! I was following advice given by eminent practitioners with very successful practices who had well-researched and published information.

My conclusion is that these practitioners' recommendations are wrong because they only look at the surface of statistics; for example, "greater fat = greater prostate disease," which seems true on the surface, but it is wrongly concluded from the research. Like urologists who say that aging causes prostate disease, these practitioners are drawing the wrong conclusions from the data.

We have to be very careful in concluding that saturated fats are one of the causal factors of prostate disease as many health advocates claim. It may well be because the fat we consume today is no longer the natural healthy fat of yesteryear.

Saturated fat as found in animal fat and coconut oil is essential to our health. It is the highly processed modern vegetable fats taken in such excess that is the culprit, not the animal fats. We are also creating harmful foods by the way we feed and house animals today (i.e., grains instead of grasses, toxic chemical supplements in the feed, toxic antibiotics, pesticides, etc.)—that is the other real culprit and not the saturated fat. Today's mainstream animal fats are toxic, and these toxins are causing our decline in health and increase in prostate problems.

We need our fat to come from healthy, free-ranging, grass-fed animals and fowl, like our ancient diets. Add to that healthy cod liver oil fats and rich fats found in salmon and coconuts—these are the foods that nourished our ancestors throughout the ages.

The pundits, both conventional and holistic, blame saturated and animal fats for our prostate disease. However, I submit that the use of quality saturated fat will be the most important decision you can make regarding fat. You can easily personally test to see if what I am saying is right for you (see Chapter 11). I bet you will find your body responds to high quality saturated fats with a big YES!

Then test other fats and what you see will surprise you.

A wonderful source of the highest quality saturated fat from grassfed cows is called ghee. It is delicious and stable without refrigeration with a long shelf life. Ghee is made from butter; it is a traditional way of preparing clarified butter in India. It ships unrefrigerated once made and is packed in jars. Ghee is a great source of the best kind of saturated fat. I love it. You can use it plain or for cooking as it has a high smoke point. See this website for more info: www.pureindianfoods.com

Avoid These Bad Fats

Avoid the modern vegetable fats except olive, coconut, and avocado oils and always use extra virgin pressings of these oils. Organic expeller-expressed sesame, peanut, and flax oils are also okay, especially in salads, but I recommend using these oils in smaller quantities or for occasional use. Avoid commercial refined varieties of oils. Stop the soy, corn, safflower, sunflower, canola, hydrogenated, and partially-hydogenated oils and margarines completely, even the health food store or organic varieties. Ignore the mainstream marketing of how healthy they are for you! For more info, read these excellent articles on fat:

- "The Great Con-ola" [http://bit.ly/qQ22bj]

- "The Skinny on Fats" [http://bit.ly/p0eBcx]

Above I advise that you should avoid margarine, so let's take a look at what goes into making margarine. Vegetable oils are heated to extremely high temperatures. This causes the oils to become rancid. A nickel catalyst is then added to the heated oils to ensure that the oils solidify. Deodorants and colorants are also added in this process.

> *"The final solidification process creates harmful trans-fatty acids, which are highly carcinogenic. Margarine contains other extremely harmful ingredients such as emulsifiers, preservatives, free radicals, artificial flavors, bleach, soy protein isolate (MSG), sterols, and hexane, as well as many other artificial and synthetic ingredients. Hexane in itself should never be consumed, as it is derived from crude oil. Sterols are estrogen compounds which can cause endocrine problems and also have the ability to contribute to sexual inversion in animals. BHT (Butylated Hydroxytoluene) is used as a preservative in most margarine products. What is really concerning about this ingredient is that it is also linked to symptoms and side effects such as abdominal pain, dizziness, nausea and vomiting."*
>
> Botes, Shona. 25 February 2011. "Why organic, raw butter will benefit your health"
> www.naturalnews.com/031497_raw_butter_health.html
> [http://bit.ly/o2eWiX] (Accessed 6 May 2011)

Eat More Fats!

Increase the amount of good fats in your diet! Yes, I said *increase* them! These were the revered foods of our ancestors. They prized the fat and internal organs of the animal for their rich nutrients. After a hunt, the internal organs were often eaten right away and raw for their richness. The lean cuts were fed to the dogs and only eaten when they had nothing else. Our ancestors knew what to eat to survive and thrive.

Dental and skeletal records show that pre-agricultural humans were taller, stronger and had no cavities compared to those after agriculture began. The amount of good fat was reduced in the diet of many as the population increased through agriculture and gave up the quality sources of nutrition.

Once our ancestors learned to ferment and soak grains, they were able to avoid the ravishes of the phytic acid in those foods. But too much reliance on grains with a lack of the good fats led to a decline in health, which can also be seen in the skeletons and dental records.

Please read more here in this fascinating book:
An Edible History of Humanity [http://amzn.to/i0wUha] by Tom Standage 2009.

> *"Hunter-gatherers actually seem to have been much healthier than the earliest farmers. According to the archaeological evidence, farmers were more likely than hunter-gatherers to suffer from dental-enamel hypoplasia—a characteristic horizontal striping of the teeth that indicates nutritional stress.*

Farming results in a less varied and less balanced diet than hunting and gathering does. Bushmen eat around seventy-five different types of wild plants, rather than relying on a few staple crops. Cereal grains provide reliable calories, but they do not contain the full range of essential nutrients...

In addition, many diseases damage bones in characteristic ways and evidence from studies of bones reveals that farmers suffered from various diseases of malnutrition that were rare or absent in hunter-gatherers. These include rickets (vitamin D deficiency), scurvy (vitamin C deficiency), and anemia (iron deficiency). Farmers were also more susceptible to infectious diseases such as leprosy, tuberculosis, and malaria as a result of their settled lifestyles...

At some archaeological sites it is possible to follow health trends as hunter-gatherers become more sedentary and eventually adopt farming. As the farming groups settle down and grow larger, the incidence of malnutrition, parasitic diseases, and infectious diseases increases."

We have been led down a false path in the interests of false assumptions and corporate profitability promoting unhealthy highly processed oils (modern oils are extremely profitable to industry).

We pay a huge price in our declining health in prostate disease and increased cardiovascular disease since modern oils replaced our healthy fats and today's animal fats have been transformed into health destroying toxins from factory farms designed to produce food with no regard to health. The Weston A. Price Foundation says:

"Saturated fats are required for the nervous system to function properly, and over half the fat in the brain is saturated. Saturated fats also help suppress inflammation. Finally, saturated animal fats carry the vital fat-soluble vitamins A, D and K2, which we need in large amounts to be healthy.

Human beings have been consuming saturated fats from animal products, milk products and the tropical oils for thousands of years; it is the advent of modern processed vegetable oil that is associated with the epidemic of modern degenerative disease, not the consumption of saturated fats."

The Weston A. Price Foundation. 01 January 2000. "Principles of Healthy Diets"
www.westonaprice.org/basics/principles-of-healthy-diets
[http://bit.ly/qrOWjX] (Accessed 6 May 2011)

Please notice that saturated fat suppresses inflammation. This is a key benefit for reducing benign prostatic hyperplasia or BPH for short, the enlargement of the prostate, which is now epidemic in the modern world.

If you personally test YES for meat, avoid big slabs of meat and eat high-quality, grass-fed, organic meat so you can ensure it is healthy for you.

Eat meat with saturated fat—avoid lean cuts! Yes, this goes against all the propaganda you have read, but remember our discussions of fat: it is the modern vegetable fats and the saturated fats from toxic animals that are the problem not the high-quality, grass-fed fats. Good saturated fat will nourish you and satisfy you so that cravings just melt away.

A simple rule of thumb for meat portion sizes is to eat a portion that fits into the palm of your hand and is no thicker than your middle finger. This allows different actual sizes for different folks. A lumberjack's hand will be a bit larger I imagine than an anorexic model's!

You can personally test for portion size to see if the palm-sized portion is a good rule for you to follow.

People become obsessive with their diets, especially health practitioner proponents: Following a "Do this, don't do that, one-size-fits-all" diet has it's dangers.

For instance, the high protein weight loss diets that are in vogue will give good short-term results. You will loose weight. But in the longer term your body will become toxic (ketosis) from such excessive amounts of protein. You are asking for trouble, like:

- *kidney failure and kidney stones*
- *cancer*
- *organ failure*
- *high cholesterol*
- *osteoporosis*

women.webmd.com/guide/high-protein-low-carbohydrate-diets
[http://bit.ly/n44Nhy]

Conclusion – A Recap of the Healthy Fats

Let's recap the healthy fats and oils. Use these as a rough guideline, adjust for your body size, and remember to personally test for compatibility and amount.

- **Saturated fats:** Animal fats in meat and in butter, ghee, and tropical oils (e.g., coconut oil and palm oil) contain primarily saturated fats. Daily saturated fat recommendation: 3-6 tablespoons.

- **Monounsaturated fats:** olive oil, sesame oil, peanut oil, avocado oil, and nuts (e.g., almonds, cashews, walnuts, pecans, etc.) contain primarily monounsaturated fats. Daily monounsaturated fat recommendation: 1-2 tablespoons (or a small handful of nuts).

- **Polyunsaturated fats:** cod liver oil, flax oil, fish oils, evening primrose oil, black currant oil, and borage oil contain primarily polyunsaturated fats. Daily polyunsaturated fat recommendation: 1 teaspoon – 1 tablespoon.

Protein

Protein is another controversial topic. We have so much invested in the notion that high protein is what we crave and need to be healthy. As discussed earlier, it is the quality fat we really need but have been told by the punditry to avoid. Worse yet we are told to use commercial toxic fats and oils instead.

With adequate natural saturated fats, your cravings for protein will be reduced substantially. It is nutrient-rich broths with the animal fat and coconut oils and butter that will make a big difference to your metabolism. Remember the dangers of too much protein already discussed.

The best solution is to test for the amount of protein your body needs through personal testing. Remember the portion size rule or better yet personally test to determine the optimal amount of protein for you.

If you are vegetarian, then ensure that any protein from dairy comes from grass-fed animals and any beans, pulses, nuts, and seeds are thoroughly soaked or fermented prior to sprouting or cooking to remove the harmful phytates.

Whole grains and beans, by the way, are excellent sources of high quality protein.

Read these two articles for more info on protein:
"Grass-fed basics": www.eatwild.com/basics.html
"Sources of grass-fed meat and dairy": www.eatwild.com

Poultry and Eggs

Choose organic, free-range products, as the commercial products are highly toxic from poor feed, confinement, and manufacturing additives that are especially harmful to your prostate.

Commercial eggs have much more omega-6 fats than organic, free-range ones, which are higher in the beneficial omega-3 fats.

Some health gurus say that eggs are one of the worst foods you can eat and others the complete opposite, like this Natural News article: Eggs - Consume this natural protein source [http://bit.ly/rjXfzG]

I recommend that you personally test to see if eggs are okay for you and how many eggs you can eat on a particular day.

I recommend reading a book called *Nourishing Traditions: The Cookbook that Challenges Politically Correct Nutrition and the Diet Dictocrats* [http://amzn.to/oF0Jni].

Despite its title, this book will educate you on the whys and hows of proper food preparation. It is a fantastic book filled with all kinds of great mouth-watering recipes, dietary information, and important phytate-reducing techniques.

Carbohydrates – Grains, Beans, and Legumes

There are some guru pundits of low-carb diets who claim that we need to avoid carbohydrates like grains, beans, and legumes at all costs. Some claim that primitive man did not eat carbs, but recent evidence shows that tubers, which are a carb, were eaten regularly in ancient times.

Today, so many of our carbs come from denatured, highly-processed grains in the form of white flours (breads, cakes, muffins, cookies, etc.) and extruded with high-temperature processing (e.g., rice cakes and packaged cereals, etc). These are deadly for the body. All the vitamins and minerals have been removed and you are left with a non-nutritious starch full of chemicals from agri-biz farming.

What about other carbs, like grains and flours? While filled with nutrients, the problem with whole grains today—even organic grains—is that the phytic acid or phytates have not been removed through traditional techniques of soaking and fermenting. These grains become difficult to digest in the body and the phytates deplete valuable minerals like calcium, iron, magnesium, and zinc. When processed properly by soaking, grains and beans are wonderful additions to the diet especially when combined with good fats like butter or coconut oil to make them even more digestible.

The phytate problem is only recently becoming known in health circles. For 35 years, the mainstay of my diet was grains and beans. I never knew the harm I was doing by eating so many phytates and losing vital minerals (like zinc, which the prostate requires to be healthy). The whole time I was adding toxins to my body!

My digestion was always terrible no matter how much I cleansed or fasted. All the while I thought I was eating so well because I was following "healthy" guidelines. Combine that with my past aversion to saturated fats and a low-fat diet and no wonder I developed an enlarged prostate in spite of my other good dietary habits, which included organic foods, lots of vegetables, and every supplement under the sun!

It is essential to remove the phytic acid in carbohydrates. Avoiding this simple step defeats the many benefits of the goodness found in whole grains, beans, and nuts and seeds. Phytic acid harms your body little by little (even if you do not notice it). Sourdough bread is a step in the right direction because of the partially fermented process. Pre-soaking the grains would reduce the phytates even more (see Chapter 8 for more info on Phytic Acid and Phytates).

If carbs are not a major portion of your diet then you may not feel the results of improper cooking with occasional use, but it is still best to soak them. It is easy to do. Soak your rice overnight or in the morning for that evening's dinner.

I believe the no- or low-carb diets are too extreme. The key is to prepare carbohydrates properly and to use the whole grain not the devitalized processed ones. Whole carbohydrates provide rich minerals and nutrients, and they are very pleasurable to eat! Just add good saturated fat like organic butter to make them even more digestible and tasty. Avoid all extruded grain products even from whole grains like rice cakes and flaked and puffed cereals, as they contain maximum phytates due to the high-temperature processing.

Many people are allergic to gluten in grains. If you are one of those, try soaking your grain or flour to see if you do better with phytate-reduced breads. The culprit could be that or the combination of the two. Reducing the phytates may make those grains more digestible for you. You can personally test phytate-reduced breads to see if you can then tolerate the gluten. Making your own with fresh made flour which is soaked properly may make you able to digest previously intolerable grain products. You can also try some of the ancient grains in the list below that are less gluten-rich like kamut.

You can find some good information on whole grains here:

- Amaranth [http://bit.ly/qTtcMp]
- Barley [http://bit.ly/ql6j7T]
- Buckwheat [http://bit.ly/pvT65Y]
- Corn [http://bit.ly/ozD59e], including whole cornmeal and popcorn
- Millet [http://bit.ly/naXkop]
- Oats [http://bit.ly/mS53c4], including oatmeal
- Quinoa [http://bit.ly/ppKKq5]
- Rice [http://bit.ly/oQgcpB], both brown rice and colored rice
- Rye [http://bit.ly/phzPQN]
- Sorghum [http://bit.ly/nj9G3G] (also called milo)
- Teff [http://bit.ly/pRW05A]
- Triticale [http://bit.ly/phzPQN]
- Wheat [http://bit.ly/osrCrz], including varieties such as spelt, emmer, farro, einkorn, Kamut®, durum and forms such as bulgur, cracked wheat and wheatberries
- Wild rice [http://bit.ly/qX34DL]

Read more about grains at these sites:

What You Should Know About Wheat [http://bit.ly/qRfjbs]

The Nutrition Source: Health Gains From Whole Grains [http://hvrd.me/p0ewc3]

NOTE: When using any recipes make sure you first follow the phytic acid reducing soaking procedures first.

For a wonderful breakfast cereal try Ezekiel Cereals [http://tiny.cc/00x15], instead of the high-heat extruded flakes and puffs that enhance the anti-nutrient phytic acid. Ezekiel Cereals are not high-heat extruded. This company sprouts the grains to reduce the phytates and then cooks them slowly at a low temperature to preserve good nutrients. They are packed with an amazing crunchy crunch to boot.

To increase the nutritive quality of grains, beans, and legumes, you may wish to sprout them after soaking. When cooking your beans or legumes after soaking, you can add a strip of kombu seaweed to further help reduce phytates in the cooking process. As an added benefit, both the soaking and the kombu reduce flatulence (farting).

Soybeans have a very high phytate content and must be well soaked and fermented to increase digestability and nutrient absorption. That means you must avoid all the processed soy milks and drinks, soy protein bars, tofu, soy flours, imitation soy meats, and soy protein supplements and drinks. Many of these highly processed commercial varieties are ridden with GMOs, pesticides, and are highly sugared.

It is okay to eat miso, tamari, and tempeh, which are from fermented soybeans. Use only organic varieties, as most non-organic ones not only are sprayed with herbicides and pesticides but are also GMO products. If you love soy milk then make it yourself by first soaking the beans, which will make this a highly nutritious food to eat.

Soy is a controversial food. Some proclaim it has many benefits and others warn of its dangers. If you follow the guidelines above you can enjoy soy without any risks. It is easy to personally test these products to be sure they are healthy for you to consume.

For more on soy, please read this excellent article: "The Truth About Unfermented Soy and Its Harmful Effects" [http://bit.ly/nY48TW]

The Cornucopia Institute - Organic Soy Scorecard [http://bit.ly/nSgHPO] provides a list of the best producers of high quality soy products. I would only eat the products ranked with 4 or 5 stars and only those products that have been soaked or fermented.

Read more about the risks of soy here:
- "Is Soy Healthy?" [http://bit.ly/nZyupH]
- "Soy Dangers Summarized" [http://bit.ly/qi3iFn]

Keeping in mind that the discourse on soy should be tempered by the insights gleaned above, you can get a complete breakdown of the many benefits of high quality carbs (i.e., grains, beans, and legumes) here: The World's Healthiest Foods [http://bit.ly/pvtTSt]

Dairy

If you want controversy, dairy is up there with fats and meat! Everyone has strong opinions on this, especially the holistic health specialists. Many blame dairy for what ails you, and they may be right!

The same sad story exists today around dairy as it does with meat and fats: the modern agricultural and processing methods and government regulations have transformed a once healthy food into a sickness-generating toxin.

The same bad practices plague dairy: modern feedlots, confined quarters, unnatural feed like grains, pesticide-ridden foods, and hormone additives and antibiotics have all wreaked havoc on milk products and the consumers who eat it. Add to that pasteurization and homogenization and the dairy foods are now unfit for human consumption.

Sure you can eat it and may not be able to trace its effects, but over time the naysayers of dairy will prove to be right. Not because dairy products in and of themselves are unhealthy foods per se but because of what we have done to these foods.

Organic raw milk from grass-fed animals is the healthiest dairy. This is the dairy of yesteryear, and if milking and dairy facilities are meticulous and clean the food is completely safe and highly nutritious.

Read more here:
- "What is Real Milk?" [http://bit.ly/nlwSbY]
- "Dairy Un-Forbidden: Discover the Virtues of Raw Milk" [http://bit.ly/qm8she]

While organic forms of dairy are far superior to the commercial ones, if they are pasteurized, as most are, then you still are not getting as ideal a food as raw grass-fed milk and dairy. Click here to find sources of raw milk and cheese: "Where Can I Find Real Milk?" [http://bit.ly/oYA1Zv]
I also suggest you try raw goat or sheep milk and cheeses.

My take on dairy: Some people have evolved to have a family heritage of being able to digest dairy easily while others (e.g., often Asians) have troubles with it, especially the non-raw varieties. So if you have not been eating dairy, go slow by first testing and then re-testing often the different dairy products you choose. Raw works great for me. I really feel its benefits.

Meat

I have already discussed meat earlier (see Chapter 5). Much of the same information is found in the sections on fat and protein (found in this chapter).

Please read this article to fully understand the definitions of grass-fed and organic meat, as there are many caveats: Ensure your organic meat is truly organic [http://bit.ly/poswpU]. In the Protein section of this chapter there is a link to help you find the highest quality grass-fed meats.

Nuts and Seeds

These are wonderful healthy foods—but there's a catch! Just like grains and beans, nuts and seeds contain high levels of the anti-nutrient phytic acid, as well as enzyme inhibitors that cause unnoticed reactions to mild reactions all the way to severe allergic reactions in some people. This is in addition to the mineral binding effect that phytic acid has, thereby reducing mineral content in the body and prostate.

For me it was the unnoticed response that gradually worsened in me. I used to eat lots of nuts and nut butters. After my prostate condition developed I became more and more sensitive to nuts until I reached the point that I would end up blocked and no pee would come out as a result of eating nuts. Cashews, almonds, pine nuts, Brazil nuts, walnuts, pecans and even sesame seeds at various times shut me down. No fun.

Now I know why: it was due to the phytates and the enzyme inhibitors. These natural components protect the nut from predators while growing and from sprouting prematurely. They need to be phytate reduced to be healthy and easy to digest. Soaking overnight, at least, in warm water with some sea salt and then dehydrating in your oven at 125-150 degrees will do the trick. This process also makes them even better tasting and crunchy. Many people sprout them but this does not reduce the harmful stuff as much as soaking does. Soaking and then sprouting also works great.

If you only have occasional small amounts of nuts and seeds in your diet and you do not have any reactions and no prostate condition, you are probably okay and can eat nuts and seeds without the reduction techniques. However, if you regularly consume nuts, seeds, or nut milks like almond milk, or nut or seed butters, then it would be best to make your own by soaking them first.

Nuts have many beneficial qualities for the prostate. Almonds are perhaps the easiest to digest, especially when soaked overnight and dried or roasted afterwards. Both walnuts and Brazil nuts can help reduce the size of the prostate and the growth of prostate cancer. Nuts need to be soaked and dried for optimum bio-availability and lack of reaction to anti-nutrient phytic acid.

Personally test all nuts to see if your body can handle them. A NO test response before soaking and drying may turn in to a YES after so doing. But even with a YES, it is best to incorporate soaking if you want the most benefit with the least amount of reaction. Beware of almonds that are not organic, as all California almonds are now sprayed and walnuts irradiated. Personally test for how many nuts to eat daily if you are sensitive to them. Do not overeat nuts.

Avoid cracked nuts, as they can go rancid easily. Watch out for nut butters, as they easily cause adverse reactions. Avoid mixed nuts and dried fruit. Certainly avoid canned, packed, and processed commercial nuts.

Pumpkin seeds have high levels of phytic acid and need to be soaked. While many health advocates claim benefits for the prostate in eating pumpkin seeds and pumpkin butter because of the zinc content, indulging regularly will be harmful unless you reduce the phytic acid.

Sesame seeds have very high phytic acid levels and this is one food where the hull is best removed. (Traditional cultures all removed them.) It is best if you buy white—not unhulled brown—sesame seeds.

I used to eat lots of sesame seeds, mostly with the hull on the seed. I ate sesame butter, gomasio (roasted sesame seeds with salt), ground up seeds in smoothies, and plain seeds cooked with rice. One night after having some sesame seeds, I had a reaction in my prostate; the seeds had caused a block in my pee tube... and misery. The next morning I personally tested everything I had eaten and discovered the culprit—sesame seeds!

It was only many months later that I learned it was the phytic acid and the hulls that were the source of the problem. It seems that traditional cultures removed the hulls. Tahini is hull-less and, therefore, a good sesame seed product, while sesame butter found in health food stores is made with sesame seeds with the hulls on—avoid sesame butter.

There are many other wonderful seeds like chia and flax seeds, both known as superfoods, but I have had reactions to them, perhaps by eating too many. Moderation, even with beneficial seeds and nuts, is essential. Reducing the toxins by soaking is highly recommended.

To read more on the high nutrient content of nuts and seeds go here:
• The World's Healthiest Foods [http://bit.ly/pvtTSt]

Sweeteners

Sugars are associated with the growth of cancer cells because sugar is food for cancer cells. This includes cancer of the prostate. Sugars create digestion problems and obesity, especially when combined with refined white carbs.

Sugar consumption has increased drastically. Our ancestors ate at most one tablespoon per day; today we consume a cup or more per day on average! Imagine those at the high end of the scale eating way more than the average.

Sugar is found now in most prepared foods. High fructose corn syrup, a highly refined sweetener, is even more deadly than sugar cane. See this article for more information:
"The Murky World of High-Fructose Corn Syrup" [http://bit.ly/r8NODZ]

Fructose and high fructose corn syrup (HFCS), found in many fast foods and processed foods, are deadly sweeteners linked to metabolic syndrome, diabetes, cardiovascular disease, and obesity. See this article for more information:
"Diabetes, Obesity and Metabolism Journal Article" [http://bit.ly/oCWGbT]

Also see Dr. Robert Lustig's YouTube video that explains the damage caused by fructose: "Sugar: The Bitter Truth" [http://bit.ly/p5E5oZ]

Avoid fruit juices, as their fructose is worse than regular sugar. A can of orange juice has as much sugar content as a can of Coke. Avoid fruit juices unless you dilute them with water 4 to 1—that's 4 units of water and I unit of juice, not the opposite!

Artificial sweeteners are no better. People use them in the hope that they are less harmful. They actually increase your sugar cravings! You are just trading in one bad habit for a worse one. Read all about the dangers of artificial sweeteners here: "Sugar-Free Blues" [http://bit.ly/nIOvmA]. The solution is to use healthy alternatives to both refined sugar and artificial sweeteners.

Healthy Sugar Alternatives:

- ✓ Real maple syrup (not imitation) - the darker it is the more nutrients in maple syrup. Choose grade B or C, or #2 or #3 (different grading systems). Maple syrup contains potassium and calcium as well as nutritionally significant amounts of zinc and manganese. Zinc is a crucial prostate mineral. So rich, dark, organic, pure maple syrup is your sweetener of choice, in moderation. You can find some here if not in your local health food store: Organic Maple Syrup [http://tiny.cc/vkyus]

- ✓ Raw, unfiltered honey—the darker the better as, like maple syrup, darker honey has more trace elements. (Cooking honey destroys its healthy enzymes.)

- ✓ Molasses

- ✓ Dehydrated sugar cane juice, sold as Sucanat [http://tiny.cc/k2uq8] and Rapadura [http://tiny.cc/lrq1c]

- ✓ Date sugar

- ✓ Organic Coconut sugar [http://tiny.cc/i915v]

Consume your sweeteners and desserts in moderation! One to two tablespoons per day is more than enough.

Air

I call air a food because 10 to 20 times per minute we are consuming air. If the air is polluted you are at a health disadvantage. Make sure your home and car are protected if you live in air-polluted cities. Air purifiers with a negative ion generator can make a big difference. Read more at this site filled with expertise: Office and Home Air Purifiers [http://www.airpurifiers.com]

Water

Our most essential "food" after air—water—heals or harms. If you haven't been paying attention to the quality of the water you drink and consume in beverages and cooking, start immediately!

In most cities, our tap waters contain chlorine, fluoride, and residues of all kind of toxic chemicals. Often tap water is not fit for human consumption. Bottled waters are not much better.

> *"The majority of bottled water on the market is no different than basic tap water. It does, however, cost 50-100 times more per gallon than basic tap. Even worse, if the water is bottled in plastic it leaches xenoestrogenic chemicals into the water. These chemicals disrupt the hormonal balance that should be present in the body. An example is bisphenol A (BPA), which is linked to neurodevelopmental problems in children. BPA can stimulate premature puberty and even lead to breast development in males. BPA has also been linked to breast, uterine, ovarian, and prostate cancers."*

Jockers, Dr. David. 19 June 2011. "Bottled Water is Hazardous to You and Our World" www.naturalnews.com/032744_bottled_water_environment.html [http://bit.ly/nC5n4R] (Accessed 25 June 2011)

The simplest solution is to use a water purifier. There are many options here. A countertop unit like Brita will remove chlorine but not much else. Aquasana [http://bit.ly/peKByu] makes highly rated and affordable filters that you can use at the sink or for the whole house.

I prefer a water distiller, perhaps because I was in the business in the late 70s selling distilled water and machines, until the Quebec government shut our business down. They did so because we were selling water for 99 cents a gallon—bring your own bottle and fill 'er up. The government didn't like that. The business was called AquaVie, the "water of life."

Some health pundits claim distilled water robs your body of minerals in the water that have been removed, or worse removes minerals from your body. I think it is mostly an argument that other types of machine makers use to promote their equipment. Water contains small amounts of minerals in general. Get them from your food! I add a quarter teaspoon of sea salt to the distilled water per gallon to add a touch back and to revitalize the water.

I prefer distillers that have a stainless steel chamber and a glass not plastic collection bottle. I use Waterwise's smallest unit: the Waterwise 4000. It is cheaper to buy at Amazon than direct from the maker. This distiller is made in the USA and distills a gallon in about 3-4 hours. You will also find less expensive ones on Amazon, but be wary of plastic ones:

- Water Distillers at Amazon.com [http://tiny.cc/7lvc1].

- Berkey Water Filters [http://tiny.cc/1c4rp] is another great highly rated water filter with many sizes for home and traveling.

An inexpensive way to get rid of most chlorine in water for bathing is to use vitamin C. Add 1-2 grams of vitamin C powder in your bath water. This is particularly useful if you want to lie in the bathtub without suffering the irritating effects of chlorine.

The bottom line on water is to personally test it to see that what you are using is best for you. If you are unsure of what type of filter system may be better, see if you can find someone who has a machine and personally test their water. When traveling I just test the bottled waters in the supermarkets to see what is best and distilled wins for me each time.

We absorb chlorine from the water when we bathe and shower—lots of it. Over time you are adding greatly to your toxic load. You can get simple inexpensive devices that you can put in your bath water or showerhead, or filter all your home's water. Check these items out at Amazon to find something that suits your needs and budget:

- Bath Dechlorinators [http://tiny.cc/xd3vp]

- Whole House Chlorine Water Filters [http://tiny.cc/1n41c]

How Much Water Should You Drink?

Most health advocates say we should drink at least 8 cups of water a day (8 oz each). They say that most people are chronically dehydrated and need more water to vitalize all the internal organs. Since our bodies are 70% water, it is essential to drink enough, they say.

While it may be true that we are dehydrated, that may have to do with our improper diets of too much of the wrong foods, laden with excess commercial salt and too many toxins. I believe that is the first place to make changes.

The recommended notion then is to flush the toxins out with water, but that may be adding to the problem:

> *"If you are drinking lots of water throughout the day, your stomach acid will become diluted, leading to acid reflux and all the other problems herein described. In addition, too much water may cause mineral depletion and imbalances, which can further contribute to digestive disorders…*
>
> *Paradoxically, over-consumption of water may also cause constipation. When too much water is added to a high-fiber diet, the fibrous foods swell and ferment in the intestinal tract, leading to gas, bloating and other uncomfortable digestive symptoms. This expanded mass may be too large to pass easily…*
>
> *So as people succumb to drinking large quantities of water, not only will they lower the acid levels in the stomach, their digestion and nutrient absorption will be compromised. Over time this also contributes to malnourishment."*

Pirtle, Kathryne. 25 June 2010. "Acid Reflux: A Red Flag" www.westonaprice.org/digestive-disorders/acid-reflux-a-red-flag [http://bit.ly/nQKXDM] (Accessed 6 May 2011)

Roger Mason in *Zen Macrobiotics for Americans* [http://amzn.to/rtgETB] describes a very similar viewpoint. While there are parts of his book I no longer agree with, this does make sense to me:

> *"It is surprising to many people to learn that we should only drink when we are thirsty. We should only drink when we feel the need to drink, when we have a true thirst. We never have a false thirst for water like we have a false thirst for food. Many dietary advocates advise drinking literally quarts of water per day whether you are thirsty or not. These people claim we're 'dehydrated'. Don't listen to this. This drink-as-much-as-you-can theory is very harmful—'drink eight glasses a day'.*
>
> *The proponents go on the theory you can flush your kidneys out like sewer pipes. Quite the opposite is true in that the more you drink the less efficiently your kidneys operate. Your kidneys are not like the plumbing system in your house. Kidneys filter, absorb, and diffuse, and thus should not be overloaded with water they don't want nor need. Drinking too much liquids overworks your kidneys so they can't do what they are designed to do. When you take in too much water the cells close up and unfiltered water is diverted to the large intestine in desperation. The water then goes to the bladder to be passed out without removing the toxins from your system. The toxins are therefore left in your body…*
>
> *ONLY DRINK WHEN THIRSTY and don't drink if you are not thirsty. Your urine should never be cloudy but rather clear with a deep yellow color to show that lots of toxins are contained in it. It is very difficult to drink when you're not thirsty. This goes against our very instincts when we drink if we don't need to."*

For me, it does feel natural to drink when thirsty, and it does not feel natural to force down the recommended 8-glasses-a-day dose. It just feels like too much when I try to follow the party line. Add an enlarged prostate to the mix and you can pee ever so frequently!

Many of the gurus on water and health fail to adjust for climate, age, body size, activity level, etc. It seems everyone copies everyone's recommendations and we are convinced we need our 8 glasses minimum! See how many people carry around water bottles drinking constantly, blindly following these dictates.

You can easily personally test to see how much your body wants. Keep in mind that it is important to always drink high quality water. Of course, if you drink caffeinated drinks and alcohol, which are diuretics, you will need to drink more to replace lost fluids.

Some claim you should never drink during meals. I think sipping small amounts of water *if you are thirsty* actually helps digestion. Also, it's best not to drink lots 15-20 minutes before and after eating so as not to dilute the digestive juices. And avoid cold water. That is harmful to the kidneys and what affects the kidneys will impact your prostate. In the East, they never drink cold water—always warm.

My take on water is to drink only when thirsty and err a bit on the side of extra rather than too little because being dehydrated will make you lethargic and tired. I include mild herbal teas as part of my daily water intake, but not any with caffeine. I also like hot water with some fresh lemon squeezed in with a little honey or maple syrup, especially first thing in the morning.

Caffeinated Drinks

You will find lots of information both for and against caffeinated drinks, especially around coffee. Some researchers say caffeine is very healthy and others say just the opposite. A simple solution is to personally test the caffeinated drinks that you regularly consume. You will know right away. If you get a YES, then do not assume it means that you can drink as much as you want. Test again to find your optimum number of cups.

In my case, I can drink caffeinated coffee only occasionally but often I get a YES for decaf. Luckily it is the taste of coffee that I like, so it does not bother me to drink decaf. Use organic coffees that use the Swiss water method of decaffeinating the beans.

Many people recommend green tea for its health benefits. Test that to see if it is okay for you and see if decaf green varieties are better. Always choose organic versions.

Beer Wine and Liquor

Fermented beers can be a wonderful beverage, especially from small homemade batches or microbreweries.

Try organic wines, as grapes are one of the most-sprayed foods. Personally test to see if you can drink wine, whether red or white, and how much.

Test any liquor you want. I find that some fine liquors I can drink a bit of on occasion without a reaction, but most times I get a NO response.

Lacto-Fermented Foods

Probiotics are live microorganisms in our foods and are proven to be beneficial to the digestive system. Probiotics improve the absorption of nutrients and promote a healthy immune system. This is a very important food group that helps immensely with digestion. It is the good bacteria and enzymes found in unpasteurized lacto-fermented foods like traditional yogurt, pickles (without vinegars), and sauerkraut that are not only tasty but they help prevent gas and irritable digestion, as well as many other benefits.

Today, many health gurus highly recommend adding all kinds of digestive enzymes in the form of supplements to your diet. There is also a trend to add enzymes like acidophilus in processed yogurts and other foods. A far superior way to get probiotics is from traditional lacto-fermented foods. These foods have been used around the world in all cultures to preserve foods and to aid digestion. They do work wonders—I can vouch for that.

The enzymes help digestion in the upper stomach, where there are no digestive fluids. Lacto-fermented foods eaten with cooked foods more than compensate for the loss of any enzymes in cooking. Some say that lacto-fermented foods are not only superfoods but are super-raw foods. Lacto-fermented foods also provide lactic acid, which further aids digestion.

Lacto-fermented foods, like natural yogurt, contain plentiful amounts of natural probiotics, which normalize the acidity of the stomach and do much more:

> *"Like the fermentation of dairy products, preservation of vegetables and fruits by the process of lacto-fermentation has numerous advantages beyond those of simple preservation. The proliferation of lactobacilli in fermented vegetables enhances their digestibility and increases vitamin levels...*
>
> *These beneficial organisms produce numerous helpful enzymes as well as antibiotic and anticarcinogenic substances. Their main by-product, lactic acid, not only keeps vegetables and fruits in a state of perfect preservation but also promotes the growth of healthy flora throughout the intestine."*
>
> Nourishing Traditions: The Cookbook that Challenges Politically Correct Nutrition and the Diet Dictocrats [http://amzn.to/nB9irS]

Here is another wonderful book filled with simple recipes to brew all kinds of delicious fermented treats:

Wild Fermentation: The Flavor, Nutrition, and Craft of Live-Culture Foods [http://amzn.to/q29P2N]

These lacto-fermented foods are great sources of probiotics and are ideal for daily eating at each meal—natural, unpasteurized versions without vinegars are the most potent:

- ✓ Yogurt
- ✓ Tamari
- ✓ Miso
- ✓ Tempeh
- ✓ Sauerkraut
- ✓ Buttermilk
- ✓ Kefir
- ✓ Cottage cheese
- ✓ Sourdough breads
- ✓ Pickles of all kinds

Use these natural forms of probiotics regularly—especially unpasteurized sauerkraut—and see the difference they make to your overall digestion.

> *"Lacto-fermented beverages are ubiquitous in traditional cultures-from kaffir beer in Africa to kvass and kombucha in Slavic regions. Lacto-fermented foods*

are artisanal products—instead of mass produced items preserved with vinegar and sugar—which taste delicious and confer many health benefits. They add valuable enzymes to the diet, and enhance digestibility and assimilation of everything we eat."

www.westonaprice.org/traditional-diets/nasty-brutish-short [http://bit.ly/o9l289]

Read more about the benefits of probiotics here:

- www.usprobiotics.org
- nccam.nih.gov/health/probiotics/introduction.htm [http://1.usa.gov/ntsiVH]

Probiotic supplements are highly promoted, but the above foods are the best way to go. If you can't eat them because of travel or other reasons, then in the short-term, taking probiotic supplements may be useful. If you are coming off a bad diet, then both lacto-fermented foods and probiotics would be beneficial. Always personally test these lacto-fermented foods to know if they are right for you and what quantities you should have daily.

Keep in mind that what your body needs does change! I had too much lacto-fermented sauerkraut it seems, because after a few months of eating sauerkraut at every meal I started to react—I tested, got a No response, and realized again that even the best of the best can turn in to its opposite with excess use. Seems like I am a slow learner! Thank goodness for being able to personally test foods and products!

Salt

Commercial salt, sodium chloride, may have the same chemical structure as sea salt but there is a world of difference. The trace elements in sea salt, not found in commercial salt, are invaluable in providing needed minerals in our diets. For example, sea salt is high in zinc, the crucial prostate mineral. This is an easy switch to make from commercial salts. It will also save you from taking an inferior mineral supplement and from being harmed by commercial salt.

Just as with wine, there are many differences amongst the sea salts you can find today, from the thick slightly grayish Celtic Sea salts to the reddish/pinkish Himalayan and Utah salts from buried seas millions of years ago to the sun-dried Antarctic pure sea salts from the currents off of Antarctica hitting the beaches of South West Africa, and many, many more!

The pinkish color that some sea salts have comes from about 60 trace minerals in the sea salt. These are ideal salts for your diet and you will find the taste far superior to bland commercial bleached and refined salt or worse yet the low-sodium salt substitutes that industry claims are better for you.

Some commercial salt has iodine added back in but sea salt already contains that and many more nutrient minerals, 60 to 80 other needed nutrients!

> *"Part of the process for refined salt, or commercial table salt, involves the use of aluminum, ferro cyanide and bleach. These are all toxic materials that your body takes in with refined, commercial salt. And because of that process, almost all the vital minerals that real, unrefined salt can offer are removed! One or two*

servings of refined salt won't send you to the grave. But continued almost daily use will avail you to the perils of aluminum toxicity. Ferro cyanide is listed by the EPA as a toxic material for human consumption. You are probably aware of the hazards to human health of chlorine, which is used to bleach the salt."

www.naturalnews.com/028724_Himalayan_salt_sea.html
[http://bit.ly/q7qRD2]

Read this article to learn about the different perils of refined salt: "Confront Salt Confusion" [http://bit.ly/o0X7z7]

Discover the world of sea salt. Try different varieties of sea salts to see what is your favorite. It is easy to find in any health store, you can also find sea salt here at Amazon: Sea Salt [http://tiny.cc/qefh4]

Fruits and Vegetables

The best advice is to eat a wide variety of fruits and vegetables, while paying some attention to seasonality and locality for your choices; these foods are more vital and have more nutrients because they are harvested closer to full ripeness. It is especially important to personally test to see whether foods from the tropics are suitable in mid-winter in northern locales. Tropical fruits are not ideal foods for daily use in our temperate climates, especially in winter.

It may surprise you to know that this winter when I personally tested for bananas I got a NO response. I only thought of testing them when I couldn't think of what was causing a prostate reaction, so I decided to test everything I ate in the past 24 hours and the culprit was bananas. I have found that something that was good for me at one point in the year changes and becomes not so good in another season.

The healthier you are the less will you experience reactions and you will be able to eat a wide variety of foods without problems. If you are in a more critical situation then testing becomes essential as your body rebuilds and doesn't yet have the strength to deal with less than ideal inputs.

Avoid fruit juices except on occasions and when you do have them it is best if you dilute them 4:1, as juices contain far too much fructose (a harmful sugar).
I bet you didn't know this about sweet potatoes/yams (nor did I):

> *"[They] ranked number one in nutrition out of all vegetables by the Center for Science in the Public Interest because they are such a rich source of dietary fiber, natural sugars, complex carbohydrates, protein, carotenoids, vitamin C, iron and calcium."*

> Walling, Elizabeth. 01 March 2011. "Nine reasons to eat more sweet potatoes" www.naturalnews.com/031543_sweet_potatoes_minerals.html [http://bit.ly/pzapa0] (Accessed 10 May 2011)

When buying local produce ensure it is organic and not chemicalized nor sprayed. Read this article for a personal and environmental health perspective: "Local and Organic Food Farming: Here's the Gold Standard" [http://bit.ly/pHLtiN]

Eat a wide variety of fruits and vegetables both raw and cooked every day. Eat raw foods at every meal; this includes lacto-fermented raw foods. Decide the proportion of raw foods in your diet based on where you live, the current season, your sensitivity to particular foods, and the results you receive when you personally test. I live in Canada, and when I personally test some tropical raw fruits and vegetables during the winter I tend to receive a NO response. Check and see what's right for you.

Download this simple produce guide to know which are the worst sprayed and least with pesticides in conventional produce:
EWG's Shopper's Guide to Pesticides in Produce [http://bit.ly/mVZ9bE]

To read more about harmful ingredients found commonly in supermarket foods, read this article: "What's really in the food?" [http://bit.ly/pAp509]

Nightshade Vegetables

Potatoes, tomatoes, eggplants and bell peppers are part of this group of vegetables. Sensitive eaters may have reactions to some of these vegetables, including prostate reactions, arthritis and rheumatism, nervous system reactions, and more. These vegetables contain harmful glycoalkaloids. Green parts of potatoes and their eyes have high amounts of these toxins. Many people are unknowingly allergic to tomatoes. The solanine in these foods can be harmful. It is best to test nightshades often, minimize their use and to stop their use entirely if you react, at least for some time period.

Oxalate Vegetables

Chives, beet leaves, swiss chard, rhubarb, spinach and parsley contain high quantities of oxalic acid. Oxalic acid binds with minerals like calcium and iron, forming urinary stones, which can easily irritate the prostate. Oxalate vegetables should only be eaten on occasion and only if you personally test positive for them.

Herbs and Spices

These items add great variety and flavor to our foods. The problem is that many can be irritants, especially if used frequently. The only way to know is to personally test them from time to time. Another danger is that people often keep them around too long and they lose their freshness and can go off, causing even further reactions. A year is about the maximum time to keep herbs and spices unless refrigerated. I have had severe reactions to many herbs and spices thinking they are used in such small amounts as herbal teas or seasonings that it wouldn't matter until I wisened up (I am slow sometimes!) and started testing them. Eat safe. Check 'em out!

How and When to Eat

Food is crucial for nourishing us. We need to learn to take more time than we are used to when preparing and eating whole foods. Food is your daily medicine and eating in a non-rushed manner is a good habit to develop.

Chewing more often than we are used to helps make the food much more digestible, so that we benefit from the high quality food choices we are now investing in.

Adjust, too, to the fact that quality food will cost more than cheapo foods that harm you. You can still save by buying in bulk, joining food coops and buying clubs, buying direct from the grower, attending local farmers markets, and start growing your own food, even on a balcony. Take a look at this website that has lots of resources for container gardening: journeytoforever.org/garden_con.html [http://bit.ly/rbGWkx]

Do you live in a tiny apartment with no balcony? You can still sprout all kinds of seeds: Sprouters [http://tiny.cc/lym2r]

In summary:

- ✓ Eat widely across all food groups.
- ✓ Eat lacto-fermented foods to help you digest more.
- ✓ Eat slowly and chew well.
- ✓ If you want to drink while eating, sip rather than drink large quantities.
- ✓ Limit desserts to one meal a day at most to lessen your addictions to sweets.
- ✓ Enjoy the rich tastes of natural wholesome foods!

In the Ayurvedic tradition, there are times that are thought best to eat that correspond with natural body biorhythms that enhance digestion. Those times are 8 am for breakfast, 12 noon for lunch, and 6 pm for supper. Eating around these times (plus or minus an hour) is ideal and avoid eating after 8 pm, as our digestive juices decline rapidly in the evening.

Seasonal Foods

Once you start personally testing your food, you may very well discover that foods from other seasons or climates may not work for you. If you choose to eat these foods even though your test response was a NO, you could be irritating your body and prostate. A good example is eating melons in winter in Chicago. Small amounts may be fine, but frequent use could easily cause a reaction. Test and you will know.

I can only eat bananas on occasion in the winter. If I ignore this and have many bananas then I have a reaction. Although we can eat out-of-season foods due to modern conveniences of transport and cooling it does not mean that these foods are ideal for us, no matter how organic, fresh, or filled with nutrients the food supposedly is. The old adage of moderation will serve you well.

Superfoods

Superfoods are a group of foods that contain extra high amounts of beneficial nutrients. The list is subjective, as there is no official definition of what is and is not a superfood. Keep in mind, what may be a superfood for one could be harmful to another. The only way to know is to personally test each food you eat. That said check some of these out: ghee, avocados and avocado oil, coconut oil, sauerkraut, miso, lemons, and green superfoods.

Ghee

Ghee, also known as clarified butter, ideally made from butter from grass-fed cows, is my current favorite superfood. Ghee has a yummy, sweet buttery taste that adds both richness and flavor to your food. Ghee is basically butter with the milk protein taken out, leaving pure butter fat. Ghee has a higher burning point than butter, meaning you can cook Ghee at much higher temperatures than butter without it burning. It's a great cooking oil.

Try some here: www.pureindianfoods.com
They have several flavors but I suggest you start with the plain version first.

Avocados and Avocado Oil

Avocados are a superfood delight and so delicious. Filled with good fats that provide excellent anti-inflammatory benefits. Avocados contain:

- ✓ Phytosterols, including beta-sitosterol (found in Saw Palmetto)
- ✓ Carotenoid antioxidants
- ✓ Vitamins C and E
- ✓ Manganese
- ✓ Selenium
- ✓ Zinc
- ✓ Omega-3 fatty acids

Read more about avocados here:
www.whfoods.com/genpage.php?tname=foodspice&dbid=5 [http://bit.ly/ncRYea]

Avocado oil has a very high burning point, so it is great for cooking and is delicious on salads. Get extra virgin, cold-pressed, organic varieties. It will cost more but Avocado oil [http://tiny.cc/ajyjo] is a superb, versatile, very healthy oil.

Want a potato chip made with healthy oils? Try these super yummy chips made with organic avocado oil: Avocado Chilean Lime Chips by Good Health [http://amzn.to/qehS7L]. As with all foods, remember not to overdo this oil. Since avocados are a tropical fruit, they are best eaten in moderation especially in winter.

Coconut oil

This amazing oil, a saturated fat, is best taken like olive oil, in its extra virgin state, which means the least amount of heat processing to preserve its optimum nutrient values. Coconut oil is perfect to cook with, use in salads, and it is also wonderful on your skin and hair. Read more here:

- "Latest Studies on Coconut Oil" [http://bit.ly/oP1tjN]
- "Latest Headlines on Coconut Health" [http://bit.ly/nH0pl1]
- "The Many Benefits of Coconut Oil and Coconut Butter" [http://bit.ly/rmiZMU]

> *"Coconut oil also helps to balance hormones, stabilize blood sugar levels and boost the cellular healing process. It is also known to stimulate the thyroid and reduce stress on the liver and pancreas. This increases metabolism which helps us burn fat far more effectively while stimulating clean sources of energy that make us feel terrific."*

> Jockers, Dr. David. 13 January 2011. "Make sure you consume enough of this super food" **www.naturalnews.com/030990_super_food_coconut_oil.html [http://bit.ly/nk2Ir2]** (Accessed 10 May 2011)

Coconut oil also provides effective and natural sun protection without having to use toxic chemicals in conventional sun block. Coconut oil protects against free radicals, providing added protection against skin cancer. Mix coconut oil with African shea butter and aloe vera for a simple and harmless sun protection formula. This combination is also wonderful as a moisturizer for your skin and hair.

Coconut water kefir is a fermented beverage especially beneficial for gut problems such as candida overgrowth. This drink is hard to find but easy to make. Go here for tips: Kefir Coconut Juice Recipe [http://bit.ly/r2NhJg]. Coconut water is also an excellent drink to use during fasting because of its high nutritional content.

Sauerkraut

This time-honored food is so beneficial for digestion. It can be an acquired taste for some people, so start slow with a small amount and use a young version rather than a longer-aged one. Avoid pasteurized sauerkraut, as the pasteurization process destroys the beneficial nutrients in this superfood. Daily use will do wonders to your gut, so it is worth acquiring the taste. Start making your own since it sounds quick and easy to do. Here are some recipes for making your own sauerkraut:

Nourishing Traditions: The Cookbook that Challenges Politically Correct Nutrition and the Diet Dictocrats [http://amzn.to/nB9irS]

Eden foods, a highly rated manufacturer, makes excellent sauerkraut if you can't find a locally made one: Eden Foods Organic Sauerkraut [http://amzn.to/oGPK0O]

Miso

A traditional oriental food, miso is a lacto-fermented food packed with great taste and benefits. Traditionally, miso is aged 6 months to 2 years. If you go to Japanese restaurants, then you must be familiar with miso soup. Unfortunately modern Japanese miso is now adulterated from its past traditional greatness, often highly processed and containing MSG, it is best to buy organic versions free from GMO soybeans and MSG.

> *"Many studies have shown the health benefits of miso on humans and animals. Benefits include reduced risks of breast, lung, **prostate**, and colon cancer, and protection from radiation...*
>
> *Miso has a very alkalizing effect on the body and strengthens the immune system to combat infection. Its high antioxidant activity gives it anti-aging properties."*
>
> Minton, Barbara. 4 February 2009. "Miso Soup: A Delicious Bowl Full of Health and Anti-Aging Benefits" www.naturalnews.com/025519_health_anti-aging_soy.html [http://bit.ly/n8r1ut] (Accessed 5 May 2011)

Miso often is made with rice or barley added to the soybeans during the fermentation process. I find the rice version (genmai miso) mild and delicious. You can find some here: Organic Miso [http://tiny.cc/0uqbt]

Here is a very quick and simple way to use Miso. I do this most days: boil water, pour into a cup, add a teaspoon or more of miso and stir to dissolve. That's it—now you have a refreshing and uplifting drink with amazing health benefits.

Lemons

Lemons contain vitamin C and bioflavonoids, plant derivatives with antioxidant and anti-inflammatory, as well as anti-cancer properties. Lemons are a superb food for the prostate.

High in potassium, lemons affect the body's biochemistry and pH levels in a positive and powerful way. Astringent in nature, lemons have an overall alkalizing affect on the body, even though they are acidic before entering the body.

I like to use a little lemon juice in place of vinegar in salad dressings. You can add it to steamed veggies, soups, sauces, dips, and even desserts. I add a bit when making applesauce.

Most mornings I start the day with some lemon squeezed into a cup of very hot water and mixed with a teaspoon of honey. Use unpasteurized honey. According to Ayurvedic practices, this drink is good for the liver, and aids digestion and the immune system. I also switch honey for maple syrup for variety. Read more about lemons here:
Lemons/Limes [http://bit.ly/neERaO]

Green Superfoods

Greens or green superfoods are highly promoted as powders, juices, and supplements. These include wheatgrass, chlorella, blue-green algae, barley greens, parsley powders, spirulina, and more. Packed with natural nutrients, vitamins, and minerals, green superfoods come highly recommended by many practitioners. I won't get into all the claims here because, in the final analysis, you will be the judge by personally testing to see if green superfoods are right for you.

As I mentioned below in my personal adventures with kale, be careful with these greens, they can cause reactions in you and your prostate. If greens test positive for you, they can be beneficial in helping you rebuild after years of poor diet habits because of their high nutrient content. You can read more here:

The Natural News Store: search for "Green Superfoods" [http://bit.ly/qyNW4k]

Green Superfoods at Amazon [http://tiny.cc/afu5f]

Pure Synergy Superfood [http://bit.ly/pkuxBI] is a top-of-the-line green product I used to take. There is quite the story of where and how it is made. Click here for more info: Pure Synergy Superfood [http://bit.ly/pkuxBI]

It may be best to take a single green product rather than a mixture of many. You could test positive for an individual product but a combination product could have something in it that disagrees with your system. So go to a health food store and start with single items to test. Then monitor over time to ensure you do not end up with a negative reaction. I still can't eat these because I react. You will know if green superfoods are right for you when you test.

Other Superfoods

Many people have their own lists of foods that contain high concentrations of valuable nutrients. Superfoods are a far superior way to get what you think you may be missing vitamin or mineral wise rather than taking a supplement. I will list some here:

- ✓ Cod Liver Oil [http://bit.ly/py6nHA] is such an important food source. I discuss it in more detail further on. It a potent food with vitamin D and omega-3s in an easy to absorb form that make it so potent.

- ✓ Manuka Honey [http://tiny.cc/git1i] - there has been lots of research on honey products.

- ✓ Swedish Bitters [http://tiny.cc/ayv3j] to balance all the tastes.

- ✓ Evening Primrose Oil [http://tiny.cc/z2p6i], Black Currant Oil [http://tiny.cc/z8u0x] and Borage Oil [http://tiny.cc/cbjfo] are special, potent oils.

- ✓ Kelp [http://tiny.cc/99om2] has a high mineral content, especially iodine, which many people are deficient in. You can find powdered kelp with sea salt as a condiment that is quite tasty.

✓ Wheat Germ Oil [http://tiny.cc/nw1vh] is an excellent source of natural vitamin E that can be added to smoothies

✓ Sprouts can be a powerhouse of concentrated nutrition. Soaking and then sprouting releases nutrients and decreases anti-nutrients like phytic acid in grains, nuts, beans, and seeds. Sprouts are a great way of having fresh greens in the winter, bioavailable vitamins, minerals, amino acids, proteins, beneficial enzymes and phytochemicals. The only caveat is that you personal test them to ensure their compatibility as with any superfoods you eat. Sprouting is easy to do right in your kitchen. Get seeds at your local health food store or at Amazon: Sprouting seeds [http://tiny.cc/h64gb]

Super Seeds

Seeds have healthy omega-3 fats and have minerals and vitamins our bodies need. Personally test these seed types before eating them, and then find the correct quantity (one tablespoon, two tablespoons, etc.). Often the best way to eat seeds is by grinding them first. I grind mine in a coffee grinder.

Chia Seeds

Organic chia seeds [http://tiny.cc/8v3sf] contain 15 times more magnesium than broccoli, 6 times more calcium than whole milk, 3 times more antioxidants than fresh blueberries, more fiber than flaxseed, plus more protein than soy, and are extremely high in omega-3 fatty acids.

As with other seeds and nuts, to reduce phytates you may need to soak or sprout then dry the seeds before consuming them. You can find some organic varieties made from sprouted seeds. I still test negative for chia, perhaps because I used too much before I knew about personally testing foods and phytates. If you get a YES response when you test, then remember to find your optimum daily amount.

Flaxseeds

Touted today by many as a superfood, flaxseeds [http://tiny.cc/1twsl] can be highly beneficial, as can the oil. I used to take it until learning about cod liver oil. Best to take flax fresh grounded in your coffee grinder. If you use flax oil, it must be refrigerated to keep its potency. I must have had too much of a good thing as I still test NO for flaxseeds even now, but you may find the seeds useful.

Pumpkin Seeds

Supposedly good for your prostate, pumpkin seeds [http://tiny.cc/luous] and its oil may be useful, but pumpkin seeds do contain phytates, so it is best to buy them whole and soak the seeds to reduce the phytic acid before eating them. Pumpkin seeds are also available as a nut butter; I used to eat it often before I knew about the phytate anti-nutrient and had to stop when I had prostate reactions. I still test negative to pumpkin seeds, including its oil. So you know what to do now! Test for yourself to see if these seeds are good for you!

Oil Smoke Points

When you cook with oil you want to make sure that you do not allow the oil to reach its smoke point. When oil starts smoking, the oil transforms and can become a carcinogen (i.e., cancer causing). That is also why BBQ'd meats that flare because the oil catches fire are hazardous to you.

Below are oil smoke points of recommended oils sorted by temperature. Oils listed in **bold** font are suggested safe oils to use daily, use other oils on occasion, and omit oils are not listed below because they are unsafe to use at any temperature (e.g., canola oil).

Temperature	Oil
225°F	Flaxseed Oil, Unrefined – *do not heat this oil!*
320°F	Peanut Oil, Unrefined
	Walnut Oil, Unrefined
350°F	**Butter**
	Coconut Oil
	Sesame Oil, Unrefined
361–390°F	Lard
	Olive Oil, Extra Virgin
	Macadamia Nut Oil
410°F	Sesame Oil
430°F	Almond Oil
	Hazelnut Oil
440°F	Peanut Oil
482°F	**Ghee**
491°F	Avocado Oil, Unrefined

Just got to have BBQ'd meat? The smell is just too much for you? Well here is an occasional compromise that can reduce the toxins. Just don't go overboard! It's the compounds called heterocyclic amines (HCA), which seem to be one of the culprits in prostate cancers, caused by cooking on the grill.

Well, a new study shows that marinating meat in special herbs sharply reduces the level of HCAs...

"The researchers marinated steaks in three different types of marinade for an hour each, and then grilled them at 400 degrees, five minutes per side. They also grilled steaks minus the marinade. Amazingly, the steaks

marinated in a "Caribbean mixture" containing thyme, red and black pepper, allspice, rosemary, and chives—showed an 88 percent reduction in HCAs. An herb marinade composed of oregano, basil, onion, jalapeno, parsley, and red pepper provided a 72 percent reduction, and a third marinade with paprika, red pepper, oregano, black pepper, garlic, and onion brought a 57 percent reduction."

Barron, Jon. 8 November 2008. "Marinated Meats Less Toxic" www.jonbarron.org/natural-health/bl080811/blog-dietary-supplements-meat [http://bit.ly/ragqEO] (Accessed 8 May 2011)

You still must avoid flare-ups from burning fat as this is a whole other danger, so cook at the lowest temperatures that you can. BBQ for special occasions only, not regular use!

Antioxidants

This is a controversial subject with many health advocates proclaiming the benefits of taking antioxidants daily as a supplement. Although, some recent research suggests that over indulging in antioxidants can have a harmful affect, this study refutes that claim: "Study Citing Antioxidant Vitamin Risks Based On Flawed Methodology, Experts Argue" [http://bit.ly/qBIdl1]

This is what the National Institutes of Health says:

> *"Antioxidants are substances that may prevent potentially disease-producing cell damage that can result from natural bodily processes and from exposure to certain chemicals."*
>
> nccam.nih.gov/health/antioxidants/introduction.htm [http://1.usa.gov/oAcD63]

Here is a summary of the supposed benefits of antioxidants:

> *"Studies over the last 20 years have shown that free radical fighters found in a certain group of nutrients, namely antioxidants, can protect against a great many free radical initiated diseases. Antioxidants extinguish free radicals!*
>
> *Free Radicals cause oxidation in the blood. Once oxidation occurs, disease can result. Antioxidants keep free radicals from causing oxidation in the blood, thus neutralizing disease. Also, stress, chemical pollution, environmental pollution, and the normal aging process increase the demands put upon the immune system.*
>
> *Studies indicate antioxidants do more than protect against free radicals; they also stimulate the immune system's response to help fight existing diseases."*
>
> www.antioxidants.net (Accessed 11 May 2011)

This article lays out the specific ones that the author believes are the best: "The vital role of antioxidants in achieving optimum health and longevity" [http://bit.ly/qPJjNx]

The realization is that all fresh foods contain lots of antioxidants and if you are eating well then you are getting plenty of them, especially if you include some of the superfoods already described in your regular diet. That said, some of you might want to add antioxidants in to your daily regime.

I would suggest foods as your primary source, superfoods next, followed by food-based antioxidant supplements. My best advice is, as always, to personally test before consuming them. I have found that most recommended antioxidants have a NO test result for me, or at best endure for a very short time, which saves me a lot of money. I must be getting what I need from my good diet—and so can you!

I will talk more about antioxidants in the section on supplements found in Chapter 9.

Cravings

I've told you about the conditions that create prostate disease, what you need to stop doing, and what you need to start doing. One obstacle that often lies in the path of making these types of major lifestyle changes are cravings.

Cravings have many causes. A deficiency in vital nutrition will easily urge you to crave certain foods. Unfortunately we end up binging on foods that only add to the problem. If you are missing enough good quality salt, as an example, you could end up eating more and more devitalized breads, cookies and cakes—all of which will add weight and make you less healthy.

Gluten, which is difficult to digest, unless the grain is first soaked, actually leads to cravings because they produce pleasant feelings and the desire for more. If you have candida and parasites in your gut, then those lead to sugar starchy cravings as food for those overgrowths.

A lack of saturated fats easily leads to cravings. Having enough of these high quality saturated fats does the opposite. We feel satisfied when we eat them and it stops the cravings. The poor quality vegetable fats found in processed and fast foods become addictive because our bodies are never truly satisfied by them (our bodies crave real food, not food-like substances).

The more sugary foods you eat, the more you will crave. Today many of our manufactured foods also have food additives in the form of artificial flavorings and preservatives, which little by little cause us to become addicted. Some manufacturers add items to increase cravings because this increases sales.

What's the solution to constant cravings and weight gain? Eat real food. Slowly, little by little, start reducing the foods on the STOP list while adding whole foods that nourish you. Make sure you get enough good saturated fats and high quality sea salts every day. Healthy foods will do the trick! Your cravings will disappear, as will pounds and pounds of unwanted fat. The Happy Zappy Prostate Diet has real side benefits: a much healthier you!

My Story, Part II: The Journey of Self-Healing

This has been such a journey of discovery and insights that will save you years of grief if your goal is to prevent or heal a prostate condition.

I have discovered powerful solutions that eluded me for the next seven and a half years, a period when I tried all I could think of.

Being an entrepreneur, I am extremely persistent, which is a blessing and a curse because I do not know when to quit. However, this gift has served me with finding the solutions to my prostate condition, and for that, I am so grateful!

I won't mention names of the healers and practitioners I tried, but know this—I spared nothing in my quest and was totally committed to the process. During the course of this period, I spared no money. I tried anything that had any possibility of success. Many of these were not in my comfort zone, but I openly embraced whatever came my way.

But failure—one after the other—seemed to be my destiny. I burned through so many alternative approaches. I gave each my all; I followed the advice of each expert to a tee. But no success! And I am talking about all kinds of great practitioners both close by or within a day's ride and, with the Internet, it was easy to have well-known practitioners, wherever in the world they may have been. I was diligent always in following their advice, but success eluded me. Some of these practitioners were very successful in their fields with published books and large practices. I learned a lot from each of them.

I never cheated along the way, eating or taking things that were not for me. The consequences were too extreme, and this meant that I was able to accurately gage whether or not their treatments worked for me. I began with acupuncture and homeopathy and moved on to a more refined macrobiotic diet.

About a month after I first saw the urologist, I got a call from the hospital to book me in to the emergency surgery. I had come to the top of the list. The booking nurse could not believe it when I told her No! I did so a second time a few months later because they thought I had lost my head and gave me a second chance.

Nobody would refuse the chance to get urgently needed prostate surgery! This happened at a time when the non-emergency waiting list was a year long. Patients wished they could be on the emergency one and here I was refusing enlarged prostate surgery! I began doing saliva and blood hormone tests. I started taking natural hormones and using topical natural hormone creams that would supposedly balance my hormones.

I had suspected at one stage that perhaps my mercury fillings were the culprit.

(There is a ton of alternative info claiming how harmful these can be to your health). I did a whole series of blood tests to find any heavy metals. The hospital asked if I had worked in the mines, as they had not done such a series of tests in a long time! The results came back to me at the low end of acceptable results. So the problem wasn't my fillings.

During this first year, I went to Montreal for a visit. I saw a good friend who also had come down with a severe enlarged prostate condition. He said he blocked every now and then and was able to use a catheter himself! I had never heard of anyone doing this himself, but he assured me it could be done. He told me to buy some catheters just in case.

I flew home and I had time for one stop in town before I had to catch the last ferry to my island home. So I ran into a pharmacy and bought a couple of them. Was I lucky I did that! Within a week I needed it.

I woke up one night, and lo and behold I could not pee. Not a drop. Here I was again at that very frightful place. I tried all kinds of tricks that I had picked up in my research from deep breathing to perineum massage to hot baths to a vigorous walk. They had been successful in some cases where only a few drops came out initially. I waited and waited in the hopes that the tricks would work, but this time was more severe and none of my attempts worked. The pain was coming in waves and getting unbearable!

So I used the catheter. Definitely not the favorite use of the male instrument. It prefers to be encased by a warm tube rather than to encase a cold plastic one! Instead of screaming in pain from a bursting bladder, the catheter brought relief at last! Thank goodness I had bought one!

Over the next years, I was diligent in trying all kinds of things. But instead of getting better I was getting worse! I tried everything that made sense. Sometimes it seemed like I was making some progress and then suddenly I would block. The worst was when I could not get any urine to flow and had to use a catheter. It was always a major setback.

As time went on I was able to find what it was that triggered the block, an acute extra swelling of the prostate. It was usually something that I ate. I saw that foods that were once fine could suddenly become something that could set me off. A good example was cashews (sometimes okay for me but often not). Of course I didn't know this until after the fact when I would trace back to find the cause.

I later learned that an antinutrient called phytates was in many of the foods that I ate on a regular basis. Often it was the phytates in the foods that was causing the blockages. Read on to the next chapter to learn more about phytates and how to prepare foods in ways that reduce this harmful form of phosphorous that naturally occurs in grains, seeds, nuts, beans, and many other foods.

Chapter 8: Phytic Acid – Why You Should Soak!

What is Phytic Acid?

Do you know that a wide range of food types contain an antinutrient that robs your prostate of its most important mineral zinc? That unknown antinutrient is what triggered my prostate condition and it took me decades to find out about it.

Phytic acid occurs naturally in grains, beans, pulses, nuts, and seeds; it is there to help the plants defend against their insect predators and prevent premature germination. As such, phytic acid, also known as phytates, is an antinutrient.

Phytic acid acts as an irritant in the body while gradually removing vital minerals over time as you eat foods containing it. Phytic acid binds with calcium, iron, zinc, and magnesium, removing them from the body.

These minerals are especially important for vibrant health, a lack of which can cause all sorts of health problems that seem to materialize later in life. Cumulative reductions in these elements over time take their toll.

In the particular case of the male reproductive system, zinc deficiencies are a real problem. The prostate requires lots of zinc to function properly.

> *"Zinc deficiency can lead to numerous health conditions, including prostate disorders which may in turn lead to prostate cancer."*
> **Zinc is Essential for Good Health [http://bit.ly/ozBxZu]**

The reduction in calcium levels also helps produce cavities and osteoporosis. Combine low levels of magnesium and you have a recipe for many diseases.
"Magnesium is Vital for Good Health" [http://bit.ly/mUd2pf]

Magnesium is an absolute necessity within our bodies, especially these days when our intake of and exposure to toxins and heavy metals is so high and occurs on a daily basis. With accumulation of toxins and acid residues, our body will degenerate and age more quickly. Simply put, magnesium is needed for the survival of our cells. A deficiency of this mineral sets the stage for cancer. It's an extremely powerful mineral with the ability to rejuvenate and prevent calcification of organs and tissues, which is what happens in old age and degeneration.
Dr. Mark Sircus' Magnesium for Life website [http://magnesiumforlife.com/]

More and more research is showing the benefits of magnesium both as a method of detoxing the body from heavy metals built up over time in the body and as a key element in the natural treatment of cancer. Most of us can use additions of magnesium. The best way to increase your magnesium intake is with a simple water-based spray applied to the skin—a very inexpensive and effective mineral to use.

> *"Magnesium does protect cells from aluminum, mercury, lead, cadmium, beryllium and nickel, which explains why re-mineralization is so essential for heavy metal detoxification and chelation as well as radiation protection. Magnesium is essential for the survival of our cells but takes on further importance now where our bodies are being bombarded on a daily basis with heavy metals and radiation."*

Sircus, Mark. 3 June 2011. "Magnesium Offers Strong Radiation Protection". www.naturalnews.com/032596_magnesium_radiation.html [http://bit.ly/nzlcaJ] (Accessed 7 June 2011)

For more information on the benefits of magnesium, see this site: Dr. Sircus' Blog - Magnesium Oil [http://bit.ly/oZn8ek]

You can also buy magnesium on Amazon: "Ancient Minerals" Magnesium [http://tiny.cc/rsaqa]

Another detriment of phytates in foods is its deleterious effect on digestion, causing all kinds of problems. Phytic acid inhibits enzymes needed for digestion including pepsin for breaking down proteins in the stomach, amylase for turning starch into sugar, and trypsin needed for digesting protein in the small intestine.

Sadly, I never knew about phytic acid until very recently. I should have known of it because for decades I was mostly vegan, and I always seemed to have digestion problems with lots of gas and bloating. I ate many phytate-rich whole grains, beans, and nuts three times per day. No wonder I developed a severe enlarged prostate condition even while eating healthy organic foods. The culprit was phytic acid! Combined with a low fat and especially no saturated fat diet and with the loss of vital zinc and other minerals, I was a breeding ground for prostate enlargement!

You can download a comprehensive article about phytates here: *Cereal Grains: Humanity's Double-Edged Sword* [http://bit.ly/pt5fno]

For another thorough article on Phytic Acid and reduction techniques, please read this article: "Living With Phytic Acid" [http://bit.ly/pWLlTm]

Phytic Acid Levels in Some Foods

The following is a list of foods containing the antinutrient phytic acid. It is not that we should stop eating these food groups but rather we must learn how to remove the phytates through proper food preparation. Otherwise we risk unexplained disease development over time. As a wise preventative measure, start changing your cooking habits with these foods now.

Food	Phytic Acid (mg per 100g)
Sesame seeds dehulled	5,360
100% Wheat bran cereal	3,290
Soybeans	1,000–2,220
Cocoa powder	1,684–1,796
Oats	1,370
Brown rice	1,250
Oat flakes	1,174
Coconut meal	1,170
Almonds	1,138–1,400
Parboiled brown rice	1,600
Barley	1,190
Whole corn	1,050
Rye	1,010
Walnut	982
Whole wheat flour	960
Lentils	779
Navy beans	740–1,780
Hazelnuts	648–1,000
Wild rice flour	634–753
Refried beans	622
Peanuts germinated	610
Pinto beans	600–2,380
Corn tortillas	448
Corn	367
White flour	258
White flour tortillas	123

Note. Measurements are in milligrams per 100 grams of weight.

From "(Part I) Whole grain toxicity - Phytic acid contained in popular foods" [http://bit.ly/qLQ2p7] (Accessed 8 May 2011)

Soaking or fermenting are the primary ways of reducing phytates, while sprouting and sourdough leavening help. If phytate-rich foods are not soaked first, the phytates remain in the food.

The Weston A. Price Foundation documents:

> *"What researchers often overlook is the fact that seed foods-grains, legumes and nuts-are prepared with great care in traditional societies, by sprouting, roasting, soaking, fermenting and sour leavening. These processes neutralize substances in whole grains and other seed foods that block mineral absorption, inhibit protein digestion and irritate the lining of the digestive tract. Such processes also increase nutrient content and render seed foods more digestible."*

http://www.westonaprice.org/traditional-diets/nasty-brutish-short [http://bit.ly/o9l289]

Go here to learn more about phytates and to get great recipes: rebuildmarket.com/catalog/phytic-acid.html [http://bit.ly/nWvnpX]

These phytate-rich foods can be real triggers for unexplained sudden prostate attacks (e.g., blockages, very frequent urinating, and more). I believe that phytates are a big part of why we have enlarged prostates and other prostate diseases, especially when coupled with our many poor diet habits and depleted commercial toxic foods.

This cookbook is a superb comprehensive work filled with great recipes and health creating information. *Nourishing Traditions: The Cookbook* [http://amzn.to/o7OMVt]

To be fair, I now offer you counter-arguments to the many articles about the problems of phytic acid in foods. I completely disagree with this information because personal testing easily confirms that phytates are harmful for me. You decide after personally testing phytate-rich foods and after reading this article: Phytic Acid Friend or Foe? [http://bit.ly/nWIYKV]

Once I started testing I realized how wrong I was when I assumed that my basic diet of grains, nuts and seeds was perfect for me. At this point I must severely limit foods that have phytates in them, even with maximum reduction techniques, as these foods result in a medium to severe reaction in my prostate. It was humbling for me to admit I was wrong for 35 years! I needed to challenge my past assumptions and really examine what foods are ideal for me right now, in this moment. It was also empowering to find the answers at long last and to heal my prostate condition!

If you are very healthy, small daily amounts of phytate-rich foods may not be harmful, as your body can deal with them. However, larger amounts over time is a recipe for health problems. That is why many vegetarian or vegan diets that use a lot of these foods can be harmful to your health over time.

Chapter 9: Supplements for Prostate Health

Over the years I took all kinds of supplements, all highly recommended for prostate health. I spent a fortune. Overall with tests, books, and supplements my monthly average was easily $1000 to $2000. All to no avail. That does not mean that supplements will not be effective for you.

I have been unable to tolerate many recommended products at different points in time. Some supplements even caused a reaction and I had to stop them. The problem with many of the products is the use of too many herbs. The theory is that more is better, but sometimes too many herbs can cause an irritation. It is best to test products to see which are best for you, and it is better to test on the individual herbs. Some of the products that I reacted to had great research and high quality ingredients (organic or wild).

By far the most important supplement is your daily food! I can't emphasize this enough. Making the right food choices is *the key to health*. If you think supplements can make up for poor food choices, you are sorely mistaken.

The complexities and bio-availability of nutrients, enzymes, naturally occurring minerals, vitamins, trace minerals, and antioxidants found in whole foods cannot be replicated in a laboratory making synthetic versions of these essential ingredients for life. Even natural supplements are a far second to the benefits of natural whole foods eaten daily.

Do not fool yourself into believing that you can make up for your poor dietary habits by supplementing your diet. Sure, in the short term if you are unable to take proper care by eating well, then supplements may have a place. But in the long term, your personally-tested optimum diet is the secret to your health and the health of your prostate!

When you do choose to supplement your diet, here are my rules of the game:

- ✓ Use bio-available natural supplements made from whole foods and herbs.

- ✓ Use freeze dried forms, tinctures, extracts, concentrated or low temperature dried forms, which are closest to the whole foods that we eat.

- ✓ Supplement on a temporary basis, not in the long term unless it is a concentrated food like cod liver oil.

- ✓ Choose organic ingredients whenever possible.

- ✓ Avoid synthetic versions found in most commercial grades sold by large mainstream retailers (pharmacies and supermarkets). The quality and digestibility of these are questionable at best, as are the possible toxins they contain.

Supplements have become a mega-billion-dollar industry. You can find a huge variety that claim benefits for your prostate and overall health. Supplements can have a varying:

- amount of active ingredients
- quality of ingredients
- organic or commercial sources
- natural or synthetic ingredients
- type of binders or fillers
- price

What to Choose

In order of importance, these are the supplements worth considering when adding supplements to your healthy diet.

Sunlight and Vitamin D

Vitamin D studies show both how deficient most people are today in this essential vitamin and that increasing the amount of vitamin D in your body reduces your cancer risk by 50% or more, including prostate cancer! Vitamin D has many other health benefits. It is the single most important nutrient for your good health. Being low in it makes you much more prone to a whole range of health conditions.

Vitamin D actually acts like a hormone in the body and is crucial for prostate health, let alone your overall health. Most men are terribly low in vitamin D, especially black or darker-skinned Americans, whose skin color was designed to withstand lots of daily sun exposure. In the winter in the US, most people are extremely deficient in vitamin D because of the lack of sun exposure. Black Americans have the highest rates of prostate cancer. Many practitioners correlate that risk with low levels of vitamin D.

We have been sold on the fact that sun exposure is bad for us. Now people avoid the sun completely, cover up when out, or use chemical sunscreens, which are actually toxic and cancer causing. Responsible sun exposure, avoiding the strongest mid-day rays, is so beneficial and needs to be done without sunscreen for at least 15-20 minutes per day and much more the darker your skin because it takes longer to absorb the needed amount of Vitamin D from the sun with dark skin. If you want to use a sunscreen during mid-day then use an Organic Zinc Oxide Sunscreen [http://tiny.cc/trzk6].

There is overwhelming evidence indicating that people benefit from sun exposure. This is by far the best supplement of all! Build up slowly if you have sensitive skin with just a few minutes and then augment until you get at least 20 minutes over as much of your body surface as possible, ideally including the prostate area. There is something to say for nudist colonies!

I urge you to become better informed about sun exposure because it is such an important issue for your health. Here are several good sources of information regarding sunlight and Vitamin D:

- *"Vitamin D is the single most effective medicine against cancer, far outpacing the benefits of any cancer drug known to modern science."*
  "The Healing Benefits of Sunlight and Vitamin D"
  [http://bit.ly/nvz8rS]

- "The sunscreen myth: How sunscreen products actually promote cancer" [http://bit.ly/rdZUm2]

- "'Epidemic' of Vitamin D Deficiency": MUHC study
  [http://bit.ly/nDdAvm]

- "Higher Vitamin D Intake Needed to Reduce Cancer Risk"
  [http://bit.ly/owZ1IW]

- "7 surprising things you're not supposed to know about sunscreen and sunlight exposure" [http://bit.ly/o6DLuy]

Here are the conservative views of the National Institutes of Health. You will learn more about vitamin D from them but, according to many new studies, their minimum doses are outdated: National Institutes of Health [http://1.usa.gov/rjIPFt]

And this article:

> *"The results of two studies published in the British Journal of Cancer and Journal of Clinical Oncology found people with higher levels of vitamin D - at the time they were diagnosed - were more likely to survive.*
>
> University of Leeds. 23 September 2009. "Vitamin D new cancer hope."
> www.leeds.ac.uk/news/article/136/vitamin_d_new_cancer_hope
>
> [http://bit.ly/nys92Z] (Accessed 30 July 2011)

Read this comprehensive information from the Vitamin D Council [http://www.vitamindcouncil.org] if you are not already convinced.

These articles should reinforce the benefits of moderate sun exposure and adequate Vitamin D supplementation when not enough sun is available.

If sun exposure cannot happen because of winter cold, due to dark, cloudy days, or because you lack the time, then the best way to supplement is with potent cod liver oil. This way you are getting your vitamin D direct from a food source rather than a manufactured supplement.

This amazing concentrated food source provides digestible fat-soluble vitamin D plus vitamin A as well as rich amounts of eicosapentaenoic acid (EPA) and docasahexaenoic acid (DHA).

> *"Cod liver oil is also rich in eicosapentaenoic acid (EPA) and docasahexaenoic acid (DHA). The body makes these fatty acids from omega-3 linolenic acid. EPA is as an important link in the chain of fatty acids that ultimately results in*

prostaglandins, localized tissue hormones while DHA is very important for the proper function of the brain and nervous system."

Fallon, S., Enig, M. 8 February 2009. "Cod Liver Oil Basics and Recommendations." www.westonaprice.org/cod-liver-oil/cod-liver-oil-basics [http://bit.ly/qD5KBX]

For more information on cod liver oil read this article: "Update on Cod Liver Oil Manufacture" [http://bit.ly/q57lS9]

Natural cod liver oil is by far the best supplement I have ever taken, and I still use it daily in the winter, as I live about 300 miles north of Seattle where it is often grey for six months or more of the year. The natural cod liver oil is fermented to increase its potency and absorbability and is mixed with High-Vitamin Butter Oil. The combination of the two produces an amazing health food in very concentrated form: Highest Quality Cod Liver Oil [http://bit.ly/py6nHA]. Capsules are what I use: Green Pastures Blue Ice Royal Capsules [http://bit.ly/njtFp8]

It is crucial that you personally test for the optimum quantity you need, and retest regularly to see if the quantity changes, especially as the seasons come and go. I needed 8 capsules per day when I started out (daily recommended dose is 2) and am now at 2 per day during the summer.

The next best choice for vitamin D is natural vitamin D3 supplements, but this is nowhere near as good as the cod liver oil, which has been time tested over thousands of years.

When buying any vitamin D, make sure that you're getting Vitamin D3 [http://tiny.cc/a3mtl] (cholecalciferol), not D2, an inactive form of Vitamin D. D2 is about 10 times less effective because it is difficult for the body to absorb and use. Vitamin D3 is fat-soluble, so it is best to take it with some fat or oily food. That's why cod liver oil is so effective!

I prefer 1000 IU because you can easily personally test how many to take and adjust easily the amount. But again, a food source, like cod liver oil, is your best choice. I took natural D3 before I learned about the benefits of cod liver oil.

Fresh Air and Deep Breathing

Getting fresh air should never be on a list, but I am putting it here because so many people today live the bulk of their lives indoors. We need fresh air to oxygenate our cells. Do deep breathing exercises or simply breathe as deeply as you can, ideally in and out through your nose.

Without fresh air daily we compromise our health. The latest research shows that city living augments stress levels. In the June 2011 issue of *Investment Executive* (page B9), the author describes "nature-deficit-disorder" as a big cause of stress, depression and high blood pressure. The solution: vitamin N for Nature! Also known as eco-therapy!

Get out to parks and the countryside whenever you can. Add green plants to your indoor environment to get more oxygen. Plants breathe in carbon dioxide and exhale oxygen, the opposite of what we do. Here is an excellent site that explains how to improve your indoor air quality with certain houseplants: Clean Air Gardening [http://bit.ly/qxRshE]

Why does it feel so good when you visit a large greenhouse? It's the excess of oxygen! There's another idea: every city has large public greenhouses you can visit for a wonderful uplifting hit of big O!

Over Supplementing

I used to take a ton of natural supplements every day following the advice of many natural health practitioners, sometimes as many as 30-35 different ones per day! In the end I realized that I was getting worse and it was costing an arm and a leg to boot! Now that I know how to personally test, I have dropped down to 2-4 supplements per day. All the other supplements keep giving me a NO test response, and these are the highest quality organic ones I could find with wonderfully convincing research and more as to why I should take them, including all kinds of antioxidants.

I am not saying you should avoid supplements beyond the cod liver oil. You just need to personally test to ensure these supplements are useful for you right now. I have spent lots of time in the health food store testing many supplements that seemed of interest. I get mostly NOs and only occasionally a YES. So save your funds by personal testing as much as possible and invest your money in the best foods you can afford. That way you will get the most bang for your buck.

Keep in mind that your body's needs and testing responses will be different from mine. Testing will help you avoid unnecessary supplements and the possible weakening effects of some supplements, no matter how fantastic the literature is on them.

One of the supplements recommended by many are the green superfoods. These supplements are really just concentrations of high content green foods. You may benefit in the short term using them, but likely over time could find these supplements harming more than helping. This is because our bodies prefer cooked greens over raw greens, which can be difficult for some body types to digest. Cooked greens are best with added saturated fats for optimum digestion.

I know this because I have had reactions (including complete prostate blockage) to the very best green superfood supplements. I never suspected that such abundantly "good" ingredients could do that until I started personally testing everything and realized I could not make any critical assumptions about the benefits of even the supposed best of the best.

If you are relatively healthy, you probably won't have negative reactions like I did, but still these products may be a waste of your money unless you test to see if you will benefit from them.

Now I personally test everything and no longer suffer the difficult side effects that I did before I instituted this practice. So with these caveats in place, I will list some possible excellent products for you to check out, ideally at your health food store before you buy.

Vitamins and Minerals

The more I learn about vitamins and minerals, the more convinced I am that it is a mistake to take them in pill form. The best way to get plenty of vitamins is through good eating habits, using sea salt, and supplementing with cod liver oil. You will get more than enough vitamins that way.

In Timeless Secrets of Health and Rejuvenation [http://amzn.to/nmUh4Y], Andreas Moritz says that we do *not* need extra vitamins and that they could actually be harmful to our health:

> *"Taking extra vitamins can be harmful if the body is unable to make use of them and is left with the additional burden of having to break them down and eliminate them. Because vitamins are strong acids, an overload can lead to vitamin poisoning (vitaminosis) which damages the kidneys, and actually cause the same symptoms that accompany a vitamin deficiency.*
>
> *Instead of filling the body up with large doses of vitamins it cannot even process properly, it would be more healthful and efficient to cleanse the body from accumulated toxins, stored proteins in the blood vessel walls, and impeding gallstones from the liver. Although taking mega doses of vitamins may temporarily increase the pressure of diffusion of these nutrients for a short time and quickly relieve symptoms, any 'benefits' may be short-lived. If digestive functions are impaired, taking extra vitamins may actually endanger your health…*
>
> *To avoid imbalance in one way or the other, you should obtain your antioxidants only from one source—food…*
>
> *Fresh fruits, vegetables, legumes and grain foods, ideally of organic origin, still contain more than enough vitamins to supply the body many times over…*
>
> *You will need to determine whether it is worthwhile to spend a lot of money on supplements that don't work, but could possibly affect you negatively…*
>
> *The common practice of producing food synthetically and making it 'healthier' by adding synthetically derived vitamins and minerals is at the root of many health problems afflicting both children and adults in the developed world.*
>
> *Synthetically derived 'nutrients' are foreign matter to both animals and humans alike. Making laboratory foods palatable and attractive does not mean they are harmless."*

I share these views after being a supplement junkie, taking recommended vitamins and minerals for years with no positive outcomes and perhaps negative ones. I gave it my best shot for years, yet my prostate just kept getting worse!

Here is an excerpt from the book *Nourishing Traditions: The Cookbook that Challenges Politically Correct Nutrition and the Diet Dictocrats* [http://amzn.to/nB9irS]:

> *"There is a large difference between the vitamins found in foods and many of the vitamins sold in pill form in our health food stores and drugstores. Vitamins in foods come with many cofactors—such as related vitamins, enzymes, and minerals—which act with the vitamin to ensure that it is absorbed and properly used...*
>
> *Most commercially produced supplements contain vitamins that are either crystalline or synthetic. Crystalline vitamins are those that have been separated from natural sources by chemical means; synthetic vitamins are produced "from scratch" in the laboratory. Both are purified or fractionated concentrates of the vitamin, which act more like drugs than nutrients in the body. They can actually disrupt the body chemistry and cause many imbalances."*

Eat good food, cleanse your body, and you will absorb what you need from your food. Personally test any vitamins and minerals you want to take. Get sun. Add cod liver oil, which is a food, to your diet.

I urge you to change your mindset about vitamins and minerals. Use the following sources of information to find foods rich in the vitamins and minerals you want. Here is a list of food sources of any vitamin or mineral you need (caveat, a few of the foods are not in my "good" list, like soy):

- www.webmd.com/diet/guide/vitamins-and-minerals-good-food-sources [http://bit.ly/qZ3pCO]
- www.mcvitamins.com/Vitamins/vitamins-in-food.htm [http://bit.ly/plbYFS]

If you must have minerals, check out these links for high quality bio-available ones:

- Eniva [http://www.eniva.com]
- Kornax [http://bit.ly/nHUIMp]

Also, whenever you consider taking a vitamin or mineral supplement, make sure it is made from natural ingredients. Those "experts" who profess that natural or synthetic ingredients are all the same need to read this article: Synthetic vs. Natural Vitamins [http://bit.ly/o9Hiwu]

The supplements may be chemically the same but the effects on the body of the synthetic supplements can be quite different and in some cases very dangerous. The same risks occur in modern foods that add synthetic vitamins or minerals to raise the nutritional profiles. Be very wary of these non-foods. Over time they have a definite health destroying ability.

Possible Supplements for You – Endogenous and Exogenous

Supplements that are found in common foods or naturally in our bodies are called "endogenous" supplements. Those that are **not** found in our bodies or in common foods are called "exogenous" supplements.

Basically, every food and their derivatives are endogenous, while many herbs are exogenous meaning they lose their benefits after 1 to 6 months and you may have reactions to them.

So when you come across a supplement or herb that you believe may be useful to you, then please personally test it and retest often. That is the only way to know if a suggestion is going to be good for you. If you get a YES response and the supplement is exogenous, know that you must stop using it at some point. I guarantee you that you will receive a NO test response at some point, and when you do just stop using it.

Some Possible Daily Supplements:

Many manufacturers use a multitude of herbs for health supplements or as general antioxidants. These are the main ones:

Supplement	Benefits
Beta Glucan	Antioxidant
Quercitin	Antioxidant
N-Acetyl-Cysteine	Antioxidant
CoQ10	Antioxidant
Lipoic Acid	Antioxidant
Food Enzymes	Digestive aid (use lacto-fermented foods instead)
FOS	Digestive aid (use lacto-fermented foods instead)
Acidophilus	Digestive aid (use lacto-fermented foods instead)
L-Glutamine	Digestive aid (use lacto-fermented foods instead)
Glucosamine	For bones and joints
PS (Phosphatidyl Serine)	Brain/memory supplement
Acetyl-L-Carnitine	Health enhancer
Flax Oil	Omega-3 fatty acids (use cod liver oil instead or Organic fish oil omega-3) [http://tiny.cc/yq2uh]
Lecithin	Protects against many diseases

Specific Prostate Supplements:

Most prostate supplements come in capsule form and some as tinctures or teas. You will find many of the below ingredients in them as well as many added vitamins and minerals and some superfood greens. The thinking is the more the better. I am not so sure about that, as it is easy to have a negative reaction to one or more of them, especially given what we now know about the dangers of vitamin supplementation by non-food sources. I find taking simpler versions gives me a YES test response sometimes when I test, while the concoctions give me a NO. You will have to test to decide.

Prostate Supplement	Benefits
Beta-Sitosterol/ Phytosterols	The active ingredient in Saw Palmetto
Saw Palmetto	The best known prostate herb
Pygeum	Another well known prostate herb
Nettle leaves	Another well known prostate herb
Pumpkin seed extract	Contains high levels of phytates, so be careful
Lycopene	Conflicting research on this one... some say it is a useless ingredient
Soy Isoflavones	Mixed reviews on this one as with soy in general with some saying it is essential for prostate health
Zinc	A crucial prostate mineral- best to eat oysters and other zinc foods (brazil nuts, wild salmon, liver, egg yolks, sea salt, dark maple syrup)
DIM	Lowers excess estrogens (eat cruciferous veggies)
Pollens	Like rye pollen and others
Small Willow Herb (epilobium parviflorum)	Common in Europe
Selenium	An important mineral deficient in our soils

If you are relatively healthy and have only minor symptoms, you may not have any negative reactions to a broad-spectrum prostate supplement, and it may work well for you. If you have a more serious condition, then a simpler version or single herb may be the way to go.

Some men get relief using Saw Palmetto. Trust your personal test results no matter how incredible the fancy marketing brochures appear! What works for you will be unique to you. Remember retest often because most herbs are exogenous and will loose their effects over time or, as I have found, often start to have negative reactions.

- Mother Nature Prostate Formulas [http://bit.ly/qyhZrV]

- Prostate Supplements at Roger Mason's site [http://bit.ly/mZn72T]

- Prostate Supplements at Amazon [http://tiny.cc/3244d]

When you see a product you like, click on it and then scroll down to read the ingredients.

If you want the most common prostate herb, then try Saw Palmetto [http://tiny.cc/m8hdy]

Some claim the whole herb is the best way to go, while others suggest you take the active ingredient in it, as that is more potent: Beta Sitosterol [http://tiny.cc/s5f73].

There can be a world of difference between a whole herb, like Saw Palmetto [http://tiny.cc/m8hdy], and an isolated and concentrated nutrient taken from it, like Beta Sitosterol [http://tiny.cc/s5f73], which often gets promoted as way more potent than the herb itself. I seriously question that assertion for it can be the interaction of different nutrients in the whole herb that is most powerful. Look at this recent article:

> *"The synergy in which phytochemicals affect the human body is complex. Synthetically produced phytochemicals, or nutrients used as pharmaceuticals, do not have the same action as those naturally occurring in the whole food. Plant foods contain a synergy of nutrients and phytochemicals that have potent anti-cancer actions, along with antioxidant and other health promoting effects on the body. The importance of these foods in the diet is undisputed; however, the reductionist medical view of turning nature's perfect food into pharmaceutical drugs misses the point. When isolating compounds unforeseen actions can occur and side effects begin to emerge where they are not seen when consuming the whole plant."*

> Hartle, T.M. 26 March 2011. "Researchers believe plant based food could be used as an effective treatment for cancer." **www.naturalnews.com/031840_plants_cancer_treatments.html** [http://bit.ly/pYBqqI] (Accessed 27 March 2011)

Dr. Andrew Weil wrote an insightful article on the differences between whole plants and the drugs that are isolated from them:

> *Using whole-plant remedies is a fundamentally different—and, I would argue, often better—way to treat illness…*

> *Human beings and plants have co-evolved for millions of years, so it makes perfect sense that our complex bodies would be adapted to absorb needed, beneficial compounds from complex plants and ignore the rest. This is an established fact in nutrition, but the West's sharp distinction between food and medicine somehow blinds us to these properties when it comes to botanicals…*

> *Plants are (usually) better than pharmaceutical drugs.*

> Weil, Dr. A. W. 19 November 2010. "Why Plants Are (Usually) Better Than Drugs." www.huffingtonpost.com/andrew-weil-md/why-plants-are-usually-be_b_785139.html [http://huff.to/pSBRSn] (Accessed 12 August 2011)

For a good tincture of just 3 ingredients, try Prostate Dr. – Native Remedies [http://bit.ly/qyIRWj]

Another good quality Ayurvedic prostate supplement is Prostate Protection – A holistic approach to prostate health [http://bit.ly/pLwY7F]

The only way you will know for sure is by personally testing each supplement. (I know I say this a lot, but if you want to save time and lots of money, then personal testing cannot be beat!)

Here is a fascinating supplement, Prostex, I just discovered doing some research.

> *"Amino acids are the building blocks of protein, and occur naturally in the body. Prostatic fluid has been found to contain particularly high concentrations of the amino acids glycine, alanine, and glutamic acid, and a special formula of these three substances has been used for decades to treat the urinary symptoms of BPH...*
>
> *While the exact method of action is not fully understood, it is thought that, like other nutritional and herbal supplements, the formula works through a diuretic and anti-edemic effect, reducing excess swelling of prostate and surrounding tissues and encouraging normal urine flow."*

"Amino Acid Therapy"
www.prostex.com/prostate-guide/amino-acid-therapy/ [http://bit.ly/qty9P5] (Accessed 12 April 2011)

Order on their site or here at Amazon, which is a bit cheaper:
Advanced Prostex [http://tiny.cc/u2c3a]

Prostate Supplement Comparison:

A company called MD Health Reports claims to rate prostate supplements by doing lab analyses. While the idea may be good, I would have liked to see who owns the site. Who is doing the investigation? Could they have a vested interest in the results? I was not able to find out anything about who they are, so be careful using the information:
www.prostatepillreport.com/index.php#land [http://bit.ly/q119EC]

That said, you might be able to get ideas from comparing different products. Certainly if you read the FAQ page by scrolling half way down, they present a fairly good review of all the prostate herbs that may be beneficial to you:
www.prostatepillreport.com/prostate-health-frequently-asked-questions.php#land [http://bit.ly/nQAk2X]

Use the information from the site to personally test which products or herbs resonate for you. That's what I do. Remember that your answers will be unique to you.

Check out this high potency phytosterol/beta-sitosterol product:
NeoProstate [http://bit.ly/nVifzC]

Here is a source for French Green Clay Capsules [http://bit.ly/oMsrBu] that is an inexpensive supplement that also acts as a cleanser to remove toxins from the body:

> *"While many people recognize the benefits of natural clays for skincare, most Americans have yet to experience the age-old European practice of including specialized French Green Clay in the diet. This special form of clay (also known as illite clay) features minerals, trace elements and phytonutrients (which give it its green color). It also absorbs unwanted substances in the GI tract, making it an excellent addition to any detoxification program."*

> www.swansonvitamins.com/SW1222/ItemDetail?n=0 [http://bit.ly/oMsrBu]

Use the following anti-inflammatory herbs in your cooking if they test YES: rosemary, cinnamon, oregano, turmeric, ginger, and garlic. Eat zinc-rich foods like oysters, nuts, and seeds. Eat salmon regularly for its omega-3 fatty acids. Eat cruciferous vegetables like broccoli, cabbage, brussels sprouts, kale, bok choy, su choy, collard greens, and broccoli sprouts.

> *"Sulforaphane from broccoli and cruciferous vegetables selectively destroys cancer cells*
>
> *Research details published in the Molecular Nutrition & Food Research journal explains the potent mechanism exhibited by cruciferous vegetables such as broccoli and cauliflower to ameliorate developing cancer cells. The active photochemical known as sulforaphane targets prostate and other hormone dependent cancer lines and leaves normal healthy cells unaffected."*

> Phillip, J. 14 July 2011. "Sulforaphane From Broccoli And Cruciferous Vegetables Selectively Destroys Cancer Cells." www.naturalnews.com/032988_sulforaphane_cancer_cells.html [http://bit.ly/qxYhlj] (Accessed 12 August 2011)

The Natural Medicines Comprehensive Database [http://bit.ly/o9lob2], which requires a subscription, is a comprehensive guide to natural medicines that includes details on interactions with other medications. Here is an example of GINKGO [http://bit.ly/mRh7Am].

Conclusion

We live in a world of great complexity and have the benefit in the West of access to a wide range of foods and supplements. The keys to health are to embrace a diet rich in nutrients, to learn how to prepare foods using time tested traditional methods that enhance digestibility and vitamin mineral absorption, and to supplement wisely with the highest quality natural ingredients that you personally test to reveal a need in your body. This way you will avoid the mistake that so many make of thinking that more is better when we are actually harming ourselves through not knowing what is best for us and our specific and unique dietary needs.

Something remarkable happened today. I was having reactions to something. I retested my current supplements and found that even these final 4 that I had been taking were now not needed any more. For the first time in 8 years I am not taking

Chapter 10: Cleansing

You can't get healthy without first implementing the STOP food list found in Chapter 5 and then doing a cleanse to help your body eliminate some of the stored toxins in your cells and organs. Cleansing is an essential step to upgrading your health and allowing your body to start to heal. In order for the nutritious foods you are eating to have any benefit, you have to cleanse so that those nutrients can be absorbed.

Cleansing and detoxification are essential for real healing. This is quite an extensive section because there is a lot to learn. Please start with a cleanse that resonates for you and that is simple to do, like taking a good herbal cleansing formula or a simple water fast. Then you can build on your success with more potent cleansing methods.

Read first the whole section. Then leave it for a day and come back and reread to see what makes sense for you. Remember to take it slow and easy.
Cleansing gets rid of old toxic build-ups much quicker than simply improving your diet. Cleansing and fasting are time-tested methods used to maintain and enhance health.

You will benefit from the healthy changes to your diet more quickly if you also cleanse your body. This way you allow prevention to become your gateway to health of your prostate.

No matter how sick your prostate is, you can heal yourself. Your body knows how; you just need to give it a chance to do that job, to heal and restore itself.

When you cleanse, especially if you have never done a cleanse before, it is possible to experience a cleansing reaction or "healing crisis." As your body starts to detox you can feel yucky. As the toxins are released you can get flu-like symptoms, aches and pains, sweating and shakes and more. This is a good sign! The detoxing is working. It just needs to get out of the body and then you will start to feel much better. You are on your way! Do not stop. Allow the toxins to get out.

If you can afford it, you can visit clinics that specialize in cleansing but that is not necessary.

Drinking extra water when thirsty can help, walking and exercising can increase blood flow, having a massage with a trained practitioner or a sauna especially a Far Infrared Sauna [http://tiny.cc/ydp2o] can assist to relieve the yuckiness. Far Infrared Saunas actually use infrared heat to help detox the body. The rays penetrate deeply, and they feel wonderful. Be careful to choose a brand that emits low levels of EMFs. Read this comparison of different brands of saunas:

- www.farnorthsaunas.com/emfr-warning [http://bit.ly/r6wYMM]

Read about the benefits here:
- www.farnorthsaunas.com/health-benefits [http://bit.ly/opVRBN]

You should be able to find a health center in your town that offers sessions with these saunas. They help you cleanse and feel great!

Some Insights

The liver, the largest internal organ in the body, is the command central of the body and the storehouse of toxins, as it constantly works to refresh and cleanse our blood. The toxins that can't be eliminated create stones deep inside our liver and gallbladder affecting our bile production, which impacts our digestion.

As a result, many of us no longer digest properly. We accumulate toxins and old fecal matter in our colon. This adds weight to our bodies, which become clogged, blocked and toxic. Your bowel movements become stinky, you have constipation or frequent loose bowels, use a ton of toilet paper when a healthy movement requires one to three small wipes at most, and you develop prostate conditions.

It is essential to cleanse to allow healing to take place. Cleansing allows the good food choices you are now making to nourish you properly and little by little allow your prostate disease to stop worsening, start to turn the tide, and with time become healthy.

Here is a simple daily practice that your liver will appreciate as it helps it to cleanse a bit each morning. Make a lemon and maple syrup or honey drink first thing in the morning: take 1/4 of a fresh lemon and squeeze it into hot water. Add a teaspoon of maple syrup or honey for a wonderful drink.

Importance of Cleansing

As we age, our ability to deal with toxins slows down. By age 40 the tiny tubes and ducts that come and go from your liver are likely getting clogged; this is similar to what happens to our arteries. This tubing is affected by undigested fats, gallstones, scar tissue, and metabolic waste. By age 50 your body may be having difficulties breaking down fats because your body is producing only a quarter of the bile required to digest those fats. Instead of emulsifying the toxins, the liver encapsulates and stores them for many years. Gallstones are common among all ages and can choke the biliary tubing.

www.allonetogether.com/LiverCleanses.html [http://bit.ly/rlVqxL]

If you feel concerned about your toxicity, use this online test to score how toxic you are:
- Toxic Screening Test [http://bit.ly/psnxcJ]

If you then want a specific analysis of your harmful mineral toxicity or healthy mineral deficiencies, you can have a laboratory test done that analyzes your hair:
• Comprehensive Mineral Hair Analysis [http://bit.ly/mYu3e5]

Each hair analysis contains a detailed 10- to 15-page report from the laboratory itself, which shows bar graph readings indicating high, low and reference range levels. The hair analysis also includes a metabolic profile, and recommendations for foods, diet, and supplements based on the test results.

Please remember to personally test all of the recommended foods and supplements before adding them into your diet. Use the test results as a guideline. Use cleanses to remove toxins and your daily diet to increase mineral-rich foods for the minerals you need. Make sure you use high quality sea salt in all your cooking and eating.

You can also start by doing "The Personal Heavy Metal Screen Test" [http://bit.ly/oPBJWU], which I mentioned earlier when we talked about mercury fillings.

You can order these metal tests at Amazon Heavy Metal Test [http://tiny.cc/gekdl] or through LifetimeHealth www.lifetimehealth.ca/category_s/2.htm [http://bit.ly/qaFcjx]

Here is a tip to use if you get this test kit. Instead of adding 4 mls of urine at one time as in the instructions, add 1 ml at a time and see how the color changes. If it changes to High with only 1 ml, then you are very toxic. If it takes additional amounts of urine to the 2 ml, 3 ml or 4 ml amounts, then you are less toxic if you get a High reading.

If you test positive for heavy metals, you can get heavy metal cleansing kits here: LL's Magnetic Clay Bath from LifetimeHealth [http://bit.ly/ooQYzP] or here: LL's Magnetic Clay Baths [http://bit.ly/qBYtQe]. You start with bathing your feet with the clay every few days and eventually build up to having a full bath.

Clay has been used for thousands of years to heal the body both externally and internally, as it binds with toxins and expels them from the body. The clay baths combined with Swanson's French Green Clay [http://bit.ly/q4zcS6] capsules will do wonders.

PectaSol Chelation Complex [http://bit.ly/quLgxF] capsules may also be useful to you. These are an advanced form of modified citrus pectin that is capable of safely removing heavy metals.

After a bit of time, you can then start one of the other cleanses that follow.

A Healthier You from the Inside Out [http://bit.ly/paM9v7] is a book with lots of information on cleanses and is quite affordable. It provides a lot of information about cleanses and may overwhelm you! But it is quite a good resource. It is described as offering,

> *"a wide variety of cleansing and detoxing routines, as well as simple ways to improve overall health and well-being. [It] also contains information on*

important health factors, such as parasites, pH balance, yeast overgrowth, friendly flora, and heavy metals, plus a recipes section and resource directory."

Here are some useful quotes from the book:

"Periodic cleansing is definitely worth the effort. A cleaner inner environment can pay off in a variety of ways—less aches and pains, clearer skin, more energy, increased mental clarity, better digestion and elimination, and a greater sense of well-being. As long as you keep your body clean, inside and out, it is extremely hard for any virus, bacteria or form of dis-ease to take hold. Some healthcare practitioners believe that almost every disease starts with an unclean colon and recommend doing some form of cleansing at least every six months, even if you are healthy.

Everyone is unique, and results from any cleansing/detoxing/fasting efforts will, of course, depend on your own personal body chemistry and current state of health. But everything is interconnected, so whether you end up doing a general body cleanse, or one that targets a specific organ or system, your overall health is sure to benefit from the process. In fact, doing something like a liver cleanse will sometimes bring about improvement in conditions that you might not even think were related, such as allergies, shoulder or back pain, etc."

Virtually all holistic or natural health practitioners will have their own favorite cleansing protocols. Cleansing falls into one or more of these methods:

- Water fasting

- Juice fasting

- Herb fasting and cleansing to loosen blockages

- Master cleanse

- Colonics

- Liver and gallbladder flush combined with colon cleansing

I will describe each of these so that you can decide which is most appealing for you. Start with something that you feel you can do easily and then move on to deeper or longer cleanses.

Water Fasting

This is a wonderful way to give your body a rest, and it is easy to do! You just stop eating—no preparation is really necessary. Water fasting was the method of choice throughout the ages by many cultures, tribes, religions and spiritual leaders. Water fasting is the simplest and purest cleansing method. You simply stop eating and drink water when thirsty. Let yourself ease into it and go for 24 hours to 5 days or more. This gives your body a complete rest from the hard job of processing your food intakes... it takes a lot of energy to digest food.

You will go through periods of high energy and exhaustion during a total water fast. If you wish to cleanse after consuming a toxic diet (which our ancestors never had to deal with—at least not with all the chemicalized foods we ingest today), simple water fasting may not allow some of the toxins to come out because they can be deep inside the body's organs and cells or caked on to the inside of the colon or as stones in the liver and kidneys. Having said that, if you have never done a water fast, then it will be a welcome new experience with many benefits.

I have done many water fasts, some of which lasted 4-5 days. They are truly restoring for the body and highly recommended. The best way to start is to go easy. After supper, do not eat until the next night's supper, thus missing two meals. The following week you could miss 3 meals.

I like to drink the lemon and honey drink described earlier. Purists will stick to water. Just make sure it is the best water you can get.

You can read any of these classic books to find out more and gain some good tips:

- *Fasting-The Ultimate Diet* [http://amzn.to/mVP3K3]

- *The Complete Idiot's Guide to Fasting* [http://amzn.to/q40d1v]

- *The Miracle of Fasting: Proven Throughout History for Physical, Mental, & Spiritual Rejuvenation* [http://amzn.to/oF6F3c]

- *The Miracle Results of Fasting: Discover the Amazing Benefits in Your Spirit, Soul and Body* [http://amzn.to/ngcCmx]

With any cleansing program you may feel uncomfortable as toxins are loosened and eliminated. This is completely normal… know that it will pass. Here are a few good articles about fasting:

- "Fast for Weight Loss and Detoxification" [http://bit.ly/o3Te7o]

- "The Miracle of Fasting - Part 1 (Your First 36-Hour Fast)" [http://bit.ly/nXRXsn]

- "Whole Body Detoxification (Part 2): Fasting" [http://bit.ly/ppjSNf]

Other ways of cleansing are designed to help accelerate the detoxing of the body.

Juice Fasting

Juice fasting involves stopping all regular foods and drinking only fresh-made juices. Green foods mixed with a small amount of fruit juices are a common approach. Juice fasting can be very stimulating, but be careful of consuming too much sweet fruit juice. Vegetable juice is much better. Always use whole natural foods, avoid premade juices, and make the juice yourself.

Many people recommend having fresh juices every day. For me the problem with that is you are not eating the whole food and you are losing the fiber. However, for a short period, vegetable juicing will be a big boost and will allow you to cleanse your body of toxins. You will feel energized doing a juice cleanse.

If you do not have a juicer machine, you will need one for this cleanse. Champion Juicer [http://amzn.to/oOzhJF] is the classic and time-tested juicer. Other top juicers can be fond here: More Juicers at Amazon [http://tiny.cc/rla5v]

The Natural News Store [http://tiny.cc/4mjac] carries great juicers. Search Store for the word "juicer."

For more information about juice fasting see this article:
"Juice Fasting Leads to Easy Weight Loss" [http://bit.ly/rkg7Jw]

Here is a juice fast you can do while still eating! It is not a pure fast but can be a great start for a newbie: "Heal Yourself in 15 Days with Health Ranger's Living Juice Recipe" [http://bit.ly/o1Uo05]

Herbal Fasting and Cleansing

I really like the Sambu Elderberry Cleanse [http://tiny.cc/doyet] and have done it many times. It comes as a complete kit with full instructions. The kit contains an uratonic tea, elderberry juice and tabs, powdered fiber (psyllium husks) to absorb wastes in the colon, and an extract of birch and juniper to cleanse the body. You can get a 5-day or 10-day kit.

The fiber mixture that you drink dissolved in water provides bulk, reduces hunger, and absorbs all kinds of toxins from the colon. The elderberry juice gives you energy and nourishment, while the other ingredients help detoxify the body.

I have always felt great after doing one of these cleanses. It is easy and completely worth the price. Flora, the manufacturer, is one of the finest suppliers in the world for herbal quality products, which are grown organically on Flora's own farms worldwide. This is a great cleanse to do, especially if you are new to cleansing.

Sambu Elderberry Cleanse [http://tiny.cc/gmsmm] product features (from their site):
- Designed For Anyone Wanting To Do A Lengthened Cleanse Of The Sinuses, Skin, Colon, Lungs, Kidneys And Liver

- Used To Release A Toxic Load From The Body

- Helpful For Anyone Wanting To Lose The Excess Weight Of Toxins And Metabolic Wastes

- Beneficial For Mucous Congestion, Sluggish Digestion Or Allergies

- Great For Those Unaccustomed To Fasting But Who Still Wish To Cleanse

Note: You can't buy this cleanse directly from Flora, but it can be found in many health food stores and here at Amazon: Sambu Elderberry Cleanse [http://tiny.cc/doyet]

Master Cleanse

The world-famous Master Cleanse uses fresh lemons, maple syrup, and cayenne to cleanse the body over many days. Tens of thousands of people have done it. It is a serious cleanse and it takes time and commitment.

Lemon Mixture Ingredients:

- 2 tablespoons fresh squeezed lemon or lime juice (approx. half a lemon)
- 2 tablespoons genuine maple syrup—the darker the better—do not use maple-flavored sugar syrup
- 1/10 teaspoon cayenne pepper (red pepper) or to taste
- 8 oz water, room temperature
- Combine the juice, maple syrup, and cayenne pepper in a 10 oz glass jar and fill with the water.
- Shake it up and drink.
- Use fresh organic lemons or limes only, and avoid canned or frozen juices

You can have this mixture many times during the day. This is all you consume for as many days as you can, usually 5-10 days are recommended.
I have never done this cleanse, but I know many people who have and who swear by it for its many benefits.

There is a lot of free information available on the Master Cleanse, but following expert advice can be very beneficial to get all the tips you can to help make it successful, especially if you want to do it for a long time. Check out one of these ebooks:

- Master Cleanse ebook 1 [http://tiny.cc/6ecfr]
- Master Cleanse ebook 2 [http://tiny.cc/nmv7s]

You can find some fine organic maple syrup here if none is available locally: Maple Syrups [http://tiny.cc/vkyus]. Remember the darker the grade, the richer and more nutritious the syrup.

Part of this cleanse involves detoxing and cleansing with clay, which has been used for thousands of years. It is a safe, fast, and inexpensive way to cleanse the body of toxins. Read more here:

- "Clay Baths: The Safe Method for Detoxing Your System" [http://bit.ly/r3geXj]
- "Criteria for Selecting a Quality Healing Clay" [http://bit.ly/nzYWcsy]

Bentonite Clay [http://tiny.cc/3o69d] can be used externally and internally. Follow the instructions in the article above.

Colonic Cleansing or Colonic Hydrotherapy:

This is a non-fasting cleanse that uses water to cleanse the colon. Done by a certified colon hydrotherapist, this is a highly beneficial cleanse. The water loosens old fecal matter in the colon and removes it from you automatically. I have done many of these and believe that it is an essential cleanse to do. It can be combined with any of the other cleanses for even greater results.

Here is what I once wrote for a brochure for a practitioner friend:

> If you are like most of us, you do not always eat ideally: not enough time in today's fast-paced life to prepare nutritious healthy meals, too many shortcuts taken, eating fast foods, processed foods, overly rich food, junk food... too much sweets, unhealthy fats, sprayed and pesticide ridden food, food not chewed properly, not enough fiber in the diet and/or not enough pure water ingested... and the list of less than ideal burdens to our body goes on and on.

> We all do it, and we pay a price in our health, feeling bloated, stuffed, lethargic, always tired and just no energy. Overweight or undernourished, depressed and just not yourself. Dragging through the day and feeling unhealthy.

> The result is a high incidence of intestinal toxicity and the walls of the colon become a sticky, coated mass. Eventually the walls of the colon become so thick with plaque that undesirable bacteria ferment old fecal material and produce poisons. These poisons are then absorbed into the body from the intestines. This is called autointoxication and plays a large part in the development of many diseases. The colon is probably our most neglected organ, the garbage can of the body.

> Common signs of toxicity include: headaches, fatigue, bad breath, allergies, pot belly, backaches, body odor, irritability, arthritis, fibromyalgia, constipation, confusion, skin blemishes, dark circles under eyes, cold hands and feet, abdominal gas, bloating, diarrhea, asthma, muscle pain, sciatica, nausea, and more.

> There comes a time when we all need a deep cleanse that actually removes the years of excess build up of undigested toxins and debris in the colon caused by our poor habits. These toxins never get a chance to be fully expelled. They accumulate in the gut—the colon—and cause all kinds of problems including gas, constipation or diarrhea in some and bloating and leaky gut syndrome and stomach aches and misery in others. When the colon, your large intestine, is filled with debris (it can expand to many times its healthy normal size), the small intestine also gets blocked and the liver cannot function properly. There is just too much undigested matter and our whole health suffers a wide array of ailments as a result.

206

To clean the body from the inside out, to cleanse the bowel or colon where it all gets stuck, nothing comes close to the amazing benefits of a colonic. A colonic gently removes layers of old dried hardened excess that coats the walls of the large intestine. By using warm water to flush it out, years of waste material are stripped away.

Like a chimney, you do have to clean it from time to time if you want your stove to function properly and safely. No matter how well you feed the fire over the years, debris cakes onto the inside of the chimney and it builds up restricting optimum functioning. In the same way, the colon must be cleared for you to digest fully and feel great. Even if you go regularly or frequently or are eating healthily now, you still have a build up of dense matter in the colon from prior years. We all do. And there is only one way to safely and fully clean it out. Unlike the chimney which cleans from the top down, the only way to do it is with a colonic—bottoms up!

A colonic uses warm water to enter the rectum and loosen and remove debris. Today's modern device contains two small tubes (one for inflow and one for outflow) joined together and inserted gently 1-2". Yes it is a minor bit uncomfortable for about 15 seconds while inserted but after that, the warm water is turned on and you feel fine. The miracle starts to happen as the water forces out the old fecal matter.

The clear tubing allows you to see exactly what comes out. As the older caked on debris is loosened and travels out you actually feel like a huge load has been lifted as you literally cleanse yourself from the inside out like you have never before. The whole process takes about 45 minutes while you lie on your back or side.

Your trained hydrotherapist knows exactly how to control the flow of the water in and out for maximum results and comfort. Trained fully, your practitioner will delight with you in the removal of your accumulation leaving you feeling like a renewed person.

A colonic will cleanse the colon of impacted fecal matter, parasites, heavy metals, mucous deposits and more. You will be amazed at how yucky this old debris can look! You will be very happy to clear it out.

Things you should know about colonics:

✓ *Colonics, invented in biblical times in ancient Egypt, were standard practice upon admission into a hospital in the West until the 1940s and is still common in Eastern Europe and Russia because of the immediate benefits to the patient. Too bad the West has abandoned this practice for pills and surgery.*

✓ *It is very discrete. You wear your tops and are given shorts with a fly in the back or a gown so you are not exposed at all.*

✓ *The initial discomfort of insertion is minimized by the small compact high tech tubing and the lubrication to gently insert it. Once in, the discomfort is gone.*

✓ *Everything is completely sanitary and clean as the machine is self-contained. The equipment is hygienic and disposable.*

✓ *Having a treatment is not embarrassing: there is no mess or odor. Your personal dignity is always honored.*

✓ *A certified hydrotherapist is very experienced and knows how to create the maximum results with your comfort always foremost—and they enjoy doing it, seeing the yucky stuff flow away! You can find a colon hydrotherapist in almost all towns and cities.*

If you have never done a colonic before, it is best to do a series of three colonics over about 10 to 21 days. The reason is that it takes several colonics to remove all the layers that have been accumulating in you for decades. This cleanse results in an immediate feeling of being renewed. I always feel great after a colonic and do 1 to 2 a year.

Epsom Salts Intestinal Cleanse:

The Epsom Salts Intestinal Cleanse from the book *Timeless Secrets of Health and Rejuvenation* [http://amzn.to/oOyISE] is another simple and inexpensive method of cleansing the colon. While this is an excellent alternative to a colonic, remember that a real colonic is the gold standard. The Epsom Salts Intestinal Cleanse is its silver cousin.

> *"Another method of intestinal cleansing uses Epsom salts. Epsom salts not only cleanse the colon, but also the small intestine. This may become necessary if you have major difficulties absorbing food, repeated kidney/bladder congestion, severe constipation, or are simply unable to have a colonic or Colema.*
>
> *For one week, mix one teaspoon of Epsom salts (magnesium sulfate) with one glass of warm water and drink first thing in the morning. This oral enema flushes your entire digestive tract and colon, from top to bottom, usually within an hour, prompting you to eliminate several times. It clears out plaque and debris from the walls, along with parasites that may have been living there. Anticipate the stools to be watery for as long as there is intestinal waste to be disposed of. Stools adopt a more normal shape and consistency once the entire intestinal tract is clean.*
>
> *This treatment can be done twice a year. In the beginning, and whenever the intestines release some major pockets of waste and toxins, you can expect gas, bloating and even some cramping. Your tongue may become covered white and be thicker than normal. This indicates increased intestinal cleansing. If you are allergic to Epsom salts or just cannot tolerate this product, you may use Magnesium Citrate, Colosan, Oxy-Powder® or similar methods of cleansing instead."*

Moritz, A. December 2007. *Timeless Secrets of Health and Rejuvenation* [http://amzn.to/n71lG7] (Accessed 14 July 2011)

Liver and Gallbladder Flush Combined with Colon Cleansing

In my opinion, this is the best cleanse that you can do! It is the ultimate cleanse because it is a deep cleanse for your liver, gallbladder and colon at the same time. I have done about 10 of these, and the results are astounding. This cleanse:

- ✓ completely cleaned my colon of caked on debris;
- ✓ removed liver and gallstones by the hundreds each time;
- ✓ changed my digestion from poor to excellent; and
- ✓ improved my bowel movements from very loose to a just-right, firm texture.

This cleanse will remove gallstones lodged deep inside your liver and gallbladder, formed over years of ingesting toxins that often do not get fully eliminated but stored away forming harmful stones. These stones, little by little, diminish the functioning of your liver, which affects so many of the body's systems, from digestion to lymph functioning. Of all the cleanses, this is the best!

Andreas Moritz (who also authored Timeless Secrets of Health and Rejuvenation http://amzn.to/oOyISE) wrote the book on this cleanse called The Amazing Liver & Gallbladder Flush [http://amzn.to/qls7Te]. I advise purchasing this book or Timeless Secrets, as it is very important to follow the instructions and timing precisely.

You can buy both of Andreas Moritz's books as downloadable ebook PDFs here: Timeless Secrets and Liver Flush ebooks [http://bit.ly/rbYdS5]

The Liver Flush involves drinking a quart (liter) of apple juice for 6 days on top of your regular eating (eating high quality foods will assist you). The malic acid in the apple juice softens the stones. On the 6th day at noon you stop eating and in the evening you take some Epsom salts to get you pooping and then you drink a combination of olive oil and grapefruit juice at bedtime to slowly force the stones out. In the morning you will have many watery bowel movements and the gallstones will float to the surface of the water for you to see. You will be amazed at what comes out! It is then ideally followed by a colonic to remove further wastes and any stones trapped in the colon's creases that did not get pooped out.

The ideal would be to do a colonic before the end of the 6th day to cleanse your colon, as well as a day or 2 after the flush, especially if you know you have digestion problems and a toxin-filled gut.

Please get the book and follow the instructions precisely. The worst that happened to me was feeling noxious during the night. Drinking a tablespoon or two of aloe vera juice relieves that symptom. So keep some aloe vera juice ready in case you need it. You may feel a bit uncomfortable at times as the stones move out of the liver, but this cleanse never made me feel bad. By the next morning at 10 am you can start drinking some juice and then eating after that.

This is the most powerful and deepest and fastest cleanse I know of and it will give you a big head start as you change your diet and give your body a chance to heal your prostate. This cleanse will help you lose weight as your digestion improves, and it is also very inexpensive. Drinking the juice is easy. Just time the 6th and 7th days to be the weekend when you can do the actual cleanse part.

The main reason I strongly recommend the Liver Flush cleanse of Andreas Moritz is because it removes a huge amount of toxins quickly form the body. Yes, you will feel it, but only for about 12 hours, and then you start to feel better and better. You will see an amazing amount of toxic stones and debris coming out as you poop. It is fast and powerful! Do this cleanse. It renews both your liver and gall bladder as well as the colon if you integrate the colonics as part of the cleanse. I cannot recommend this cleanse highly enough! There are too many important details to follow for me to list them all here. Get the book.

The Amazing Liver & Gallbladder Flush [http://amzn.to/qls7Te]

The Liver

This section explains why the liver is so crucial to cleanse. To consider the importance of cleansing, we must first understand the organs, in particular the self-generating liver. According to Chinese medicine, the liver is the most important organ; it is where emotional *dis*-ease is held. It has multiple roles and jobs in the body.

First, the liver is the major filtering system for the blood, filtering out the internal and external toxins and waste that circulate in your body. This includes microorganisms that can cause infection as well as alcohol. The liver filters nearly 100 gallons of blood every day! Your cells benefit from this by being able to get more nutrients. If you didn't have a liver to remove these pollutants from the blood, you would die within hours.

Second, it is in the liver that fat-soluble chemicals are converted into water-soluble chemicals, which are then excreted from the body via the bile and urine. Not only that, the liver produces the bile that transports these chemicals. It makes a liter or more of yellow-green liquid bile every day, which is then stored in the gallbladder. It's actually the bile that breaks down the fats you eat. So, if you eat fat or protein, the gallbladder releases stored bile and squeezes itself empty. The bile travels to your intestine to help metabolize and assimilate the fat you ate.

If the liver is malfunctioning, higher levels of LDL (the bad cholesterol) and lower levels of HDL (the good cholesterol) could result. A malfunctioning liver can also result in blocked arteries, high blood pressure, heart attacks, strokes, cellulite, extreme weight gain and the inability to lose weight.
The liver also produces chemicals and hormones! 13,000 of them! These include cholesterol, testosterone, and estrogen.

The liver helps support and maintain good digestion, fat metabolism, and immune response in a very critical way. If you experience digestive problems like abdominal bloating, indigestion, constipation, blood sugar problems (like hypoglycemia), depression, allergies, skin rashes and/or recurrent headaches, you may have a toxic liver. Your liver also regulates your blood sugar levels and helps to prevent dangerously high highs and low lows.

The liver is a lover of vitamins A, D, K and B12. It stores them and helps to prevent your bones from becoming brittle. What else does it do? The liver manages over 50,000 enzymes, which help maintain a state of health.

If you are not yet ready to do the liver flush then you could try Colonix [http://bit.ly/onK7yi] for cleansing the liver. It costs a bit but has many good testimonials. Be sure to click on the pictures to see how yucky the stuff can be that it gets out of you! This could be a good way for you to start cleansing before doing a full liver flush. It may be cheaper at Amazon:
• Colonix at Amazon [http://tiny.cc/yijc5]

While this list of cleanses offers many choices, it is not a complete list. There exist many herbal supplements that you can take that will help you cleanse your liver, but I have had reactions to some I have tried over time. Once I learned how to personally test, the herbs tested NO for me. Herbs may have had some benefit but also may not be optimal. If you are going to use herbs, then do personally test them before, so you are sure that you are getting what you need without reactions.

During the last two years, because I was so clean inside from all the cleanses I had done, my body acted as a barometer. I could quickly feel the results of things I ate or supplements I took. My discomfort, peeing frequency or blocking would tell me right away if something I did was off the mark.

And it was not an allergy but in some ways was a direct reaction like an allergy to an irritant. Often the food would be okay to eat several months later, especially after learning how to reduce phytates found in many grains, nuts and seeds.

Most people would not notice the subtle reactions that I was able to detect. The effect of the wrong foods or supplements could lead to more irritation and inflammation of the prostate, resulting in a build up over time and then BPH. It is important to recognize the causes and address them early on.

Discharge

This is the word I use to describe part of the process of cleansing where we eliminate toxins from our body. You can see it on your tongue, in your bowel movements, in aches and pains that mysteriously appear, in lower-back and kidney pain, in headaches, in swollen toes, and more. These discharge symptoms are unique for each individual (my toes swelled once for several days while I was fasting. I could barely walk I was discharging so much!); remember that these discomforts are actually a good sign of progress. The yucky stuff has to come out and sometimes it hurts a bit (or more!). Know that it will pass.

There are layers of healing, and it does not happen all at once. But know this: you are progressing and making your whole body much stronger. Your rewards will come. Be patient and easy on yourself, and when you are done your cleanse you will feel wonderful, you'll have lost weight, you'll feel lighter and freer and be much healthier!

Stomach Acid

If you notice that your digestion still suffers after you have done cleanses, improved your diet, added sauerkraut or digestive enzymes, then it could be that you have too low an amount of hydrochloric acid in your stomach. Often this happens as people age. Mistakenly antacids are prescribed only making conditions worse! You can supplement temporarily with Betaine Hydrochloric Acid [http://tiny.cc/0tssl].
Read this article for tips on what to do:
"Heal Leaky Gut Syndrome By Restoring Stomach Acid Levels"
[http://bit.ly/roGo3G]

Dry Skin Brushing

This is a superb daily practice to detox the body. Skin brushing removes lots of toxins and stimulates the lymphatic system, a vital part of our daily detoxification. Many lymph nodes are adjacent to the prostate. Read this article for more insights:
"Dry Skin Brushing: A Natural Way to Detox" [http://bit.ly/r44BNe]

Emotional Cleansing and the Prostate

Larry Clapp of *Prostate Health in 90 Days: Without Drugs or Surgery* [http://amzn.to/qEGzzg] reminds us of the body-mind connection and the theory of how emotions are held in our bodies. There is a huge body of research in this area. As with any illness, emotions shouldn't be ignored when on the path to health.

Here's what Larry Clapp has to say about emotions and prostate cancer:

> *"Emotions are another largely ignored cause of prostate cancer. Our unreleased or 'stuck' emotions create energy and eventually physical blockages, called adhesions, in the body, which hamper circulation. The muscles become rigid in order to keep the emotions suppressed.*
>
> *How do our emotions restrict the flow of blood and oxygen to the prostate? This gland is the center of male emotions concerning sexuality. All of our emotions and judgments around sexual inadequacy, immorality, feelings of guilt, anger, and stress are stored in the tiny muscles and other tissues of the prostate, restricting blood flow...*
>
> *Various toxins can harm the prostate, including the many chemicals we're exposed to at home and work: in pesticides, smog, tap water, coffee, tobacco, alcohol, and food preservatives. Parasites, bacteria, and viruses can also add to our toxin load. Ideally, the liver, kidneys, lungs, skin, colon, and lymph glands expel toxins from the body. But when these internal garbage disposals are overwhelmed, the toxins pile up in the body, weakening the immune system, interfering with endocrine glands, hampering the body's ability to utilize*

vitamins and minerals, upsetting body chemistry, and setting the stage for disease.

Most medical doctors aren't concerned with toxins, primarily because they know little or nothing about them or the harm they do, and because they don't register on standard medical tests. General lifestyle also contributes to the health or illness of your prostate. Exercise promotes circulation and relieves tension in the body, which greatly facilitates a healthy prostate. 'Uptight' men have a higher incidence of prostate cancer, again related to the flow of blood in those tiny arteries.

Clapp, Larry. *Prostate Health in 90 Days: Without Drugs or Surgery* [http://amzn.to/qEGzzg]

Furthermore, there is increasingly more evidence that reveals the power of the mind—our expectations—affects our ability to heal ourselves or not. Scientific experiments have proven that it is the expectation that heals and not the drug itself. This is a profound breakthrough basically invalidating modern medicine's love affair with drug treatments! Read this pivotal article by Andreas Moritz:

"My lifelong assertion that much of medical science is literally wishful thinking has now been confirmed by new, groundbreaking scientific research involving the, so far, underestimated healing power behind patient expectation. The study, entitled 'The Effect of Treatment Expectation on Drug Efficacy: the Analgesic Benefit of the Opioid Remifentanil' may completely crush the principles upon which medical science has built its case, to date. Yet, this finding may also open the door to an entirely new way of treating disease …

Instead of instilling death fright in a patient, a doctor ought to help the patient to develop hope-filled expectations that can then translate into the necessary biochemical responses in the brain and heart that are required for the patient's body to actually and fully heal itself. On the other hand, telling the patient that he (or she) is suffering from a terminal illness introduces a factor of expectancy that is undeniably capable of executing the doctor's unintended death sentence."

Moritz, Andreas "Research Reveals the Healing Power of the Mind" www.ener-chi.com/positive-expectation.htm [http://bit.ly/pgszZi] (Accessed 28 April 2011)

Summary

Cleansing is an essential part of your toolbox of changes to bring into your life if you are serious about healing. Time tested and powerful, cleansing has been done over thousands of years by people in all cultures. All animals when they are sick fast with only water or cleanse by eating different wild herbs or grasses to help them eliminate.

Fasting and cleansing will aid your overall health, set the stage for your prostate to heal, and it has the added benefit of losing unwanted weight! Remember that your prostate is deep inside and acts to remove toxins in your sperm, so it requires your body to become a cleaner vessel if you want your prostate to heal. So start with cleansing now and see the benefits of rejuvenating you whole body.

I could never eat onions without you know what kind of a reaction. I loved them but if I ate some, even just a bit well cooked to make them more digestible, watch out! Talk about noise! NASA could have hired me for their new rocket ship fuel! It was that bad.

Now look at what happened. Last night I ate a whole cooked medium sized onion. Not one peep came out of me in 24 hours! Impossible but true.

Talk about the power of cleansing. That's what did it! Cleanse and change your life!

My Story, Part III: Fasting, Cleansing and Diet

I did lots of fasting the first few years and that seemed to help while I was fasting! Unfortunately the fasting did not change the overall condition.

Then, in a later period when I did major body cleanses, I did see positive results until something again triggered a reaction. This was way beyond an allergy because these were foods I had eaten all my life with no problem but for some reason they could cause a reaction and stop me from peeing. Once even kale from my garden did it!

All during this time of great challenges, I knew there was something I was missing; something there that I did not see that was the unexplained factor that was the cause.

I knew my body was so clean from all the cleanses I had done, from my diligence in impeccable eating with no bad habits. I remember once I had a cookie that my friend baked fresh and sold at the island farmers market. It was delicious with all natural ingredients, but that was the night that blocked me so bad I couldn't get the catheter through the last inch! I had to call the ambulance and it took 5 hours to get to the hospital!

Still there were many times when my symptoms just seemed to get worse or not show any improvement, no matter how diligent I was following the health advice of the practitioners I was working with at the time.

Many recommended products I could not tolerate at some point. Some even caused a reaction and I had to stop them. The problem with many of the products is the use of too many herbs. The theory is that more is better. But sometimes too many can cause an irritation. Some of the products that I reacted to had great research and super high quality ingredients, organic or wild.

You see, because I was eating better than anyone I knew and had such a fine-tuned system, I could detect what triggered me or irritated me at the extreme.

What I didn't see or realize was there was an underlying condition that kept my tongue so sore and coated with white in the morning. It just didn't make sense with the great diet I was on of all-natural ingredients, all cooked by me, often food from my garden, all organically grown. You can't get better than that!

Yet still I was suffering and getting worse! Yikes, what was it? What was the secret that was eluding me?

Oh how happy I am to at last know! So what was the culprit? I knew it was there somewhere and the clue came finally from an unlikely source: a mainstream doctor with a wide knowledge. This doctor was a temporary replacement on the island for one day that I happened to see to get back some new test results. He advised that I be careful about grains. I know now that it was the phytates in them (and in other foods as well) that was the cause of my enlarged prostate!

Still there were many times when my symptoms just seemed to get worse or not show any improvement, no matter how diligent I was following the health advice of the practitioners I was working with at the time.

I would find myself needing to use the catheter 4 to 6 times per year, with many very close calls in between where I got lucky and, drop-by-drop, I was able slowly to release.

But those drops were so painful. It felt like the urethra was on fire. That is one of the symptoms of an extreme enlarged prostate. So little urine passes that the bladder is spasming from inability to empty.

When it came to following my diet recommendations, I never cheated because the consequence was just too painful. So I never deviated. But even so, no success.
That just made me more open to approaches that I had not yet tried. Every new attempt was done wholeheartedly. I prayed, I surrendered myself. I did every thing I could.

During this period, I was working on the biggest business venture of my career as an entrepreneur and there were times when stress was a major factor. So part of my search involved ways of managing that stress better. From attitude to meditude, I did what it took to be in the "now." I took up new practices. They helped with the stress, but not my prostate.

During a full on military funeral ceremony for the father of a key employee that I was attending, I blocked and could not pee. Nor could I leave. The next 2 hours were an agony as I waited for the funeral to finish. I would run to the nearby bathroom and try, but never any luck. When it was over, I realized that I had not taken my emergency prostate kit with me. So we had an hour's drive to get back to my business partner's home. I was trembling in agony when I tried to insert the catheter. It took 3 tries to get it through. Never again would I travel without my catheter kit available!

Once on the way home from taking care of my mother in Montreal in 2009, I had to urinate on the plane but couldn't. I was able to wait till we landed between flights. I went to the men's room where I was able to use a catheter. It wasn't a great place for this because it's not easy to be sterile, which is necessary if you don't want infection problems.

Jump ahead to Chapter 13 if you'd like to learn more about catheters. The next section in the book delves into personal testing. If I had been able to personally test foods and products years ago, then I would have been able to evade all of my prostate problems! Read on, give it a try, and see if it will work for you.

Chapter 11: Personal Testing and the Prostate

I have mentioned the use of this testing technique throughout the book because it is so important to be able to test whether something is healthy for you to eat or use. To recover from a prostate problem it is important that you know what helps and harms the healing process, and this is different for each person.

Wouldn't it be wonderful to have a reliable way to KNOW that? And to just KNOW that you know! Well, there are simple techniques you can learn that tap directly into your inner wisdom.

We all have that internal guidance system. It comes with being human. In an article titled "The Intelligence of Your Cells," [http://bit.ly/o5p4Qj] Dr. Bruce Lipton [http://www.brucelipton.com] states that the conscious mind is capable of processing 40 nerve impulses per second. The subconscious mind can process 40,000,000 nerve impulses per second! Hence, when you personal test, you tap into your inner knowing and bring it to conscious awareness.

The problem is that many of us have lost the ability to tap directly into our inner knowing. Modern life disconnects us from our roots with nature and puts stresses of all kinds on us. The list of reasons that we are disconnected goes on and on. How many times in your life have you said to yourself, "I'm full, I shouldn't eat any more," and then found yourself dishing yourself up yet another plateful of food? You knew that you didn't need more food, but you didn't listen to your body and ate more anyway. In the West, we have trained ourselves to stop listening to our bodies' signals and needs. The discomfort from being overfull and overfed is ignored. We ignore the feedback mechanisms that are meant to keep us healthy and in balance. Personal testing gives you a way to tap back in to that inner wisdom, to learn to listen to what is right for you in this moment.

When you personally test, you are connecting with your inner intelligence. This will help you choose foods and products that are truly health enhancing to speed you on the path to recovery and heal your prostate. Some readers may scoff at the techniques for personal testing, possibly because they feel it is not scientific. What I can tell you is this: It has worked for me and for thousands of others—there is no cost or drawback to giving this a try. With an open mind, try the techniques outlined in this chapter. Try it in the quiet comfort of your home, with no one watching, and see what happens. If these techniques work for you, then you have gained an unparalleled tool that will facilitate your healing and save you time and money. There is nothing to lose and everything to gain.

All I can say to you, dear reader, is that this skill has saved me from countless agonizing experiences and has speeded me to recovery from a very unhappy prostate. If you are able to put aside your doubts and skepticism and give this an honest try, I believe it will do the same for you.

What is Personal Testing?

There are three basic ways to personally test foods and products to see if they are healthy for you: muscle testing with a partner, personal muscle testing, and testing with a pendulum. All three involve learning to center into your body's natural energy, which then gives you the answer you are seeking. All you are doing is tapping into your personal energy awareness or bio-energy. We all have the ability. It may take some people more time to develop the skills, but luckily there are three basic ways to do personal testing, one of which will work well for you.

I call it "personal testing" because you are testing whether something is beneficial for you or not. It has other names as well: muscle testing, behavioral kinesiology, body tuning, energy testing, energy awareness, bio-energetic testing, bio-resonance, pendulum testing, personal dowsing, and more.

Personal testing can quickly let you know:

✓ whether a food is good for you or not

✓ whether a supplement is conducive to your health or not

✓ whether a medication or herbal remedy is good for you or not

✓ whether a bodycare product is good for you or not

✓ whether a household product is conducive to your health or not

✓ how much of an item is optimum to take

In case you think that tapping into your body's natural energy is all hokey-pokey and razzle-dazzle, let me tell you I love chocolate. I have not been able to test positive for months and months. I go into the health food store and test the organic chocolates they sell and I always get a NO, no matter how much I wish for a yes! I gave up testing for about a month and lo and behold I am now getting a YES for a small amount of 85% dark organic chocolate.

If you allow your inner energetic wisdom to lead, it will guide you clearly on what is best for your body, for your optimum health in the "now." There are no theories or facts about what you should or shouldn't eat.

Please be patient with yourself as you attempt to learn to personally test foods and products. It takes a bit of time, but with persistence you will develop a skill that is invaluable to have for your health. Attempt to approach this with an open mind or you will just sabotage yourself.

How to Personally Test

I will describe three basic personal testing techniques that you can use:

1. Muscle testing with a partner
2. Personal muscle testing
3. Pendulum testing

Once you master a technique, it means you have the ability to tune into your inner knowing about what is best for you. You may simply know the answer without using testing techniques as your awareness develops and you strengthen your natural instincts and intuition. Eventually, you won't need to apply the test anymore to know what is or isn't beneficial for you.

Personally, since I am a very visual person, I love seeing the results of a test and find pendulum testing my favorite. Others who may be more attuned to sensations may find personal muscle testing to be their favorite, while others may enjoy and find they get the best response when testing with a partner.

Whichever test you end up attuning to, let yourself practice more and more and tell your inner skeptic to take a sabbatical while you test drive the testing, because the benefits are so worthwhile. Giving this a try can save you a lot of personal anguish, pain and help prevent prostate attacks. It will also save you a lot of money by avoiding buying products that may be wonderful for others but not for you (at least at this time), and you will be able to design your own perfect diet not based on some expert's advice (including me!).

I offer you these three methods so that you can find one that you like. There are slight variations on each. Just develop the skill with whichever works best for you. Okay, let's begin!

Muscle Testing with a Partner:

Also known as behavioral kinesiology, this test requires two people, you and your partner who will test you. The environment should be quiet and calm.

1. Both of you stand. Your left arm should hang down comfortably at your side. Your dominant arm (for most people it is their right arm) extends outward in a horizontal position with your elbow fully extended. (If you are left-handed, reverse the arms.)

2. Your partner should stand behind you. Close your eyes and relax your mind. Your partner then places her left hand on your left shoulder to keep you stable, and the fingers of her right hand on top of your right arm over your wrist. Some prefer to face each other but I think it is best to avoid visual contact.

3. Your partner will say, "Resist," and then to press down quickly on your arm, while you try to resist the pressure. Your partner should do this firmly and smoothly. It is not a contest but rather a way to notice if the arm remains strong or weakens.

4. Your arm muscle will test strong in this neutral state. If you are in an emotional state or under the influence of drugs or alcohol, it is not a good time to test as you could get mixed results.

5. Now we want to test something true. Your partner will ask, "Is your name [insert your name]?" Your arm should remain strong, which is a YES response.

6. Now your partner will ask a question that will give a negative response, such as, "Is your name Mary?" Your arm will become weak and will descend when pushed down on, which is a NO response.

Now you are ready to test a food or product. Hold the food item in your non-dominant hand (for most people this is the left hand) against your prostate area or solar plexus. Then repeat the arm test. If the product is good for you, your arm will remain strong; if your arm is weak and it collapses, then the product is not good for you at this time. Now you have your answer!

In the case of a supplement that gave you a YES response, you then want to know how much to take or to eat. Here is what to do. Start with one capsule in the palm of your hand and test again. If you get a YES, then try 2, then 3. Keep testing until you get a NO. The last YES is your dose for the day. You could take that amount spread over the day (e.g., take one supplement three times if you have three capsules as the daily dose).

In the case of a food like eggs that tested YES, retest with one egg then 2, and so on, to see how many you can eat.

It is wise to retest an item every day to ensure it is still valid or that the dose doesn't change; this is especially important when you begin using new products. For example, I started testing a new supplement that gave me a YES response. The label advised 2 capsules per day, but I tested for 8! I obviously needed that supplement (cod liver oil)! That dosage lasted for a week. Through repeated testing I started to reduce the dose per day; my current stable dose for that supplement is 2 capsules per day.

You will have to practice the testing until it becomes easy and natural to you. It is necessary to have an open and calm mind when you do muscle testing. Remember your inner critic is AWL (away with leave)!

This Muscle Testing with a Partner Video [http://bit.ly/oezgEk] is a good video to watch because it demos the basic technique.

Your arm muscles will respond to a particular item either with weakness or with strength, so long as you test properly. Many products that seem irresistible based on their nutritious contents and marketing will test NO. I find that some wonderful products do this. If you test NO for a product that seems to have many "good" ingredients, it may be because one of the ingredients does not resonate for you. Trust your test results. Move on to something else. Your body may not be able to process or digest it properly, and you do not want a prostate reaction.

Personal Muscle Testing

If you don't have a partner to help you, you can still muscle test alone. There are two ways to do this:

Standing Method

Stand in a relaxed manner and repeat the word "YES" to yourself. Allow your body to move or swing you forward. Now repeat the word "NO," and you will find your whole body moving backwards. Thus, by holding a food or supplement against your prostate area, you will either tilt forward or backward, depending on your body's response to it. Does it resonate or not?

Try the name test: My name is [use your name]. You should swing forward a bit - YES. Then say something false: "My name is [use someone else's name]." The opposite now – NO. You don't need to make the statements aloud—silently is fine. The idea is to train your mind for truth and falsehood, YES and NO. Just practice this for a few minutes a day until it works for you.

Try some seemingly obvious items: see if Coke gives you a YES or NO and then try an orange or carrot. You are ready to test now!

Here is a video for the Standing Personal Muscle Test [http://bit.ly/nblk7F]

Finger Method

Hold the thumb and first finger of your left hand so they make a circle (reverse if you are left handed). With the index finger of your right hand, you place it inside the circle and say YES, then pull it briskly outward (towards where your thumb and index finger are connected). You should test strong (YES), and you will not be able to open the circle. Now do it with NO and your finger should open the circle. Do the same Name test as above to get your YES and NO responses. Now you are ready to test.

You can then hold the product you want to test against your prostate area or sternum using your arm while you then use your fingers to test. If it is a negative product, your finger will open and exit the circle.

Some testers use different fingers. Use what seems best for you. Here is a video for the Finger Personal Muscle Test [http://bit.ly/nP3NU1].

Pendulum Testing

Pendulum testing is my favorite, and I also believe it can be the most accurate method if used correctly. Pendulum testing requires the use of a pendulum to see your YES and NO responses. What I particularly like is that there is a way to ensure you do not get a false test, like a false positive. Learning that technique will ensure optimum accuracy of your results.

Pendulum testing amplifies your body's awareness and responses to what you are testing.

While a pendulum can be made out of virtually any object that you can hang off of a string, there are better and more responsive pendulums that you can purchase. I believe that getting the best pendulum is well worth the price of around $30.

You will instantly break-even the first time you go to buy a supplement that is supposedly great for you and you test and get a NO. You will then have recovered the price of the pendulum, and it's free sailing from then on! I can honestly say it has been the best purchase I have made in my entire life, both because of the money it has saved me and because of the anguish of health reactions I avoided. Pendulum testing has been central to my growing health.

To avoid false positives and personal reactions to the device itself, select a pendulum that mimics the shape of the body's energy field, which is egg-like. This eliminates many pendulums offered for sale in shops and Internet sites. The most responsive and accurate device is called the Perfect Pendulum.

The people who make and sell Perfect Pendulums are experts in the field of personal energy testing with decades of experience, and I highly recommend these, as they are the very best. These pendulums teach whole-body energy awareness, and once you master using the pendulum you can then graduate to using your body or hands as the testing device, even more accurately than the above methods. I still have a personal liking for seeing the responses, so I use my pendulum every time I test.

I can easily test with an old nail, nail clippers, or exotic drop-shape pendulums with points on the bottom. I have used them all, but none come close to the accuracy and ease of a Perfect Pendulum. The detailed instructions that come with the Perfect Pendulum are equally as valuable as the pendulum itself. These instructions describe how to use the Perfect Pendulum for different kinds of testing that I have never seen done accurately with the other testing methods. Keep in mind that you cannot ask just any question when testing with a pendulum. This technique requires that you request a direct Yes or No response.

Being made of opaque stone, the Perfect Pendulums are more accurate than glass, wood, plastic, or other materials, which helps to avoid switching errors (i.e., when your energy switches back and forth, which will affect your testing responses).

This information is from the Perfect Pendulum [http://bit.ly/m7J913] website:

*"**Learning to use the Perfect Pendulum***

(from the 12-page instruction booklet free with each Perfect Pendulum)

1. *Hold the chain between your thumb and index finger, with the small ball in your palm.*

2. *Deliberately swing the pendulum backwards and forwards with your wrist dropped rather than straight.*

3. *Have the flat palm of your free hand facing up.*

4. *While watching your pendulum, touch your thumb and index finger together—this is called **acceptance mudra***

   - *If your pendulum veers into a circle, this is your YES direction*

   - *If it doesn't, open your fingers, wait a few seconds, start the pendulum swinging back and forth again, then close thumb and index finger again while watching your pendulum. Each time you do this, you are clearing your bio-energetic testing circuit*

- *Continue doing this until you get a change of direction with acceptance mudra*

Once you have found your YES direction, you should also practice your NO direction. This is exactly the same process, using acceptance mudra again, but, this time, with your palm facing down.

Please note: it's very important that you generate your YES and NO directions with the acceptance mudra. Other techniques, such as writing YES and NO on different pieces of paper or asking yourself questions, should not be used.

"Testing for switching - the self test

Before doing any sort of energy testing (with your pendulum, a muscle test etc.), you must first establish whether your energetic 'testing circuits' are flowing properly. Your energies can 'switch' often during the day, perhaps as a reaction to a food, a person or being in a certain place. So it is very important to check yourself before using your body as a testing instrument—which is what you are doing when using a pendulum. Many people use pendulums without checking to see if their body is working properly and hence get false or variable results. You can only evaluate the correctness of your answer using a pendulum, if you know that you are reliably getting a 'YES' or a 'NO'.

To do the Self Test, place the Self Test mudra—the thumb pointing out between the two middle fingers of your closed fist—against your heart center. The heart center is approximately two inches up from the bottom of your sternum (breast bone).

A NO means 'not switched', no problems, you can test. A YES means you are switched and must unswitch your circuits before you can use the pendulum or do a muscle test."

Perfect Pendulums Information [http://bit.ly/m7J913]

If you test "switched", just follow the instructions on the site to unswitch. Now that you can get a YES or NO, this is the way I test a product or food. I hold the item against my prostate area and test by swinging the pendulum forwards and back and then it will give me a YES or NO by the direction it then rotates. It's as simple as that.

Below I share with you two videos I made demonstrating personal testing. Before you see these videos, I want to caution you that the motions of your pendulum may be very subtle at the beginning. The turning won't be as strong for you as you see in these videos demonstrating how I personally test foods and products. It may take time for your responses to become as powerful as mine, but even a small movement yes or no is enough to get your answer.

- Part 1: Pendulum Personal Testing - Part 1 [http://bit.ly/ogcAmJ]

- Part 2: Pendulum Personal Testing - Part 2 [http://bit.ly/p52bDv]

Occasionally, you will get a neutral response, neither a yes nor a no. Nothing happens or what happens is unclear. That means exactly that: the product is neither good nor bad. If you are healthy, then use that product in moderation. If you have a health condition, then I would not use that product unless you feel there is a good reason. When you are stronger, then it will not matter as much. Retest that item later if you want to use it again.

If you find you are having difficulties learning to personally test products then go to Food Energy Awareness Solutions and Training [http://www.feast.realhealth-online.com] for an online consultation with the experts. These experts can help you learn with specific tips or by testing the foods and supplements that you want. Stephen and Lynda Kane are exceptional in this area. They are the ones who taught me and are the makers of the pendulum that I use.

One amazing technique you can use with the Perfect Pendulum is to personally test for something using a picture of the product if the item itself is unavailable to you. This is great for brochures or even online while looking at the product. It works the same as testing a product through a container (e.g., holding a bottle of wine and testing to see if you could have some of it).

Try to Set Aside Your Skepticism

Time and space do not exist in this mode... I know, it's a bit too wacky for you and over the edge. This writer is too much!

I know it is surprising, but this approach has consistently worked for me. Many times I've tested a product in a health food store inside its bottle, and then re-tested the same product at home with the actual capsule in my hand, and I got the same response.

Personal testing has also worked on something that I sure wished was a yes, but I got a no response. It was a super sounding prostate supplement, and I wanted to try it, but No means No so I passed on it.

I have bought on many occasions from the Internet on yeses and they tested the same when they arrived. The last time I did it, I tested the package without opening it after I got it all wrapped from the post office. Then I tested it in the bottle. All times were a yes, including the pill itself. If I take a supplement that came back as a "No" when I did a personal test, then I feel it on my tongue or prostate usually within hours.

If you have concerns about a bias or having an agenda, then consider muscle testing with a partner (as shown earlier in this chapter). If you have concerns about people seeing you attempt this in a store, try the Finger Method (also shown earlier in this chapter), as this approach can be very subtle. It looks like you're fidgeting, and no one will even notice you doing it.

I know it is hard to put your skepticism aside, but you have nothing to lose and a lot to gain. Try it and see! This has worked like a charm for me and saved me a ton of dollars, and I hope it works for you too!

Personal Testing Theory

So what is the theory behind personal testing? It works on the same principles as acupuncture—energy flows and centers in the body drive your personal energy testing. You tap into that by using the methods presented.

If you want to learn how this works, read more here: "Energy Medicine" [http://amzn.to/qCsgUo] or "Muscle Testing" [http://tiny.cc/2g1fb].

How personal testing works through a closed package or bottle is a mystery to me, but again it does work. I can live with uncertainty about how it works because it has proven, without a shadow of a doubt, to work for me. It removes all the guesswork from my choices about other experts' recommendations. I just personally test each item and get my answer.

Testing Tips

When you get a yes for something new, retest it again regularly to ensure that product is still good for you, especially if you have many sensitivities or if you are healing. You can calm your mind by placing your tongue up to touch the roof of your mouth behind your top teeth. When you get good at testing, it will only take a few seconds to get a response.

Remember no matter how "good" for you a food or supplement is, whether recommended in this book or elsewhere, if you have too much of it, then it can easily change to "bad" for you! It has happened to me many times—with ghee, miso, sauerkraut, saw palmetto, selenium, greens, flax oil, and more!

As you cleanse and detox and start to heal, your sensitivity to foods and supplements goes up. Your body knows what it needs. Set aside your opinions and personally test (and retest). You will then know what is healthy for you to eat or not. As you get healthier and your sensitivity diminishes, you find that you have fewer reactions.

Conclusion

Personal testing will revolutionize your health by going beyond the advice and recommendations of others no matter how qualified or eminent they are. Testing goes beyond the selling points of a product or the ideas someone else has for you about what you "need" or "should" eat.

Each one of us is so unique that we need these tools to KNOW what is best for us. It is easy to learn one (or more) of these tests, and this skill will empower you to make the right health decisions for you.

Have you been totally confused by all the conflicting health information out there? No more! You can now test and know. What a leapfrog from where you were before!

You can take all the good advice that comes your way and put it too good use by testing and making decisions based on your true knowing.

Personal testing will revolutionize and empower your life! Learn it! (If personal testing is not for you or you find it too difficult, here is an option for you. Take this survey of symptoms [http://bit.ly/r6h6tB]. The company will then test 115 foods to find your culprits.)

A while ago I had some coconut butter that I used to cook some sockeye salmon. I had bought a jar and had been using it for 2 weeks. Everything seemed fine, but then something subtle changed... I must have been using it too often even though I did not notice anything amiss.

Next day was difficult for me. I had to urinate constantly all day sometimes going many times in an hour. Obviously I had had a reaction to some food and the reaction was in my prostate. I was able to find the culprit by personally testing the foods I had eaten the day before.

Had I been more alert, I would have tested before using the coconut butter, but I forgot. At least I was able to find the cause after the fact and learn a lesson or two!

When I had first learned of my enlarged prostate, my reaction would have been more severe. I would have blocked and had to use a catheter whenever I ate something that triggered a strong reaction. But because my overall prostate health was improving, my reactions at that time were not as severe.

It is important not to add irritants over time. We all have them, and most of us are unaware of them. Eating these irritants causes a slow erosion of our health over time. That is why personally testing foods often (even daily) is so central to your health.

Testing allows maximum prevention (and healing) by being aware of which foods can cause you irritations in the prostate.

I have to admit, it does take time to recognize reactions like I have learned to, and it also takes time to trace it back. It is well worth the effort to train yourself with personal testing. By identifying your riskiest foods and avoiding them, you can begin healing your prostate.

Today, now that the culprit has passed, I am fine, and the urgent peeing has gone AWL (away with leave)!

Chapter 12: Hormones and the Prostate

As we have discussed earlier, the prostate gland is very sensitive to hormones, in particular **testosterone** and **estrogens**. Because of this, the prostate easily reacts to artificial chemicals in our diet that mimic hormones, especially the estrogens.

You can find these toxins in our food, toys, plastics, bodycare and household products, cans, and in the air and drinking water. The amount of toxins we are exposed to every day takes its toll on our prostates.

That is why it is so essential to improve one's diet by reducing the toxic load intake and by cleansing to help eliminate possible past toxins from our bodies.

Let's start with simple terms. While men and women share the same hormones, the proportions are vastly different.

Male hormones = testosterone (part of the androgens)

Female hormones = estrogen (estradiol and estrone)

DHEA (dehydroepiandrosterone) is an endogenous hormone (made in the human body). DHEA is easily converted into other hormones, especially estrogen and testosterone. Regular exercise increases DHEA production in the body.

The main and most well-known **androgen** is testosterone, produced in the testes of males. Females produce trace quantities of androgens, mostly in the adrenal glands, as well as in the ovaries. Androgen primarily stimulates or controls the development and preservation of masculine characteristics.

If the proportions of hormones get out of normal range, then disease can result. In the case of the prostate, low levels of testosterone coupled with high levels of estrogen easily affect the prostate and other sexual organs, causing lack of libido, erectile difficulties and prostate conditions, especially enlargement.

Most men's testosterone levels fall as they get older, so increasing the levels to youthful amounts can do wonders for your health. As men age as testosterone falls, estrogen becomes dominant instead of testosterone.

In *The Natural Prostate Cure* [http://amzn.to/r7ib38], Roger Mason writes:

> *"Youthful levels of the androgens (testosterone, androstenedione and DHEA) protect you from prostate illness, and supplementing low testosterone and androgen levels helps you cure your illness.*
>
> *Men have smaller amounts of estrogen until the age of 50, when male levels rise. Female levels fall at this age, and men commonly have more estrogen than women! This is a dangerous situation, obviously, as the testosterone to estrogen ratio is now reversed. The reversal of this ratio is the key to understanding not only prostate disease, but many other male illnesses...*
>
> *Testosterone is your friend (and excess estrogen is your enemy)."*

Hormone Testing

Saliva testing is the best way to know what your hormone levels are so that you can develop corrective action. It is easy to do. You just order a test kit and when it comes provide a saliva sample that you mail to the lab. They then send you the results.

You can order a hormone test right from ZRT, a highly reputed lab [http://bit.ly/qoF2QU].The best and most accurate is the hormone saliva profile test of "Five (5) Tests: Estradiol (E2), Progesterone (Pg), Testosterone (T), DHEA-S, and morning Cortisol (C1)."

When you do a saliva or blood test for your hormones, do not take anything that could affect the test—avoid taking any hormones, antihistamines, or liquor and make sure any medications you use will not affect the results. The forms do ask you to report any of these and they may be able to adjust the results accordingly. It is best to avoid substances that will throw off the test if you can. If you will be taking multiple hormone tests in the future, it is wise to test at the same time, as hormones fluctuate during the day.

It is actually cheaper to order the test from Roger Mason's site, Hormone Test Kits (Saliva) [http://tiny.cc/uedeq], than from ZRT Lab, because he discounts it. You can easily add additional hormones to test to the two he provides after your test kit arrives.

Once the results come, do the following:

   ✓ You want your test results to be in mid range, nowhere near the extremes.

   ✓ Study the book *The Natural Prostate Cure* [http://amzn.to/r7ib38] for more insights on what to do.

   ✓ If your estrogen levels are too high, then the diet recommendations of cruciferous vegetables like broccoli, cauliflower and kale plus the supplement DIM (Diindolylmethane) are excellent ways to naturally reduce these excess female hormones.

   ✓ If your estrogen levels are too high then also take progesterone (see below).

   ✓ If your testosterone is too low, you have a choice of 2 ways to raise it:

      a. If DHEA is also low, then take 25 mg of DHEA. But you must monitor your hormone levels at least every six months, as it is possible to have negative reactions to DHEA supplements (rising estrogens). Personal testing will confirm.

      b. get a natural 3% testosterone cream from a compounding pharmacist (Compounding Pharmacist Locator) [http://bit.ly/om1pwx]

I have tested my hormone levels using both saliva testing and blood testing, and both produced similar results. I used testosterone cream for about a year with some benefits. I have stopped using it since I personally tested NO for using the cream.

You can do blood spot testing at ZRT labs [http://bit.ly/pRLKDZ] for other hormones.

Another very useful hormone for both men and women is **progesterone**. It protects men from excessive estrogens, so if your estrogens are high, then use a natural progesterone cream to help you. It is safe to use and has no toxic side effects. It also helps to counter the effects of stress in our lives. A jar will last a long time because you use just a bit at a time.

All men over 50 can benefit from using Progesterone cream (of course it must test positive for you, but I bet it will if you use a natural product).

Here are two excellent choices for natural Progesterone cream made with organic ingredients. See which one you like best:

- NatPro – Natural Progesterone Cream [http://bit.ly/oEFRTH]
- Kokoro – Natural Progesterone Cream [http://bit.ly/osi1Zg]

This is another cream formulated by Roger Mason; it is not organic, but less expensive: MyGest - Progesterone Cream [http://bit.ly/quzte2]

Here is a way to boost testosterone and balance your hormones using a potent form of natural testosterone from pine pollen from pine trees. Read about it here: "Pine Pollen - Boost testosterone and balance hormones" [http://bit.ly/p2KFbB]

You can buy it inexpensively here. I would go for the tincture:
Pine Pollen (Pinus massoniana) Tincture [http://bit.ly/p7XBWl]

The Sunshine Hormone

Remember, as discussed earlier in Chapter 9, how important it is to get sunshine on your skin to get crucial Vitamin D. This vitamin acts like a hormone and is crucial for prostate health. If you can't get sunshine, then cod liver oil is the first choice followed by natural Vitamin D3 supplements. Always personally tested for the amount.

Capsules are what I use: Green Pastures Blue Ice Royal Capsules [http://bit.ly/qsbQk0]

Liquid forms of cod liver oil: Highest Quality Cod Liver oil [http://bit.ly/oo59mf]

Melatonin

This hormone, known for better sleep, has many underrated benefits, especially for longevity and the strength of your immune system. Furthermore, the prostate contains melatonin receptors vital for prostate health.

Roger Mason in *Zen Macrobiotics for Americans* [http://amzn.to/o0Hpps] says,

"Melatonin levels fall from the time we leave our teenage years and keep falling until we have almost none left by the age of 70. The most important benefit is influencing how long we live by regulating our internal aging clocks. Mice simply given melatonin in their drinking water lived one third longer than control mice. Imagine theoretically living to 100 rather than just 75 by taking two dollars worth of melatonin every month. It is important to take melatonin only at night as we do not produce this during the day. "

In his book, *The Natural Prostate Cure* [http://amzn.to/n61OrK], Roger Mason also says,

"It also boosts the immune system, and may be the most powerful of all known antioxidants. According to new research, melatonin promotes good cardiovascular health, exhibits preventive anti-cancer properties, and could help make other cancer therapies more powerful. It is remarkably safe and non-toxic, without any known side effects... Men with prostate cancer were found to have low melatonin levels... and melatonin is an effective treatment for cancer. "

Read more about melatonin here: "Melatonin is the Super Sleep Hormone" [http://bit.ly/pV6g5z]

Test for your optimal amount of melatonin [http://amzn.to/pfsq4E]. Start with 1 mg per night just before bed and then increase if you personally test yes for more.

Summary

When considering hormones and your prostate health, this is what you'll want to focus on:

- ✓ Stop the toxins!
- ✓ Eat really well—high quality, fresh, organic real foods.
- ✓ Cleanse to remove old toxins.
- ✓ Saliva test your hormone levels.
- ✓ Reduce estrogen levels and raise testosterone.
- ✓ Use progesterone for stress and for reducing estrogens.
- ✓ Remember the vitamin D hormone—get sun on your skin or take a natural supplement.

Chapter 13: Prostate Attack!

Triggers of Prostate Attacks

A prostate attack happens when you have a sudden surge of symptoms worse than any you have had or you now discover you have a prostate problem. Ouch! Usually a prostate attack means you are having extreme difficulty urinating or can't at all! Something actually triggered the sudden shut down. You were having prostate problems but perhaps not serious enough to cause a major problem (e.g., frequent peeing, waking at night, some hesitation). But now something has happened and you had a huge reaction shutting you down.

Yikes! You are standing to pee and nada drop to be! And you just gotta go something fierce!

First of all, let's look at what triggers a sudden inability to urinate?
It most likely means you ate something that you are reacting to or took a cold medication or antihistamine sometime in the past 24 hours and are having a body reaction.

Avoid medicines that can affect the prostate like antihistamines, decongestants, and anti-depressants. If you already have an enlarged prostate condition, these drugs can push you over the edge and you can find yourself in shut down mode!

Alcohol, especially hard alcohol, and even wine or beer can trigger acute prostate swelling. Limit alcohol to 1-2 drinks per day at most. For some people marijuana can also trigger a prostate attack.

Too much of a food, superfood, or supplement (no matter how "good" or "healthy" it is) that you have been eating over time—especially if it contains phytic acid—can trigger an allergic reaction of swelling in the prostate.

Also if you drank too many liquids before bed, you have added stress to the bladder during the night.

This is why learning to personally test items to ensure your compatibility is so key. Nobody wants a prostate attack!

What Triggers the Attack?

Usually the triggers will be something you ate that day (most likely at lunch or supper), an antihistamine, or a new medicine. To know for sure, personally test everything you can think of, everything you ate no matter how "good" it theoretically is—even test fresh organic foods and small things like herbs or nuts. Test everything until you find the culprit.

In all my prostate attacks, I have always been able to trace the trigger back to something I ate or a supplement I reacted to. It could even be a small amount of something like the oil, a rancid spice, some mold, or even a trusted food that I began reacting to out of the blue.

Sensitivities to different foods come and go as you are on the path back to health. The important thing is to find out what caused it so you can avoid it until you personally test okay again for it.

Here are Some of my Triggers:

When I speak about triggers, it does not mean that each time I ate that item it would result in a prostate attack, but at a particular time it did. The items listed below will give you an idea of some common triggers.

- Too many greens, whether powdered or fresh vegetables; in my case, my own garden kale, and super green powders are triggering. I have had a bit too much of them, thinking they were all good! Greens can be hard on the body, so cooked is often better and have them with butter to soothe them, especially if you have a sensitivity to these foods.

- Green powders. Make sure you test and retest often. I forgot and, woops, blocked one night.

- Oils like canola and safflower (now I know better and I avoid these).

- Nuts like almonds, cashews, etc., especially before I learned about phytate reduction.

- Sesame seeds.

- Unsoaked grains.

- Chocolate cookies

- A piece of bagel that I ate, which had a moldy taste.

- Some herbal teas.

These above-mentioned foods are things I have to pay attention to and since I am in the healing process I cannot assume because I personally tested YES once that these foods are always a YES. As you get healthier, your reactions will reduce. Just remember that a reaction that causes an attack is not your normal state of health. No need to panic and rush for the latest surgeries or interventions.

So be vigilant, find out what your triggers are, personally test often, AND AVOID THE CULPRITS (for now). The triggers will lessen and you will find your tolerance will come back,; you may also learn how to prepare foods so as not to have a reaction.

What To Do When You Have a Prostate Attack

If you wake up and find yourself under a prostate attack and urination is difficult, painful or impossible—don't panic! There are things you can do, the crisis will pass, and then you can take corrective and preventive action. Here is what to do.

Relax and Breathe

If you were awakened, lie down again and try to make your prostate area relax. Sometimes while asleep you force "not peeing" (of course) by not waking up, and this holding back can traumatize your prostate and the bladder sphincter if you are having a reaction to something. So relaxing can give these parts of your body a chance to reset. By relaxing and breathing, even just a bit, sometimes the spasm or intensity will ease and allow some urine to flow. Don't push as that creates stress in the prostate. Breathe deep and allow some relaxation even if it hurts badly.

It may help to have a plastic pee bottle instead of having to head to the bathroom. If you can get a little to pass, you may be on your way. Lie down again and repeat. Relax. This process can allow a bit more to come out. Sometimes that is all you need to do and more and more will come out over the next 30 minutes to an hour, and then you should be okay.

Let the waves pass and relax, knowing that letting go and getting all your muscles to loosen up will help. After a minute or two get up and sit down to pee to see if you can release a bit. If you are lucky and something starts to come out, that is a very good sign, even if only a few drops come out (or course you want to let a ton more out!), but getting any amount is a great beginning. It may hurt like hell as you pee, like a burning fire… try to breathe and relax no matter how painful it is.

Lie down again. Relax, relax and breathe, breathe and relax. Wait and relax. When relaxed and the urge to go comes again in a minute or two, then again go and see if some more comes out. If lucky, a little more will come out. It is better to sit and relax than to continue standing and trying to pee.

It could take a dozen or more of little pees before you are empty, little by little letting go. Usually the pees will get better and better at some point releasing more. You repeat these steps but do not go back to sleep until you have a complete empty feeling. It can take an hour or two for you to finally empty your bladder.

If you still have urine in your bladder, avoid going back to sleep. Going back to sleep too soon can cause a further reckoning an hour or two later, and it is worse if you did not completely empty your bladder. If you drank a lot of liquids in the evening, then staying up a while longer may be wise. This avoids the blocking conditions that often arise while asleep. You may be tired, but once you are flowing it is best to keep the channels open by staying awake.

The ideal: Do not go back to sleep. Get up no matter how tired you feel. I have made the mistake of thinking the crisis has passed too soon and awoke again an hour or two later with a worse problem.

Know this: The crisis will pass. This is not a normal state of affairs for your prostate. You are having a strong reaction. Just get through it.

Other Helpful Tips

If the above does not work, get a hot water bottle and fill it with the hottest water that you can without burning your skin. Lie down and place it on your pubic bone and lower abdomen/stomach area. A thin towel may help to avoid burning. Relax as much as you can. The heat can have an almost instant effect and can help the relaxing and releasing.

This process may allow some urine to start flowing when you go pee. Keep at it for a few more minutes, giving the heat a chance to penetrate. Pee a bit, lie down with the hot water bottle again, breathe and relax, and soon you will release some more. Once you get a few drops to pass, it often will lead to more, little by little.

If you can have a bowel movement, do so as this will release pressure on the prostate through the rectal wall. Even a bit of pressure reduction can make a difference to help the prostate relax and release.

Repeat the hot water bottle application and relax. Hopefully you will experience some opening. Keep saying to yourself, "Relax and release. Relax and release. Relax and release. Breathe deeply, deeply and relax."

You can also massage the perineum area between the scrotum and rectum with some oil, ideally castor oil, while lying down. Try pressing deeply on the spot about 1 inch from the rectum towards the scrotum in the perineum area. This spot is the closest to the prostate. Massage and press that whole area.

Walking may help if lying down doesn't. Try movement and light exercise like sun salutations from yoga. Being vertical may help but could be putting too much downward pressure on the bladder sphincter. You will just have to see what works.

Another method is the sitz bath procedure. Twenty minutes with your lower body in hot water with your legs and upper body out of the water. Then do another sitz bath for 5 minutes with cold water. You may need to reduce this time to 5 minutes hot and 1 minute cold if the pain is too intense.

Catheters

If all of the above fails, then use a catheter if you have one. I will explain how to do that later in this chapter. If you do have prostate symptoms, you should always have a male catheter kit on hand when traveling or at home for emergencies. It is far less stressful to do it yourself than going to emergency rooms and waiting and waiting. It is much easier and less painful than you may imagine. I provide complete recommendations and instructions for you on how to do it in the "All About Male Catheters" section below.

Obviously, if you do not have a catheter and no urine is coming out, then seeing a doctor or going to the emergency room is the solution. Know that there is no danger of bladder eruption for quite a long period, even up to 2 days. The pain may be extreme but you have time to get help.

Be aware that something triggered the attack. If you can figure it out—now or in the morning—then you will have good information about what not to do again and you can avoid repeating the experience.

All About Male Catheters

I was buying catheters at a pharmacy a few years ago, and the pharmacist said he sells lots and lots of them now. This was unheard of before. (My Dad was a pharmacist and I worked alongside him for years… we didn't even have catheters then, only condoms hidden away in a drawer and only to be sold discretely!) Today many, many men are dealing with an enlarged inflamed prostate.

Do you remember the story of the Spartans at Thermopylae? A small band of elite warriors held off the tens of thousands of the invading hordes at the pass and saved Greece from takeover. They were able to accomplish this because it is fairly easy to block a pass.

The urethra tube that empties your bladder flows through your prostate and even the smallest amount of blockage can shut the pass down completely or weaken the flow to a painful trickle.

I will explain all this to you, as I have had the joy of inserting catheters at least 3 dozen times. I'll share all of my tips with you.

The first thing I want to share with you is that using a catheter sounds way worse than it actually is. If you have heard horror stories then know that it does not have to be like that for you.

If you get the right size (thickness of tube), the right type, and you know how to use it, then the pain is minimal. In fact, it is more a discomfort than a pain. What is painful is the fact that you can't pee and because of it you are in distress. In a matter of minutes you can find release and, oh what a feeling that is! Believe me!

What is a Catheter?

A catheter is a tube, in this case a urinary catheter, designed to get the urine out of your bladder when you need assistance because your prostate is shutting down the prostatic urethra—the part of the pee tube that goes through your prostate from the bladder and then out the penis. (A urinary catheter is any tube system placed in the body to drain and collect urine from the bladder.)

The process of inserting a catheter is known as catheterization. "Clean intermittent catheterization" (CIC) is the technical term in the literature for self-use of a catheter or the self-catheterization that you do at home.

Catheters come in different lengths for males and females and in different thicknesses or gauges (diameters). Thinner ones are used for children and thicker ones for long term use so that they do not clog with debris or blood clots. A male catheter is longer than a woman's because it has to travel through the penis to get to the bladder. So male catheters are about 12 to 16 inches long.

Catheters come in different shapes at both ends depending on its use. Long term use requires that the inserted tip be held in place while inside the bladder and not be easily removed or dislodged while sleeping or moving. This is done by being able to make a little balloon on the end by pumping it up from the external end that has two openings, one for that function and one for the urine to exit. When inflated, the balloon keeps the catheter securely in place. They are called Foley catheters and are often used for patients in hospitals who need a catheter put in place for a longer period of time.

These Foley catheters at the external end are then attached to another flexible tube that goes to a bag to collect the urine, holding about a liter or quart. They can be attached to a device beside the bed in a hospital or to your leg with a strap so you can walk around.

What Types Are There?

There are several very specialized types of catheters but, for our purposes, there are two versions of catheters for men: internal and external catheters.

❖ Internal catheter = Stopped. Can't Go.

❖ External catheter = Going. Can't Stop.

The internal catheters are used to help you pee when your prostate blocks your pee tube. The external catheters are for situations in which you do not want to have to run (or can't run) to the washroom to pee (e.g., traveling or at a ball game), or if you have a sudden urgency that you can't control. It is like a condom with a tube at the end that goes to a small bag on your leg. You go when you have to and can empty the bag later. Condom catheters are a very convenient device with no pain and peace of mind.

Here we focus on the internal catheters, because those are the ones we need to use to pee when we're blocked. There are basically two types of internal catheters:

- single use catheters (also known as short-term or intermittent catheters) are removed after you have emptied your bladder, and
- long-term catheters (known as indwelling catheters or Foley catheters), which have the balloon function at the end.

If you have a block and need to pee, what you want is a simple, single-use, male catheter. You can buy them at your pharmacy, medical supply store, or online (see the sources listed below).

But first let me explain more about these single-use, internal male catheters.

For your emergency use, you want to get 12-gauge catheters. These are quite thin. Fourteen-gauge is acceptable, even 16, if that is all you can find. Boys use 10s. They come all the way to 28 gauge (ouch!).

Now there are two kinds of single-use catheters—very flexible and a bit stiffer. They each have an advantage. The flexible ones are very soft and pliable, which is nice but may be a bit harder to insert all the way through. The stiffer versions allow an easier transit during the last stage through the prostate and into the bladder. I have used both and I recommend having both available. They are very inexpensive.

Now here is a good tip. Buy some Xylocaine or Lidocaine ointment in a tube. Some Xylocaine brands come with a special cone applicator cap that you insert the tip into the opening of your penis and squeeze some in (you can do this with just the tip of the tube if it comes with no special applicator). It lubricates the catheter and acts as a desensitizer so you barely feel the catheter going in.

Lubricated catheters are relatively new. These are the Rolls Royce of catheters because the lubrication makes them easy to insert! The whole catheter is lubricated. They just glide right in! Yup, these are the catheters to use! They do not need any Xylocaine unless you feel extra lubrication is needed. I was so pleased when I used those the last few times I needed a catheter. I wish I had had them before! They are worth the extra price.

Tip Tips!

There are two types of catheter tips: straight-tipped catheters or Coudé (French for elbowed) catheters. The Coudé ones have a 45° bend at the tip to allow easier passage through an enlarged prostate. This angled part is only about 1/6" long. I like these because it helps get through the last bit of the prostate. But straight tipped ones are fine too. It is just a matter of preference. But both or either will work just fine.

You can read more about catheters here:

- Urinary Catheters [http://1.usa.gov/oGOwzu]

- New York Times Health Guide - Urinary Catheters [http://nyti.ms/q0RJWK]

My Catheter Choice

My first choice is the SpeediCath lubricated Coudé catheter. It is more expensive than others (about $3 to $4—I paid $10 when I first found them!), but the ease of application in an emergency is well worth it. I have used $1 catheters and they work but nowhere near as easily and they are uncomfortable to use. Be extremely careful when buying catheters and ensure they are sterile, which has been built into the package design of these SpeediCath beauties.

I will describe how to use the cheap ones later on, but the SpeediCaths are more than well worth the extra price for the hopefully rare occasions that you will have to use them. They take the trauma and worry away, believe me, because I have had difficulties getting the cheap ones through the last inch or two on several occasions.

I once failed and had to call an ambulance. It took me 5 hours to get to the emergency room. Please don't skimp here! I will share tips on the cheap ones in case that is all you have, but these SpeediCaths (either Coudé or straight) are the ones to buy. Period.

Read what the company says about these catheters:

> *"The **SpeediCath** family represents a new generation of hydrophilic-coated catheters. What makes these catheters exceptional is their coating. Pre-hydrated, smooth and even, the SpeediCath coating creates minimal friction when inserting and removing the catheter. This makes catheterisation more comfortable and reduces the risk of urethral micro-trauma – even if you have to self-catheterise for a lifetime.*
>
> *Among SpeediCath's other unique features are:*
>
> - *pre-hydrated catheters that are ready-to-use right out of the pack. No need to bring water and no wait*
>
> - *polished eyelets that are gentle on the urethra minimising discomfort and the risk of micro-trauma*
>
> - *PVC and phthalates free"*
>
> www.coloplast.com/products/urologyandcontinencecare/speedicath/features_benefits/pages/featuresbenefits.aspx [http://bit.ly/qH8GZq]

All true! I really wish I had had these from the start!
Don't skimp to save a few bucks here.

What You Need for Self-Catheterization

Here is a list of items to create the minimal Prostate Kit. You really won't need the optional items, but I list them in case you can't find the SpeediCaths. If you want other less expensive catheters, go here: Other Catheters [http://bit.ly/oLfTcM]

Minimum Prostate Kit:

- ✓ 1 SpeediCath catheter lubricated: SpeediCath Coudé [http://bit.ly/r5qZev] Intermittent Catheters or Straight-Tip SpeediCath [http://bit.ly/qiCGDF]. Choose 12 gauge 14" (*#28492 - 12 FR, 14" Length*) catheter. Buy several so that you have back-ups for the car, home, work, travel bag, etc.

- ✓ 6– 10 Alcohol Prep Pads [http://bit.ly/qaLEJ9]. You can get 200 for a few bucks.

- ✓ Xylocaine (very optional): Xylocaine Ointment Tube [http://bit.ly/niVyUT] *or* Lidocaine [http://tiny.cc/hqyu6] With SpeediCath, you really do not need these, but if you are worried, then get some.

✓ KY jelly (also very optional)

✓ A plastic ziplock bag to hold all the items together as your emergency prostate kit.

I have listed the optional items in case you can't find the SpeediCaths, as they are useful for lubrication and comfort if you are using a more generic kind of catheter.

If you want other less expensive catheters, go here: Other Catheters [http://tiny.cc/q298n]

For home use:

✓ The same kit as described above, but you can substitute a bottle of alcohol with kleenex tissues that you wet for sterilizing in place of the Alcohol Prep Pads.

✓ Include 2 towels.

Tip: Add a SpeediCath catheter to your first aid kit.

How to Insert a SpeediCath Catheter:

For a visual demonstration, you can go here to watch a video of how to use these catheters. When on the page, choose "Male using SpeediCath" on the left side of the page:

Animation Showing Practical Steps for Using a Catheter [http://bit.ly/o7rLit]

Inserting a SpeediCath at Home:

1. Gather all the above items, which you should have ready in a kit in a ziplock bag plus the towels and a plastic collection bottle for the urine. A liter or quart size is adequate.

2. Wash your hands really well then wash your penis with the glans pulled back.

3. Decide where to do the job. I really prefer lying down leaning up, which is different from the video. Why? Because unlike regular users who use catheters every day (perhaps because of a spinal cord injury), you are in trauma by now, having tried everything, and still you can't release. Lying down helps you relax and is less stressful than standing or even sitting (which is a good second choice). You do not have to be in the bathroom for this.

4. Lay a protective towel under you and another to the side where your bottle will be to place the external end of the catheter tube to collect the urine.

5. Place the items from the kit on the side towel.

6. Pull back the tab on the back of the catheter package to expose the sticky part. Attach the sticky part to the bedframe or side table within easy reach and pull

down on the pull-tab enough to expose the catheter top without touching anything inside.

7. Take the bottle of alcohol, remove the cap and pour some onto the kleenex or open the swipe pads. The goal now is to sterilize everything. Always remember that what you touch from now on must be wiped clean before using. And you must re-wipe your fingers if you touch something not yet sterile! Be very careful so as to avoid the risk of possible infection through careless use.

8. Sterilize your hands and then the top of your penis with the glans pulled down. Using the alcohol, wipe your hands again.

9. One hand (your dominant one) now takes the catheter out of the package by gently taking the top of the exposed catheter, pulling it out of the package and without touching the lower part guides the catheter tip into the opening at the tip of the penis while the other hand holds the glans down, tip opened and the penis vertical up from the body. It won't be an erection at this point ☹

10. If the catheter by accident touches anything, then wipe the spot with a clean kleenex with alcohol on it or a pad. Then reinsert. Be hyper careful at all times that what goes into the penis is sterile.

11. The catheter is stiff enough to hold its length as you insert it.

12. Once in at the top, slowly push it and it will glide its way through quite easily and with only minor discomfort. Just push gently inwards and down.

13. Remember to breathe deeply and relax! You are almost done! Continue to push it through.

14. After 8-10 inches you will be coming through the prostate to the entrance to the bladder

15. The sphincter muscle that keeps the bladder shut now has to relax enough to let the catheter through. So if you feel any resistance, STOP pushing. Finesse is the key to success now and the smooth tip will be helping you out.

16. You basically want to knock on the door and give a bit of time for the sphincter to relax and open. Wait a good few seconds.

17. Push gently. Never force. If it seems blocked here is the trick to that. Twist the catheter with your fingers maybe a quarter of a turn or more and that will help find a way through. Keep twisting and very gently pushing until it slips through the last little bit. Most of the time it will go through without any problem. But you now know what to do just in case. I was taught this technique by a great emergency room nurse who explained that "finesse is the trick." Oh had I known that! I had been forcing it and it didn't work (causing blood to come out) and that was why I was there in the emergency room. **FINESSE - GENTLE - TWIST**. You will succeed easily with this trick (if you should need it). I didn't need it after I discovered the SpeediCaths. They are just so good! If

at any time even before this last bit you encounter resistance then pull back a bit and use the finesse turning trick to help the catheter through.

18. Once you pop through into the bladder (and it will seem like a lot of the catheter has disappeared inside—leaving 3-6 inches outside), suddenly urine will squirt free from the external end. Just put your thumb against the end and place it in the bottle. Then push the catheter a little further so that it is well inside the bladder.

19. Keep the bottle as low as you can beside you so gravity works to void the bladder.

20. You should now be emptying and feeling such a wonderful sense of relief. Aaaah! Oh so good! At last relief!

21. Job well done! Keep holding the catheter in place so that it doesn't slip out a bit.

22. Just lie there and feel the blessings of this little device that just saved your life!

23. The bottle will be receiving more and more of the urine, slowing down eventually to a trickle.

24. Relax and empty. Oh feels so good now!

25. After a few minutes or so—there is no rush—and no more urine flows, then slowly remove a bit of the catheter towards the neck of the bladder. That may release the last bit of urine near the neck of the bladder.

26. When done pull the catheter all the way out and discard beside you.

27. Rest a bit before clean up.

28. Sleep if you can.

29. There is no need to worry now, because the act of putting the catheter through seems to open the channel and keeps it open after it is out. Soon, you will have your first pee. It may burn a bit as the ammonia in the urine touches any part that may have been irritated by the catheter but this should be very minor as these are such good catheters. Any discomfort will soon pass as the day progresses.

30. If you do not know the cause, do your detective work and figure out what caused the prostate attack. Now is the time to personally test all that you recently ate.

How to Insert Other Catheters

Lie down with your prostate kit that has a simpler un-lubricated catheter. You will need to be more careful with sterility because more handling is involved. Be meticulous to avoid infection. In all my many uses I never had a urinary tract infection problem because I was always careful to keep everything sterile.

1. As above wash hands and penis and then lie down with kit beside you. Hopefully you will have KY, Xylocaine, or another lubricant.

2. Sterilize everything—the tube, the cap, the penis. I use many pieces of kleenex with alcohol as I do all this.

3. Remove the catheter from the package by touching only the external end. The package is not sterile so discard.

4. Wipe your fingers again with alcohol and then the catheter and place on several flat pieces of kleenex beside you.

5. Wipe first the KY or xylocaine tube and then open it. If there is a special applicator tip, wipe it and place it on the tip of the tube with your sterile fingers. If not, then wipe the tip of the tube really well with alcohol.

6. Wipe your penis tip area and glans with alcohol to disinfect.

7. Hold your penis with one hand and pull back the glans and open the tip.

8. Insert the tip of the tube and squeeze some lubricant or xylocaine into the penis.

9. Wipe the tube and tip again for reuse. Wipe fingers again. Wiping always with fresh alcohol on tissue. Always remember to keep everything sterile.

10. Grab the catheter and wipe that again at the tip area up towards the external end.

11. Then apply some lubricant or xylocaine to the catheter tip up maybe 3-4 inches, being careful to avoid the openings where the urine will enter. Never use vaseline—it is oil based and it could block the tip openings for urine entry into the catheter.

12. Now you are ready to insert the catheter into the tip of the penis making sure not to touch the catheter to anything but the entry into the penis.

13. Once inside, you start to push gently.

14. You can wipe the tube after the first few inches with kleenex and alcohol to make sure it is sterile as you push it through and can add some more lubricant or xylocaine if you want.

15. Then follow the above instructions, paying special attention to being careful and turning the catheter to help it find its way home into the bladder.

16. Go gently and slowly. If there is any spot where it does not want to go further, then do NOT push! Instead use finesse to twist the catheter until it can find a way through. **FINESSE - GENTLE - TWIST**.

17. Once you pop through into the bladder (and it will seem like a lot of the catheter has disappeared inside you), suddenly urine will squirt free from the external end. Just put your thumb against the end and place it in the bottle. Then push the catheter a little further so that it is well inside the bladder.

18. Keep the bottle as low as you can beside you so gravity works to void the bladder.

19. Now follow SpeediCath Steps 20 to 30 above.

During the day, you may feel more of a burning sensation as you pee due to irritation. It will pass in a day or so. That's why I love the SpeediCaths because the lubrication on the whole tube is much gentler on you and is superior to the tubes of lubricants—it is hyper slippery.

Note: It is possible over the next while (days to weeks) to pass some blood and blood-colored urine or even clots of blood from possible trauma of using the catheter or debris from the prostate. This condition will pass and is not cause for alarm unless you get steady amounts of fresh blood, which is a serious concern. Then seek medical help. Steady amounts of fresh blood should not result from regular use of a catheter.

Using a Catheter Away from Home

One day you may need to use your kit in a strange place. The procedure is the same except you may be sitting at a public toilet. Just use your lap for your instruments. Be so very careful of good hygiene and sterility here. Pay attention to everything you touch. Anything that goes onto the tube or catheter must be sterile before entering the penis. Use your alcohol pads here. Just place your thumb over the external end and then direct it so it can empty into the toilet once it starts.

I had to do this at an airport washroom once between flights as I blocked in mid-air. It can be done there and anywhere if you take your time, go step-by-step and pay attention to the details.

A catheter is a lifesaver! It does the trick of relief beautifully!

Here is one last and very important tip:

When you block and have tried some of the suggestions to release and they are not working, it can be best to decide early on to use the catheter rather than wait too long. The longer you wait the more traumatized you become, and it can be difficult to follow the steps if you are shaking all over.

Relief is at hand and it is not hard to do. So, decide to use the catheter earlier rather than later if you seem to be so blocked that you are not making any headway. It's a blessing waiting there for you if you need it.

External Condom Catheters

As I said above, these catheters are used for occasions where you know you may have troubles finding or getting to a bathroom, or do not want to be interrupted by frequent or urgent urination. Truck and taxi drivers, long-distance travel, sports events, and other occasions are just some possible users or uses of these wonderful devices.

They go over your penis like a condom, and have a tube at the end to drain into a bag. The trick is to keep them from falling off or getting loose so that they leak or do not work properly.

Size Matters! This is where an honest measurement of your favorite part must be accurate! Cheat and call it longer or thicker and you will leak! If the external catheter is too small, it may hurt you over the time it is on. Go here to download a sizing chart: Merlin Medical Supply Sizing Chart [http://bit.ly/prVa3E]

Now that you know what the right size is for you, I will explain how they work and help you choose what kind to buy.

You have several choices of external condom catheters, all of which attach to a drainage bag with a tube. They come in rubber, polyvinyl or silicone. They're attached by double-sided adhesive, a latex inflatable cuff, jockey's type strap, or foam strap. They're disposable and really shouldn't be used for more than 24 to 48 hours. Reusable ones are available.

Always remember with any catheter that there is a risk of infection and even external catheters can cause skin irritation: there is adhesive inside that sticks to the skin of the penis and wraps around it.

Here are step-by-step instructions for using external condom catheters:

1. First, wash your hands.

2. Next, gather your supplies: correct-sized condom catheter, leg drainage bag with tubing, clamp, manicure scissors, soap, wash cloth, towel, and protective ointment.

3. Use the manicure scissors to cut back the hair at the base of the penis. This prevents it from being caught by the adhesive.

4. Remember, the penis and surrounding area must be cleansed thoroughly with soap and water. Dry completely before applying a new catheter. This is crucial because if moisture is left inside the condom, bacteria can grow. Bacteria can cause a urinary tract infection. You don't need that on top of your prostate problem!

5. Sometimes, you might find the adhesive used inside the condom catheter causes irritation to the skin on the shaft of the penis. In the case, avoid using the condom catheter until the irritation is gone.

6. Urine can irritate the skin, so use a protective ointment and let it dry until sticky.

7. Tightly roll the balloon-like part, the condom sheath, to the edge of the connector tip. Next, put the catheter sheath on the end of your penis, but there should be about 1/2" space between the two tips: the penis tip and the connector tip.

8. It's easiest if you let your penis stretch as you unroll the condom smoothly. When done, gently press it to the penis so it sticks.

9. Connect the tip to the tube to the urine bag and strap the bag to your thigh.

10. For removal, clamp the tube closed to prevent spillage. Disconnect the tubing, unstrap the bag, and remove the condom by rolling it forward. Then empty the pee bag.

Click here for more info: Managing Urinary Incontinence With Catheters [http://bit.ly/pUsKfP]

Different men have different levels of activity. Therefore, urinary drainage storage bags come in various sizes. So, for example, men who are still active can get a smaller bag.

Want to read more about them?

- "What is a condom catheter?" [http://bit.ly/pLeP7H]

- "How to Care For Your Condom Catheter" [http://bit.ly/pWF3DJ]

As you have read, there are many types of external catheters. You will have to read more and explore to find ones that work best for you. The best idea is to try several types and see what works for you.

Sources of External Condom Catheters

- Top of the line external catheter [http://bit.ly/phxJpb]

- Best seller and inexpensive external catheter #1 [http://bit.ly/oaKjsB]

- Best seller and inexpensive external catheter #2 [http://bit.ly/nYIypQ]

- Search for other brands: put *condom catheters* into search field: [http://bit.ly/oOeANx]

These internal and external modern catheter devices have enabled men to have more freedom than ever before and peace of mind for special times or emergencies where sudden blockage occurs. Be prepared if you have any symptoms of a prostate problem. Get a kit together so if an emergency happens, you can handle it safely. In fact, a catheter should be part of every first aid emergency kit today, as well as knowing how to use it.

My Story, Part IV: Highlights and Lowlights of the Past 7½ Years

Many of the alternative therapies and approaches I tried sure seemed to make sense and may well work for you dear reader. I tried dozens!
But none worked for me. During this intense time period, I had many harrowing moments:

i) The Ambulance

Going to the hospital by ambulance after not being able to get the catheter through after 2 tries and drawing blood. I was just too blocked and didn't know how to get the catheter through the last inch into the bladder.

Whenever I blocked afterwards, I was scared. Would I be able to get the catheter through or would I have to call the ambulance again? There were times when it took three tries before I succeeded. I always felt like a beached whale after an episode like this. I'd be weakened and fragile for the whole day while I recovered and hoped it would not happen again.

Never knowing when the next attack would come is part of what makes this condition so horrific. Thank goodness I learned about finesse with catheter insertion and the new lubed catheters.

ii) The Blood Clot Episodes

In early summer 2010, about a half a year after the first time I had blood clots, I had a much worse event! I started passing blood clots but in much bigger amounts than the first time. I would have freaked out had I not had the prior experience.

The clots came in waves. One evening and night were the worst. I was peeing into a bottle so I could see what came out better. So many clots came within just 30 minutes that when I poured it down the kitchen sink to look at it, the clots completely blocked the drain sifter and no liquid could get by!

That happened once more during the same night. By morning the crisis had passed and just a few small clots came and then I was fine. YIKES! That was scary! (It was probably clots formed from using the catheters over time, given the problems I had). I have since learned some tricks to avoid catheter insertion problems, which I shared in Chapter 13 of this book.

And then I started to block again with many close calls and actual complete shut downs where I had to use the catheter 3 times in 2 weeks. I was getting worse! So I decided it was time to see the doctor again, 7 years after the initial problem showed up. I was desperate at this point… no progress. I had not yet made my breakthroughs. Knowing what I know now, I would not have embarked on all these tests!

iii) Back to the Urologist

I was sent at my request to a top urologist in Victoria that was recommended by a friend. He conducted a complete series of tests, starting with a blood and urine test that came back fine.

Then an ultrasound. This found something on my kidneys that the doc wanted to check further for cancer.

I agreed to a CT scan. I was desperate and had not yet made a breakthrough. It showed the kidneys were fine but my prostate was so enlarged that he now wanted to do a cystoscopy (a camera up the penis through the urethra) and biopsy because 3 other radiologists agreed that there was cause for alarm. They could see from the CT scan that my prostate was way too big for the TURP procedure that I had been on the emergency wait list for previously seven years ago.

So that was scheduled and happened. I waited for the results. I was not worried about having prostate cancer because I just knew I didn't. But I was concerned that I would have to have some kind of prostate surgery beyond the more simple TURP.
He explained that most likely it would have to be an open surgery (a prostectomy), the most complicated operation and requiring an incision through the lower abdomen—much more invasive than the transurethral TURP. But first, he had to know if cancer was present.

Next came the tests. Several days later he called to say, "No cancer." I scheduled an appointment with him for the following week and went to see what he thought best to do.

At the meeting, he said that he had thought that I was in constant need of using a catheter every day. After I described the low frequency of its usage he did not recommend surgery unless my symptoms got worse.

I was real pleased with his suggestion of not doing surgery! He recommended and gave me samples of Avodart (standard prostate meds with real side effects and risks) to help reduce the size of the prostate gland and improve urine flow. I didn't take those pills since they personally tested no.

Well concurrent with all this, I had gone to see my local doctor on the island when the ultrasound results came in. The normal doctor was away and a locum was in his place. He took over 40 minutes to explain what he saw in the conclusions and not to worry about doing the CT scan. He then went on to explain to me some dietary suggestions! This was an amazing doctor! He opened my eyes to something I had overlooked that eventually led to a major, major breakthrough and the start of my real healing at long last!

iv) Other Symptoms

Between 2008 and 2010 or so, a new symptom emerged. My tongue! It started to be coated with white and had raw lesions on the tip. They were not canker sores and did not go away. They diminished a bit, but most of the time they were quite red and often very sore. It felt like my tip had been sand papered with very rough sandpaper.

In 2010, my symptoms were the worst they'd been:

- frequent urination, sometimes every 2-5 minutes during an hour or two, and often at least 2-3 times per hour.

- difficulty peeing, slow start, dribbling, incomplete emptying

- waking up 5-8 times per night to urinate (sure hard to sleep like a baby when you have to go all the time... ah diapers!)

- waking many times during the night and nothing comes out or only a drop or two with an intense burning sensation and the pain of not being able to release. Sometimes it finally happened and, little by little, a teaspoon at a time, I was able to release and finally after a couple of hours I could pee maybe 2-3 ounces or a 1/4 of a cup or 75 ml.

- maximum pee amount 100 ml (about 1/2 of a cup), but mostly much, much less

- tongue problems as described above

- the worst was total blockage and catheter use

v) Log entry:

December 21, 2010, I slept 9 hours and woke only once peeing 300 ml, a record for me in 7 1/2 years on both fronts!
Oh how happy I am now to have had the breakthroughs I did, which I share in the book with you dear reader! I finally, after seven and a half years, started to heal!

Chapter 14: Natural Prostate Treatments

Now that we've discovered the many causes of prostate disease, started changes to our diet, initiated cleansing to clear out the old toxins, added personally-tested high quality food, prostate supplements and superfoods to optimize our diet, we are ready to look at specific treatments that can help our healing. Combining the above steps with some of the following prostate treatments will help you make big strides forward on the path to healing yourself.

Some of these treatments may seem simplistic and some may seem "out there," but I believe an open mind will lead you to one or two treatments that may be highly beneficial. I have had experience with some and will share my insights and comments. I offer some treatments that I have not had time to explore in case something rings a bell for you.

I begin this chapter with natural prostate treatments for overall prostate conditions, including cancer. At the end I of this chapter I focus on specific natural prostate cancer treatments.

Good Prostate Habits

This list will help you to alleviate some of your urinary symptoms if you have a prostate problem:

- ✓ During the day and evening, get up from sitting and move a bit each hour—sitting puts pressure on your prostate and irritates it.

- ✓ Get physical exercise—movement prevents stagnation.

- ✓ Pee when you have to go, because holding it in will irritate your prostate if it is enlarged.

- ✓ Ejaculate regularly—this also helps stagnation by moving fluids through the prostate.

- ✓ Stop drinking at least 2-3 hours before bed—this puts less stress on your bladder during the night and increases your chances of sleeping without waking (or has you waking less often).

- ✓ Reduce or stop consuming caffeine and alcoholic drinks—they are diuretics (increasing the volume of urine released into the bladder) and increase your need to pee during the night. Caffeine and alcohol also irritate the bladder sphincter and the prostate, making it tighter and harder to release when you got to go. You can personally test to see if you can handle the drink and if you receive a YES response then test to determine what amount is okay. I find I often get a YES response when I test for a small glass of red wine.

- ✓ Urinate before going to sleep. If you do awaken to urinate, having a pee bottle may be faster than going to the bathroom and may help you fall back to sleep easier.

✓ Sit to pee if you can, because it relaxes the prostate and bladder more than standing.

✓ Avoid over-the-counter antihistamines and decongestants. They can cause the bladder sphincter to tighten, sometimes drastically as we have mentioned.

✓ If you feel you have not fully emptied your bladder, a second pee will come soon so wait.

✓ Know the signs of prostate conditions. Make changes before they become extreme.

✓ Pain in the prostate area could be any of the three prostate conditions: enlargement, infection, or cancer. Make the changes recommended in the book now!

✓ If you have recently used a catheter or prostate massager (perhaps too vigorously), it is possible that you will find blood in your urine or blood clots. You are eliminating scarring, residues, or debris. It will pass—do not panic. If this becomes a stream of fresh blood, seek medical attention immediately. On three separate occasions over a year I passed blood and clots mixed in with the urine over 2-3 days. Some of the blood was dark red and some fresh. It passed and all was well, although at the time it did worry me. This occurred some time after I had used a catheter and had some difficulty passing it through the prostate, which may have caused scarring.

Some Prostate Products

There are many interesting herbal prostate products on the market today.

Some from India are time tested. In India they use many herbs unknown in the West. One useful Ayurvedic herb is called Ayurstate [http://bit.ly/q13kAw]. You can order from India Herbs or it may be cheaper from Amazon (less freight charges) depending on your location: Ayurstate for Prostate Care [http://amzn.to/pJA5hi].

- Prostate Protection [http://bit.ly/pLwY7F] is another well-known Ayurvedic product.

- Prostate Dr. [http://bit.ly/qyIRWj] is an excellent tincture for prostate health and prevention with just three key plant sterols or herbs. I like tinctures for their direct absorption.

- I also really like this very high quality tincture, Men's Formula [http://bit.ly/qEcGyG], by Baseline Nutritionals.

- Brassica Tea [http://bit.ly/qyXuxo] is a way to get your broccoli benefits for your prostate in tea form!

You know the hint... personally test.

Some Prostate Treatments

These are ways to help alleviate symptoms over time.

Broccoli Treatment for the Prostate

Cut up ½ lb or 250 grams of broccoli, stems and flowers, and boil in 4½ cups of water for 5 minutes. Drink half the broth on an empty stomach in the morning and the other half in the evening. After 7 days stop for 3 days and resume 2 more sessions like before, for a total of 21 days of drinking time.

I have tried this and felt it helped me. Basically what you are doing is getting a concentrated fully natural hit of cruciferous vegetables the basis for the supplement DIM. But it does take some effort. To read more about this treatment go here: "Broccoli Treatment" www.geocities.com/iastr/eindex.htm [http://bit.ly/ov9NlN], click on "Broccoli" on the left menu and then click on the "Broccoli Treatment" link in the second paragraph.

Sitz Bath Prostate Treatment

A sitz bath uses the time-honored method of alternating hot and cold water over the prostate area by using a sitz bath commode (or another way of isolating that area) to concentrate the heat and cold to that part of the body. The heat causes expansion of the blood vessels and the cold contracts them. The effect causes lots of blood to flush the area and can remove toxins as a result.

Hydrotherapy, or water therapy, has been used for ages. Look at the hot steam baths and natural hot springs in Europe. They are hugely popular.

You can use a sitz bath commode, which fits over the toilet to catch water overflow. I am not sure if you can get maximum coverage of the prostate to make it effective doing that but others recommend them.

You can get commodes at a good pharmacy or medical device store or here at Amazon: Sitz Bath Commode [http://tiny.cc/1jp9i]

Here is the basic procedure for a sitz bath:

- ✓ Fill the commode with hot water that is a comfortable temperature for your wrist. Too hot is dangerous.
- ✓ Add 1/2 cup of epsom salts to the water.
- ✓ Sit in the sitz bath for 6 minutes. If possible, add hot water as it cools, this also moves the water so that it does not stay stagnant against your skin.
- ✓ Alternate with a second commode that has cold water and sit in it for just one minute.
- ✓ Repeat this process 2 more times.

While doing this, it is important to do kegel exercises where you squeeze your prostate—like when you squeeze the stop-pee muscle in mid-stream. Do this and hold for several seconds on your out breath and then relax. Repeat kegel exercises often in both the hot and cold water. This causes debris to move out of the prostate, which will have been loosened by the fresh blood flow.

Here is my variation instead of using the commode:

Get the largest food cooler you can, 2 of them. Put them in your bathtub. (If you only have room for one, then put the hot one in the bathtub.) Fill the cooler 1/2 way with hot water (a comfortable temperature for your wrist), add the Epsom salts and sit in it. Your lower torso will be nicely covered.

Then have a handheld shower turned on to a hot trickle to add to the water and keep it nice and warm. Also remember to move by rising up and down a bit to move the water around your prostate area. Do your kegel squeezes and hold. Then go into the coldest water you can. You can keep it nice and cold by using the shower handheld to keep it on your prostate area (the lower tummy above your "equipment"). Six minutes hot: one minute cold. Repeat 2 more times.

Once you figure the process out you will actually find it quite effective and invigorating, especially if you are experiencing uncomfortable symptoms. Follow with a shower. This is also a good remedy for a prostate attack.
Read more here: Prostate Symptom Relief [http://bit.ly/obyNeS]

Herbal Sitz Bath

Take a warm bath in which you sit in water up to your waist. Add rosemary essential oil for pelvic circulation.

Anti-Inflammatory Oil Application

Mix St. John's Wort with the essential oils of rosemary and lavender. Apply directly to the perineum area to increase circulation and reduce inflammation.

Castor Oil Pack

Castor oil comes from the seeds of the castor plant. It is a very thick oil and penetrates deeper into the skin than any other oil. It has been used for centuries, both internally and externally for its therapeutic and medicinal benefits. Read more about it here: Castor Oil's Many Forgotten Uses [http://bit.ly/quIrMJ]

A castor oil pack is an effective way to apply the castor oil directly to the affected area so that it can penetrate deeply to remove toxins. It will increase circulation to the area and speed up healing. In our case the pack will be applied to the prostate area. The ideal is to do both the perineum area and the prostate area just below the bladder.

The oil is very thick so you need to prevent it from getting on your bedding. Follow the instructions below.

Castor Oil Materials

- Wool flannel cloths, enough to fold over to a thick pad to cover the perineum (between the anus and testicles) and another for the front prostate area. You can alternate areas every second night instead doing both at the same time.

- Plastic coverings (plastic wrap to contain the oil).

- Hot water bottle or electric heating pad.

- 2 old towels—one to protect your bed under you and the other on top of the pack.

- Natural castor oil. Buy at your health food store or here: Natural Castor Oil [http://tiny.cc/spc1w]

Castor Oil Pack Procedure

1. Soak the thick cloth with castor oil. It should be saturated but not dripping wet.

2. Place the pack on the prostate area (or areas).

3. You can wear an old pair of underwear (not a bad use for those dead ones!) on top of the pack to protect everything. You can skip the plastic this way if you want.

4. Cover the pack with plastic and place a hot water bottle or heating pad over the pack.

5. Cover with a towel to keep the heat contained.

6. Leave the pack on for 30–60 minutes. Use the castor oil pack for a week.

7. You will need to add a bit more oil each time to your cloth, which you can store in a jar and use over and over again.

8. Store the pack in a cool place or refrigerator until next use.

9. Remember the oil does stain, but the stains can be removed with baking soda.

10. You can rub excess oil into your hands and skin, as it is very good for skin and hair (known to thicken it).

Modified Hot/Cold Castor Oil Pack Version

Do the castor oil pack as described for just 10 minutes. Then remove the heat and apply an ice pack for 5 minutes. Alternate between hot and cold for about an hour. You may need several cold packs on hand as well as a heating pad to retain enough heat. Alternating like this will increase circulation to the prostate area to allow healing. This is also useful for prostate cancer.

Ginger Compress Prostate Treatment

Ginger compresses have been used for centuries (and more) to treat pain, inflammation, swelling, stagnation, and stiffness. The ginger compress increases blood circulation dramatically to areas where stagnation exists, and thus can help dissolve hardened accumulations of fats, proteins, minerals, and stones.

In the case of the prostate, we treat the area similarly to the castor oil treatment except we use moist water heat and ginger to break up stagnation in the prostate gland.

> *"STRONG HEAT. Strong heat will dilate the blood vessels and thereby it will activate the movement of stagnated fluids. Strong heat will also melt or soften mucus stagnations and fatty accumulations and will tend to break up mineral crystallisations. Strong heat has the further advantage of penetrating deeply into the body. Thus a ginger compress can exert its influence deep inside the body, even within solid organs such as the kidneys and liver, or within the lungs.*
>
> *GINGER. Due to its nature, ginger easily penetrates into the body... Because of its penetrating nature, ginger will also disperse stagnated... substances such as mucus and fat accumulations. Ginger will further increase local circulation because it opens the blood vessels.*
>
> *As a result of this double effect, thick liquids in the body start to liquify, heavy deposits start to dissolve, stagnated liquids begin to move again, and gradually all treated tissues become cleansed and nourished with fresh blood. That is to say, tissues will gradually rejuvenate, soften and revitalize."*

Van Cauwenberghe, Mark, M.D. "Compresses, Plasters and Packs" home.iae.nl/users/lightnet/health/messages/ginger.html [http://bit.ly/p7UI71] (Accessed 29 March, 2011)

Items Needed

- 1 gallon filtered water
- A large pot
- 6 inches ginger root (nonorganic is fine) to make 1/4 cup finely grated ginger
- Grater
- Cheesecloth or thin cotton bag
- 2 small towels for soaking
- 1 big towel to hold the heat
- 1 pair of thick rubber gloves
- Hot plate to keep the water hot while doing the treatment (optional)

1. Put the water in a large pot and bring to a boil.

2. Grate the ginger into a bowl to retain all the liquid. Use the fine side of the grater for best results to get maximum amount of ginger juice.

3. Place the contents of the bowl of ginger into the cheesecloth or cotton bag. Tie tightly.

4. Once the pot is boiling, turn off the heat and once the water is quiet, squeeze the ginger bag into the water to get the juice out. Then add the bag and any juice left from the bowl into the pot.

5. Add two of the towels folded into the pot and cover for a minute or so.

6. Use your rubber gloves to remove the lid from the pot, grab a towel and wring it out.

7. While lying down, hold the ginger towel close to the prostate area (the lower abdomen, pubic bone area) and little by little touch but do not allow the skin to burn and then when hot as possible but cool enough not to burn, place it on the skin and then cover with the dry towel to hold the heat in place. The ginger towel should be folded to about a 6"-8" square to concentrate the effort at the prostate bladder area.

8. After several minutes the heat will cool down, so remove the ginger towel and cover the area with the dry towel while you replace and exchange ginger towels in the pot and repeat the procedures. If you have a hot plate, place the pot on it to retain the heat.

9. Alternate the two towels for about a half hour.

10. You can save the ginger water. Just don't boil it and you can reuse it for additional ginger compresses.

You will have to do a series of these ginger compresses over a week or two for best results. They are extremely effective at loosening debris and stagnation. Your prostate will love it!

Herbs and the Prostate

Herbs can detox and cleanse the prostate gland, reducing swelling, and inflammation by dissolving toxins within the gland.

Pumpkin Seeds

Pumpkin seeds have been used in many cultures to treat BPH and prostatitis. They may also help cure prostate cancer. Pumpkin seeds are rich in zinc, a mineral for prostate health. Remember to soak the seeds to remove the phytates.

Stinging Nettle

This herb is very popular in Europe to treat BPH, or enlargement of the prostate. It is often combined with saw palmetto to relieve enlarged prostate symptoms such as urgency to urinate, incomplete emptying, and the constant urge to urinate.

Pygeum

This is another well-known prostate herb. Many studies show its benefits for an enlarged prostate.

Peppermint

Peppermint—not spearmint—acts as an anti-inflammatory to the prostate. It is a useful tea.

Saw Palmetto

There are lots of studies showing that saw palmetto is a preventative and it also helps to reduce prostate symptoms. Sterols are the active ingredient in saw palmetto, which is often used in supplements.

Gamma Linoleic Acid (GLA)

GLA is found in evening primrose, borage, and black currant seed products. It is an immune stimulator and anti-inflammatory.

Turmeric

This curry spice and herb is an anti-inflammatory. It is available in capsules.

Other Prostate Herbs

Herbs can detox and cleanse the prostate gland, reducing swelling and inflammation by dissolving toxins within the gland. Try some of these:

- ✓ Cleavers herb
- ✓ Thuja leaf
- ✓ Juniper berries
- ✓ Corn silk
- ✓ Willow herbs (*Epilobium parviflorum*)- very commonly prescribed in Europe.
- ✓ Great hairy willowherb (*E. hirsutum*)
- ✓ Uva ursi leaves
- ✓ Horsetail (*Equisetum arvense*)
- ✓ Sweet and spotted Joe-Pye rhizome (*Eupatorium purpureum and E. maculatum*)

✓ Rye pollen

✓ Queen Ann's lace (*Daucus carota*)

✓ Yellow and white sweet clover herb (*Melilotus officinalis and M. alba*)

Herbal Prostate Tea

Bell Prostate Ezee Flow Tea [http://bit.ly/rrZEnr] is an herbal prostate tea that many men swear by.

Chinese herbs

You will find many Chinese herbs for the prostate if you search for them. I would look for a product that contains some of these herbs. You may find slightly different spellings for them, as they are all translations.

"1. Saw palmetto

Saw palmetto has been used for over a century in traditional Chinese medicine in treating pain in the lower back, inflammation and enlargement by inhibiting dihydrotestosterone, thereby reducing its stimulation for cancerous cell multiplication.

2. Patrinia (Bai jiang cao)

Patrinia helps the body get rid of prostate inflammation and damp heat that exists in the body. In Chinese medicine damp heat in the prostate could be caused by bacteria infection, drugs and other conditions such as a habit of eating hot, spicy or greasy foods.

3. Lu lu tong (liquid amber)

Lu lu tong has the ability to improve qi and blood circulation. It also helps to reduce the abdominal, back and knee pain caused by damp heat as well as difficult urination because of bladder or prostate inflammation.

4. He shou wu

He shou wu contains several derivatives of tetrahydroxystilbene. These antioxidants and anti-inflammatory compounds may act as an estrogen, reducing levels of circulating male hormones such as DHT that fuel the growth of prostate cancer.

5. Niu xi (Achyranthes)

Niu xi contains triterpenoid saponins and sitosterol that possesses anti-inflammatory effects in both enlarged prostate and prostate cancer inflammation. It also helps to nourish the kidney liver and reduce symptoms of damp heat and difficult urination as well as stiffness and pain of lower back.

6. Gui Zhi (tokoro)

Gui Zhi is used for urinary tract disorder that pertains to ying qi levels which is the main cause of prostate inflammation. It also is used as a tonic and blood purifier.

7. Astragalus root

Astragalus root is a sprawling perennial legume. The Chinese medicine uses the dried sliced or powdered root of the plant to enhance immune function by increasing the activity of certain white blood cells, which increases the production of antibodies. It also helps to increase the body's resistance to infections, to heal the allergies, and to raise and renew the vitality.

8. Che Qian zi (plantago seed)

It is mainly used for stone strangury caused by lower burner damp-heat, such as the symptoms of aching pain in the lumbus and abdomen, poor urination or with hematuria, and urinary tract stones.

9. Vaccaria seed

It is used to reduce pain and stiffness in the lower back, drain excessive damp heat, invigorate blood and treat difficult urination."

"Prostate Health - How to Treat and Prevent Enlarged Prostate with Chinese Herbs" prostatehealth05.blogspot.com/2008/09/prostate-health-how-to-prevent-enlarged.html [http://bit.ly/p6hD4W] (Accessed 1 April, 2011)

Chinese Herbal Products

Chinese Prostate Pills [http://bit.ly/nuuu7f] contains quite a few Chinese herbs listed above (4, 5, 6, and 8) as well as other herbs. This product seems very promising. Read on their site to learn more about the Chinese herbs used. Here are some other Chinese herbal products:

- Chinese Prostate Supplement [http://bit.ly/nFvNXP]
- Chinese Herbs for Prostate [http://bit.ly/r4kBjW]

There is a long tradition of herbal healing in China passed down over the generations. If you live near a Chinatown, then I recommend that you see a Chinese herbal doctor. Just go into various herbal stores and ask them for a Chinese herbal doctor. They will direct you. I have done this on several occasions.

The Chinese herbal doctor will take your pulses to learn your condition and examine your tongue and more as well as ask you questions about your health and diet. From that examination, the Chinese herbal doctor will customize a herbal product for you. It will be weighed and mixed with a variety of herbs with instructions on how to simmer them to make a tonic to drink over the next week or two. Depending on your condition, this can be a very effective treatment for your prostate.

If you do not live near a Chinatown, then you could get an email consultation at Dr. Shen's Chinese Herbs and Medicine [http://bit.ly/r4kBjW] (scroll to the bottom of the page at the link).

Herbs combined with hydrotherapy or oil packs can be quite a combination to aid your healing. These work differently from strong medications, which often have dangerous side effects. Herbs work slowly, cleansing and rebuilding, and are more subtle in their effects, but they do have a powerful impact over time.

Guided Digital Medicine

This is a novel approach to prostate diagnosis and treatment that combines the interconnectivity of toxicity, infection and EMF radiations on prostate conditions. Dr. Yurkovsky's bio-energetic medical system toward prostate disease combines important knowledge from both conventional and alternative medicine but also physics and laws of complexity known for their efficiency in solving many scientific and technological problems. It is called Guided Digital Medicine.

"Physics views all life as primarily energetic vibrations from every cell to the entire body, and views disease as change in normal vibrational or cellular field patterns. This crucial concept leads to overcoming some current limitations in medicine:

1. Its inability to determine true causes of chronic disease because neither the laboratory nor the imaging tests are capable of obtaining this information from the internal organs and tissues themselves which are ultimately the primary site of all diseases.

2. Its inability to be truly effective in removing these toxins or infectious agents from where it counts the most – the internal organs themselves.

The first question can only be answered through bio-energetic diagnostic tuning directly into internal organs and tissues themselves. Using vials which contain various toxicological, infectious, radioactive, electromagnetic and other pertinent morbid agents, known to cause prostate illness, Guided Digital Medicine is able to find the precise culprits and thus to determine the most effective types of homeopathic treatments.

Besides harmful factors as bad diet, other unhealthy lifestyles, and individual genetic predispositions to disease, the three most fundamental factors in all chronic diseases have been determined by Dr Yurkovsky. These are:

#1.   <u>Heavy metals</u> with mercury being the most ubiquitous of these. Mercury commonly lodges in the prostate and in numerous internal organs and because of this widespread intoxication, its effective treatment is not easy to achieve with prevalent chelating methods.

#2.   Infectious <u>agents</u> with sexually transmitted diseases, E. coli, and candida family fungal infectious being the most prevalent ones.

#3.   Electromagnetic <u>fields and their deadly radiations</u>.

Each one of these is being confirmed by scientific literature as increasingly playing a big role in chronic diseases, including cancer. Concerning these Big Three, bioresonance testing and clinical experience over some 20 years has also confirmed that:

1.   They cause a mutually self-sustaining effect on one another:

a) magnetic fields are well-known to interact with all metals. This interaction greatly undermines the body's ability to release toxic metals as mercury, lead, cadmium, aluminum and others.

b) EMF radiation, at the same time, directly undermines physiologic functioning of the organs and blood chemistry itself by distorting their normal energetic field codes which represent foundations of health. Among the organs affected by EMF, besides target or sick organs such as the prostate are also organs of the immune system.

2. *Even more alarmingly, electromagnetic fields can directly stimulate the growth of infectious agents. This immuno-suppressive effect is already on top of direct immuno-suppressive effect of heavy metals residing in the immune organs.*

3. *These immuno-suppressive effects of electromagnetic fields and heavy metals render chronic infections, including the ones of prostate, as incurable where even if their symptoms may improve in the short-term following antibiotics or alternative antimicrobial treatments, they are all bound to regain ground in the long-run.*

4. *But these silent and deadly interactions are not ending here. Chronic infections, themselves, can worsen morbid effects of both heavy metals and electromagnetic fields. This, in its turn, heightens the pathophysiologic effects and retention of toxic metals with both EMFs and metals suppressing immunity further. The resultant augmented immuno-suppression leads to sustainment of the current infections and acquisition of new ones.*

Thus, this vicious deadly cycle never ends unless effective measures are undertaken." Yurkovsky, Savely. www.yurkovsky.com/prostate (Accessed 27 July 2011)

Chapter 15: Prostate Cancer Treatments

From all the readings I have done, prostate cancer results from years (or decades) of making poor diet choices, coupled with high levels of emotional stress and exposures to toxins. Prostate cancer does not just happen out of the blue.

That's the bad news. The good news is that with this knowledge you can reverse prostate cancer and destroy your tumors by doing the opposite—by making healthy choices and cleansing your body of the old. Of course many will disagree with me, especially those with a vested interest in the conventional medical view of the world as well as those who financially benefit from selling you procedures or products. Not that I have anything against financial well-being, but do believe the sanctity of the individual's health should always come first.

I do not want to minimize the dangers of disease. To me it has been a wake up call to change, to discover what I can do to heal. This path is not for everyone.

More and more you hear about and read the stories of people surviving cancer through natural and alternative methods. There is just too much anecdotal evidence to dismiss it as quackery, which is what the powers that be describe them as. Since there is no money to be gained by these non-patentable foods, herbs, and procedures, no proper research has been done and no "proof" exists as to their true effectiveness. Hence you are on your own to learn and discover what is best for you.

Now, don't let your doctors convince you that you need to screen for prostate cancer. They may not know it's a waste of time unless they keep up with the latest research results, and it is also possible that the doctor, hospital, or insurance company benefits from administering the screening procedure.

Prostate cancer screening is a complete waste of time, money, and your emotional comfort. There is a huge 20-year study written up on March 31, 2011, in the **British Medical Journal**:

> **_Objective_** _To assess whether screening for prostate cancer reduces prostate cancer specific mortality..._
>
> **_Conclusions_** _After 20 years of follow-up the rate of death from prostate cancer did not differ significantly between men in the screening group and those in the control group._"
>
> BMJ 2011; 342:d1539. 31 March 2011 "Randomised prostate cancer screening trial: 20 year follow-up"
> www.bmj.com/content/342/bmj.d1539 [http://bit.ly/nFbUSD] (Accessed 4 April 2011)

The British Medical Journal article titled "Randomised Prostate Cancer Screening Trial: 20 Year Follow-Up" [http://bit.ly/nFbUSD] concluded that those screened for prostate cancer and those not screened showed no difference in the rate of death (i.e., PSA screening has no benefit).

Here is one more study to pay attention to before deciding if conventional treatments are for you:

> *"The various forms of prostate cancer treatment -- from surgery to radiation to hormones -- can all have long-term effects on men's quality of life when it comes to sexual function and urinary problems."*
>
> Reuters. 12 May 2010. "Prostate Cancer Therapies All Affect Quality of Life." www.reuters.com/article/2010/05/12/us-prostate-cancer-idUSTRE64B5EA20100512 [http://reut.rs/qj6Akd] (Accessed 4 April 2011)

We have already talked earlier about the uselessness of screening and in particular PSA screening, as well as the risks of biopsies. The safest assumption to make is that you will have or already have some kind of prostate disease happening in your body. The best solution then is to start now to make the changes that inhibit the conditions from starting or worsening by reversing them if underway.

Since all recent studies now show no added life expectancy whether you have invasive surgeries or not, the best approach is a natural one based on the advice in this book. You have everything to gain and nothing to lose.

What you don't eat is as important as what you do. Stop your junk food habits. Many natural therapies indicate that consuming sugar in its various disguises needs to stop, as sugar creates an acidic host in the body for cancer cells to grow and multiply. So stop feeding it. Wisen up about everything you eat, drink, and put on your body. Make optimum choices as part of the new health-conscious you.

Making better healthy choices, getting adequate Vitamin D and A through high quality cod liver oil, stopping the toxic onslaught, cleansing your body, rebuilding your body with vital and nutrient-rich foods, exercising regularly, lowering your emotional stress levels through some form of quieting or meditation, getting adequate sleep, supplementing with hormones if needed and mineral rich prostate herbs, and doing various natural prostate treatments—that's what you need to do to ensure your prostate health.

What comes next are very specific natural prostate cancer and broad cancer treatments to add to the above guidelines. I have chosen the ones that have been time tested and show real positive results. It is essential that these treatments are built on the new foundation of healthy choices because **your daily food intake is the MOST POWERFUL MEDICINE OF ALL.** Your input equals your output. Begin with a solid footing first!

Natural Prostate Cancer Treatments:

Sunshine and Vitamin D

We have already said how crucial vitamin D is. It alone can reduce your cancer risk by 50%. Get sun on your skin and, if you can't, take the highest quality cod liver oil you can find.

> *"In prostate cancer cell lines, vitamin D stimulates the tumor-suppressor genes that increase the production of proteins that slow the cell life cycle."*
>
> The Vitamin D Cure [http://amzn.to/qgcYTy] by James Dowd and Diane Stafford

Read this article that new research says we need about 4000-8000 IUs per day: 8000 IUs of Vitamin D Daily [http://bit.ly/qYJ9zz]

Omega-3 Fatty Acids

Lots of good research on omega-3s. Most men are very deficient in them and have way too much omega-6s in their diet:

> *"Just how good are fish oils, flaxseed oils and other omega-3s at preventing prostate cancer? According to the experts quoted below, they may represent some of the most powerful anti-cancer nutrients available today!*
>
> *Read this large collection of quotes on omega-3 oils and prostate cancer, and you'll learn how boosting omega-3 intake while reducing omega-6 intake can help halt prostate cancer tumor growth and end the chronic tissue inflammation that ultimately contributes to prostate cancer."*
>
> NaturalNews.com - Adams, Mike. 20 April 2009. "Omega-3s - Fish Oils, Flaxseed Oil and Prostate Cancer "
> www.naturalnews.com/026085_fish_oils_omega-3s.html
> [http://bit.ly/oYZcaB] (Accessed 5 April 2011)

That's another good reason to take cod liver oil, which is full of omega-3s.

Aloe Vera

Aloe or aloe vera is a remarkable herb. You can use it as a juice or gel for prevention or as an herbal medicine for cures. It is one of the most powerful and naturally occurring antioxidants available and seems to enhance vitamins A, B, C, and E.

Aloe vera reduces inflammation. Used topically aloe is well known to ease inflammation of joints and can reduce arthritis pain. Used internally, it reduces inflammation throughout the body from the inside out. People who drink aloe vera for two weeks begin to experience a significant reduction of inflammation symptoms. For a list of studies and references, visit: Google Scholar's Aloe Search Results [http://bit.ly/ogFPdI]

NaturalNews.com has many excellent articles on Aloe: The Aloe Vera Miracle [http://bit.ly/nNmHNu]

Aloe Vera and Cancer: Many articles have been written on this subject. Aloe gel helps boost the immune system while destroying cancer tumors. Please use these links to decide if using Aloe makes sense to you for prostate cancer. It is easy to personally test it.

"New book reveals secret Brazilian Aloe recipe for curing cancer using just three ingredients" [http://bit.ly/oWwPmA]

Aloe and Cancer Books [http://tiny.cc/ztclz]

Google Scholar has many references to Aloe and cancer. Perhaps its benefit is in part due to the ability of aloe vera to stimulate the immune system:

- Google Scholar Search Results for Aloe Vera and Tumors [http://bit.ly/q3yYjq]

- Google Scholar Search Results for Aloe Vera and Prostate Cancer [http://bit.ly/rfS8eV]

Hot Pepper Treatment

Capsaicin, the part of the pepper that is *hot*, kills prostate cancer:

> *"According to a team of researchers from the Samuel Oschin Comprehensive Cancer Institute at Cedars-Sinai Medical Center, in collaboration with colleagues from UCLA, the pepper component caused human prostate cancer cells to undergo programmed cell death or apoptosis.*
>
> *Capsaicin induced approximately 80 percent of prostate cancer cells growing in mice to follow the molecular pathways leading to apoptosis. Prostate cancer tumors treated with capsaicin were about one-fifth the size of tumors in non-treated mice.."*
>
> Vanderboom, Russell. 15 March 2006. "Pepper Component Hot Enough to Trigger Suicide in Prostate Cancer Cells" www.eurekalert.org/pub_releases/2006-03/aafc-pch031306.php [http://bit.ly/qgYxEl] (Accessed 29 July 2011)

Chili peppers also fight inflammation, provide natural pain relief, have cardiovascular benefits, clear congestion, boost immunity, prevent stomach ulcers, help people lose weight, and lower the risk of Type 2 diabetes. See this article for more info: Chili pepper, dried [http://bit.ly/nDfZNU].

Green Tea

Green tea inhibits the growth of prostate cancer cells:

> *"The polyphenols in green tea help prevent the spread of prostate cancer by mobilizing several molecular pathways that shut down the proliferation and spread of tumor cells, while also inhibiting the growth of blood vessels that*

supply the cancer with nourishment, according to research published in the December 2004 issue of Cancer Research."

www.whfoods.com/genpage.php?tname=foodspice&dbid=146 [http://bit.ly/q27IJX] (Accessed 4 April 2011)

It may be best to use decaf green tea. Your testing will tell you.

Ellagic Acid

Ellagic acid in red raspberry seeds promotes prostate cancer cell death. The American Cancer Society's Complementary and Alternative Cancer Methods Handbook [http://amzn.to/pVX51H] states,

> *"Ellagic Acid has been found to promote cell death in destructive cells ... and prevents the binding of [toxic substances] to DNA and strengthens connective tissue, which may keep [harmful] cells from spreading."*

The best way to get Ellagic Acid is from raspberries. Read the info at these sites on their supplements to see which you like best:

- Ellagic Acid Supplements [http://www.ellagicdirect.com]

- Ellagic Acid Extract [http://bit.ly/orB5qH]

- Ellagic Ultra [http://bit.ly/ro5lv2]

Antioxidants

Antioxidants—found in fresh fruits, berries, vegetables, and superfoods—can help treat cancer. Eat lots in a wide variety of colors.

> *"'Antioxidants have been associated with cancer reducing effects—beta carotene, for example—but the mechanisms, the genetic evidence, has been lacking,' Dr. Lisanti said. 'This study provides the necessary genetic evidence that reducing oxidative stress in the body will decrease tumor growth.'."*

Graff, Steve. 15 February 2011, "Jefferson researchers provide genetic evidence that antioxidants can help treat cancer" www.eurekalert.org/pub_releases/2011-02/tju-jrp021011.php [http://bit.ly/pDyADC] (Accessed 28 March, 2011)

Other Foods That Can Help:

✓ **Red clover**

> *"Researchers at Monash University in Victoria, Australia found that an active supplement derived from red clover helps prevent prostate cells from advancing to cancerous stages (Cancer epidemiology, Biomarkers and Prevention, Dec 2002). The researchers involved measured the PSA (Prostate Specific Antigen) level, The Gleason score (grade of cancer), serum*

testosterone, incidence of cancer cell death, and excreted isoflavone levels before and after treatment. The supplement used was found to be particularly effective in fighting early-stage cancer cells and cancer cells were killed off five times more frequently than was the case in the control group."

healthrecipes.com/red-clover-cancer-treatment.htm [http://bit.ly/pxW44B] (Accessed 28 March, 2011)

✓ **Laetrile or B17**
How laetrile or B17 from apricot seeds kills only cancer cells
Laetrile and Information on B17 [http://bit.ly/n5rPkq]

✓ **Sodium Bicarbonate and Cancer**
Sodium Bicarbonate - Rich Man's Poor Man's Cancer Treatment [http://bit.ly/rfaSAA]

✓ **Magnesium and Cancer**
"Magnesium and Cancer Research:

Magnesium chloride is the first and most important item in any person's cancer treatment strategy. *Put in the clearest terms possible, our suggestion from the first day on the Survival Medicine Cancer Protocol is to almost drown oneself in transdermally applied magnesium chloride. It should be the first not the last thing we think of when it comes to cancer. It takes about three to four months to drive up cellular magnesium levels to where they should be when treated intensely transdermally but within days patients will commonly experience its life saving medical/healing effects. For many people whose bodies are starving for magnesium the experience is not too much different than for a person coming out of a desert desperate for water. It is that basic to life, that important, that necessary."*
www.magnesiumforlife.com/medical-application/magnesium-and-cancer/ [http://bit.ly/r3w6Fr] (Accessed 7 June 2011)

More on the benefits of magnesium? See: Dr. Sircus' Blog post on Magnesium Oil [http://bit.ly/oZn8ek]

You can buy it at Amazon: "Ancient Minerals" Magnesium [http://amzn.to/qP8I9z]

✓ **Modified Citrus Pectin**
"MCP is a highly effective neutraceutical that promotes cellular health and prevents the growth and spread of aberrant and abnormal cells throughout the body."

www.dreliaz.org/recommended-product/natural-cancer-support [http://bit.ly/nnILEW]

✓ **Melatonin**
As discussed earlier under the section Hormones, melatonin has been proven excellent in combating cancer.

✓ **General resources for more information:**

- Quotes about Prostate Cancer from the world's top natural health / natural living authors [http://bit.ly/nQ4NRZ]

- "Knowing Your Cancer Curing Options" [http://bit.ly/n1cCE1]

- "Hops Compound May Prevent Prostate Cancer" [http://bit.ly/oWjwVi]

- "Beat Cancer on a Shoestring Budget" [http://bit.ly/qZ0Xw1]

Sites Dedicated to Natural Alternative Cancer Treatments

You will find a whole world here: treatments, approaches, testimonials and insights. Prostate cancer is such a personal journey as is healing any dis-ease. To my way of thinking, optimizing your diet through personal testing after stopping the toxic input and starting a cleansing program will form the most important part of your healing.

It can be quite overwhelming to sort through all the alternative approaches with their possible conflicting ideas. Focus on cleansing and your diet. When you are well on your way with that, then you can look at some of these. Remember that prostate cancer is very slow to grow so you do have time on your side to get the basics done first.

Be careful in what you choose. Only do so with something that very strongly resonates for you. You can personally test an approach using a book, printout, or image of the treatment. There is no one-size-fits-all answer, but there is a right answer for you at this point in time.

In my opinion, the site Cancer Tutor [http://www.cancertutor.com] has the best review of alternative cancer treatments. The examination and classification of the different therapies are clearly defined for the type of cancer and its stage, a crucial distinction when choosing the best protocol. So examine the Cancer Tutor [http://www.cancertutor.com] site first and then look at these next two sites:

- Healing Cancer Naturally [http://www.healingcancernaturally.com]

- The Cancer Cure Foundation [http://www.cancure.org]

Here are some books to check out:

- *Cancer Is Not A Disease - It's A Survival Mechanism* [http://amzn.to/q9p5e6]

- *Outsmart Your Cancer: Alternative Non-Toxic Treatments That Work* (Second Edition) With CD [http://amzn.to/pW2sot]

- Alternative Cancer Treatments: Books [http://tiny.cc/47u6b]

Prostate Devices

In this section, you will find special products designed to help ease your prostate symptoms. Some are particularly good for prostatitis or an enlarged prostate. I have not tried them as yet so I cannot vouch for their efficacy.

- ✓ **Prostate Cushion** is a special cushion to relieve pressure on your prostate while sitting:

  Prostate Cushions [http://prostate-cushion.com]

  Other Prostate Cushions [http://tiny.cc/5yqfw]

- ✓ **Prostate device to wear** claimed to reduce the size of the prostate

  Prostate Treatment Device for Prostatitis and BPH [http://bit.ly/oniKLH]

- ✓ **Prostate bicycle seats** help relieve the pressure of sitting on a bike seat that normally puts a lot of pressure on the perineum and prostate areas.

  - Amazon's Prostate Bicycle Seats [http://tiny.cc/mqor9]

  - Prostate Relief Bicycle Seats [http://bit.ly/pCQ2GL]

  - The SEAT [http://bit.ly/qYJ3v7]

  - Spongy Wonder Bicycle Seats [http://www.spongywonder.com]

  - Comfortable Bicycle Seats by Spiderflex [http://www.spiderflex.com]

  Here are discussions about various ways of finding a good seat:

  - "Bicycle Seats Explained" [http://bit.ly/qmxOtd]

  - "What is the best bicycle seat for prostate relief?" [http://bit.ly/om5lEx]

  - "Does bicycling cause prostate or testicular complications?" [http://bit.ly/n1vxUV]

- ✓ **External Prostate Massager:** Just by sitting on this device your prostate gets an external massage:

  The Prostate Cradle [http://tiny.cc/wcrvd]

- ✓ **The Dribblestop Male Urinary Incontinence Clamp** is an external clamp that gently applies pressure to the top of the penis, as well as the urethra on the underside to effectively control bladder leakage: DribbleStop [http://bit.ly/n9CQOI]

Conclusion

Prostate cancer can be reversed by making the lifestyle changes described in this chapter and throughout this book. Letting your fear take over and this allowing the worried views of the medical establishment to proceed immediately with their programs to attack the body must be countered with your courage and inner knowing that reversing the causes leads to a healthy solution.

There is a bigger picture. Disease or illness has a blessing in disguise if we choose to see it. It can force us to take stock of our lives, to change lifelong habits that no longer nurture us and to embrace an inner journey to wholeness. Healing oneself has many challenges. It is not always an easy path.

It is easy to stumble along the way. There are highs and lows. The key to realize is the trend line, sloping upwards, getting better bit by bit over time. A greater acceptance of oneself and an opening of the heart to let go of fear and resistance to what is—this new awareness then allows healing to happen more and more. This too is the mindset that sometimes allows "miraculous cures" to happen. Too many documented cases cannot be dismissed when this happens—cancerous tumors shrinking, people recovering suddenly from incurable diseases.

Do not let information overload overwhelm you. Simply start with diet changes, cleansing, and work on reducing stress (which I describe in Chapter 17)—these are your keys to success. Then you can add some supplements if they test positive for you. Use some of the techniques in the next chapter to work on any emotional issues that can drive dysfunction in your body/mind. Many, many people have healed themselves from cancer, and you can be one of them!

Chapter 16: Energy Healing Methods for Prostate Health

One methodology of healing that is on the leading edge that you may want to explore, especially for prostate cancer, is called energy healing or energy medicine. Energy healing can include all kinds of practices that focus or channel energy by your hands, a practitioner's hands, or other methods to move the flow of energy in the body. Founded on ancient principles of meridians and energy centers in the body, such as acupuncture, today's methods include and often go beyond those to new methods that can have profound healing effects on some.

> *"Energy Healing is an holistic approach to facilitating the return journey to health. It involves tracing the cause of any suffering through the physical and emotional symptoms to its roots deep within our psyche.*
>
> *Our natural flow of energy always moves towards perfect health and well-being. However, when faced with difficulties in our life which we find too painful to accept, we tend to hold this unresolved energy... This creates blockages in our energy field which then depletes our vitality and can lead to ill-health and suffering."*

"What is energy healing?"
www.energyhealing.co.uk/what-is-energy-healing.php [http://bit.ly/phEA7n] (Accessed 20 April 2011)

The problem is that the effects of most of these methods are subjective and cannot be fully verified by science. Nevertheless, too many people claim good results to dismiss them outright.

Read more about energy healing here for a good overview:
"Energy Medicine" [http://bit.ly/ow8Xs3]

Donna Eden has been teaching energy medicine for decades, has had untold successes, and now has about 500 practitioners who she has taught worldwide. Donna Eden is the original Western energy healer and has integrated many ancient practices into her unique form. Check her out and read her books. Her amazing stories reveal the power of energy healing:
• *Energy Medicine* with Donna Eden [http://bit.ly/r0JuRX]

You can watch Donna Eden's 5-minute daily energy routine here:
Donna Eden's Five-Minute Routine [http://bit.ly/qrtdSr]

The healing codes have helped many sufferers with this new method that focuses your own energy in specific ways using your fingers to direct energy to speed healing and reduce the impact of stress on your body.

> *"The healing codes are a branch of alternative medicine that centers on the human energy field for healing. Energy medicine is the new arrival in healing that doesn't make use of conventional medicine or require you to take*

pharmaceutical drugs. Instead healing is made possible through subtle, non-physical means.

It may seem too good to be true, but even medical doctors are amazed by its effectiveness and **you don't have to believe in it for it to work!**

Dr Loyd, ND, PhD made his discovery in 2001 when he was looking for a solution for his wife's severe clinical depression. For twelve years she had visited specialists and tried every remedy under the sun.

This miraculous study led him to the conclusion that his discovery not only healed depression and other psychological issues but also an array of physiological disorders. He soon found out that the code could be used to allow the body to heal itself regardless of the illness...

After stumbling upon this unexplainable blueprint, Dr. Loyd used Heart Rate Variability (HRV) scans, which proved overwhelmingly positive, and he found that in eighty percent of individuals, it took less that twenty minutes after self administering the codes to bring their out-of-balance stress levels back to in-balance levels.

So to be more precise, The Healing Codes [http://bit.ly/oHo2YV] are the only precise scientific healing method that:

- *Reduce inner stresses and remove the root cause of all emotional, physical and mental health conditions without the need for medical interventions, drugs or surgery.*

- *Make your body almost immune to disease by opening the cells of the body and changing them from defensive to growth mode.*

- *Make recovery and good health a certainty rather than just a possibility by activating the three key components of healing concurrently."*

www.thehealingcodes.com [http://bit.ly/oHo2YV] (Accessed 20 April 2011)

It can be expensive but has a long guarantee time for you to try it out.

The Tapping Solution

The Tapping Solution [http://bit.ly/mPDx1I] is another modern method of energy healing that is recommended by many well known writers and experts, and it is much less expensive.

EFT: Healing the Emotional Roots of Disease

"EFT (Emotional Freedom Techniques) is a simple yet remarkable healing system that reduces the stress that underlies much disease. It has proven itself successful in many scientific studies. It works on a variety of health issues, psychological problems, and performance issues, even those that have been resistant to other methods. It can be learned and applied rapidly, which has contributed to its popularity among millions of people."

www.eftuniverse.com (Accessed 20 April 2011)

What is Qigong?

"Although the term "Qigong" was coined in the 20th century, the origin of the practices that now constitute Qigong predate recorded history. Qigong is self-initiated moving meditation consisting of a combination of movement, self-massage, meditation and breathing.

Qigong practice puts the body into the relaxation/regeneration state (the relaxation response) where the autonomic nervous system is predominately in the parasympathetic mode. Qigong can be done anywhere, anytime.

It is excellent for stress reduction, prevention of illness, dealing with chronic illness, healthy and active aging, and longevity. Practicing Qigong is as simple as doing the three intentful corrections (adjust the posture, breath, and mind)."

www.qigonginstitute.org/main_page/main_page.php [http://bit.ly/nCGbby] (Accessed 20 April 2011)

An easy-to-follow combination of controlled breathing, focused concentration, and simple movement, Qigong is the grandfather of Chinese medicine, Tai-chi, acupuncture, Shiatsu, and Reiki.

Books and research papers are filled with the health benefits of Qigong, such as:

- Improve your metabolism, digestion, and elimination. Qigong is great for weight control, youthful appearance, and balanced energy.

- Stimulate the lymph system. Qigong builds a stronger immune system so that you become less susceptible to flues and other viruses and recover faster if you do get sick.

- Improve your circulation. Qigong alleviates conditions such as arthritis and chronic fatigue.

- Retard the aging process by giving your organs an "inner massage" to restore your body systems to healthy functioning.

- Reduce tension, blocks, and stagnant energy by increasing oxygen supply to your tissues.

- Lubricate your joints for pain-free movement and greater flexibility.

- Soothe the nervous system to feel contented and serene.

Spring Forest Qigong is an advanced form of Qigong designed specifically to accelerate the natural healing process of the body. Read more about its benefits and how it was discovered and brought to the West here: Spring Forest Qigong [http://bit.ly/pruF4d]

What is Mind-Body Medicine?

"Mind-body medicine uses the power of thoughts and emotions to influence physical health. As Hippocrates once wrote, 'The natural healing force within each one of us is the greatest force in getting well.' This is mind-body medicine in a nutshell."

www.umm.edu/altmed/articles/mind-body-000355.htm [http://bit.ly/othbPq]
(Accessed 20 April 2011)

"To quote Dr. Richard Schulze: "There are no incurable diseases, none. Take responsibility and be willing to change, and you can heal yourself of anything." Stop focusing on your disease, concentrate on creating health - the effect is powerfully beneficial. View your illness as a gift towards discovering the healthy natural lifestyle. You're focusing on health. Your focus determines your future."

Stehle, Angelika 29 March 2011 "Think health, not illness" www.naturalnews.com/031874_cancer_diagnosis.html [http://bit.ly/p52a2G] (Accessed 29 March, 2011)

Chapter 17: Stress and the Prostate

Chronic, overwhelming stress may be the number one plague of modern life, causing or magnifying all sorts of health conditions. The impact of stress truly shows the power of the mind and emotions on the body.

How does stress work?

> *"Stress activates a chain of hormonal events that was originally designed to protect our ancestors from wild beasts. We've all heard of the fight-or-flight mechanism. Consistent mental and emotional stress fires up this response system and keeps it active in an ongoing way. The results are staggering. Here is what the Mayo Clinic has to say:*
>
> *'The long-term activation of the stress-response system—and the subsequent overexposure to cortisol and other stress hormones—can disrupt almost all your body's processes.'*
>
> *If you don't get a handle on your chronic stress in a personally noticeable way, such that you can feel the difference in your body each and every day, rest assured it is doing damage daily. Low stress people live longer. Highly stressed people live shorter lives."*
>
> Bundrant, Mike. 30 March 2011. "The number one health destroyer is all natural" www.naturalnews.com/031890_chronic_stress_health.html [http://bit.ly/pHBX2y] (Accessed 18 April 2011)

Stress takes a staggering toll on our bodies, contributing to a weakened immune system and a wide range of chronic health diseases, including prostate conditions. In addition, the impact on life expectancy is huge. Highly stressed people loose as much as 10 plus years. Stress affects just about everyone to various degrees.

Natural stress arises in response to a danger. This is healthy because it fires up your alertness and survival mechanisms. But chronic stress of the mental and emotional kind is altogether different. It just keeps you in the same stress response mode of over exposure to cortisol and other stress hormones. Over time you pay a huge price. So add stress to the list of causes of prostate conditions.

For more information, please go to the Mayo Clinic's website on Stress Management [http://bit.ly/obG2iO]

Chronic stress easily impacts the prostate. Stress causes the body to tighten up. As a result the flow of blood and energy gets restricted and grows worse over time. The prostate relies on tiny blood vessels for nutrition and cleansing, and the constrictions caused by chronic stress takes its toll, setting the stage for prostate enlargement and possibly prostate cancer.

> *"The prostate and bladder neck are both rich in nerves that respond to adrenal hormones. These hormones are often called stress hormones because stress, whether physical or emotional, triggers the sympathetic nervous system (SNS). Exposure to stress on a daily basis can result in chronic over activation of the*

SNS. The result for the prostate is that the smooth muscle of the gland remains in a state of chronic tension, squeezing the urethra and bladder neck. This then makes urination more difficult."

"Stress"
www.realage.com/check-your-health/mens-health/enlarged-prostate-bph-reducing-stress [http://bit.ly/pUm8bM] (Accessed 18 April 2011)

Another type of stress arises in men who already have a prostate condition. This stress manifests in urinary difficulties in day-to-day life. Frequent urination becomes problematic when away from home. Look at what this Harvard Medical School article had to say about stress and the prostate:

"Men with benign prostatic hyperplasia (BPH) often find the condition stressful. It's easy to see why. Urinary urgency that triggers a frantic hunt for a bathroom will jangle the most placid gent, and nighttime urination that interrupts sleep can only add to mental distress. If they're under stress, some young men with normal prostates can also find it hard to urinate; doctors call it paruresis or the "shy bladder syndrome."...

Harvard Health Publications. "Stress and the prostate" www.harvardhealthcontent.com/69,N0408a [http://bit.ly/pVKdFs] (Accessed 8 May 2011)

Here is a reminder of some simple steps that help you live with BPH, reducing the stress caused by bothersome symptoms:

✓ Reduce your intake of fluids well before bed.

✓ Limit alcohol and caffeine. They make you pee more.

✓ Avoid decongestants, antispasmodics, and antihistamines.

✓ Diuretic meds for high blood pressure or heart problems can be problematic.

✓ Urinate when you have to or earlier as holding will stress the bladder over time.

✓ Learn the location of the bathroom when away from home or office before you really need it.

✓ Choose aisle seats on airplanes, theaters, and sporting events.

A third type of stress occurs in men diagnosed with prostate cancer. The risk of dying from cardiovascular disease or suicide increases after getting the diagnosis. It must be the shock of the news. Sadly the disease itself is rarely fatal.

"Men newly diagnosed with prostate cancer are at increased risks for cardiovascular events and suicide.."

Fall, K., Fang, F., Mucci, L. A., et al. 2009. "Immediate Risk for Cardiovascular Events and Suicide Following a Prostate Cancer Diagnosis: Prospective Cohort Study"
www.plosmedicine.org/article/info%3Adoi%2F10.1371%2Fjournal.pmed.1000

197 [http://bit.ly/n7Ki7X] (Accessed 18 April 2011)

If you are newly diagnosed with prostate cancer, then follow the advice in this book to change your conditions and work on ways to reduce stress (see info below). Calming your mind rewards your body and the automatic reduction in stress will help you to heal.

Stress and What to Do About it

Now that we know the impact of stress on our prostates, let's look at what to do about it. This article in the Washington Post reveals the many pluses of lifestyle changes:

> *"Eating better, exercising regularly and cutting stress apparently can slow the progression of early prostate cancer, according to the first study to provide direct evidence that lifestyle changes can fight the common malignancy."*

> Stein, Rob. 11 August 2005. "Diet, Exercise and Reduced Stress Slow Prostate Cancer, Study Finds" www.washingtonpost.com/wp-dyn/content/article/2005/08/10/AR2005081001882.html [http://wapo.st/pwR9hU] (Accessed 18 April 2011)

Stress Reduction and Relaxation Techniques:

Stress management and reduction begins by learning more about what stresses you so that you can find ways to a more peaceful life. We all need to adopt techniques that can help us minimize our toxic stress loads. Accepting the fact of stress in our lives is the first step.

Stopping to breathe deeply helps to center you and focus your energy inwards thus raising your energy levels. You can do this any time you become aware that you are feeling stressed. So start to breathe deep! Right down to the very bottom of your diaphragm. In and out deeply. Slow it down a bit. Breathe in and out through your nose. Deep breathing will instantly calm you.

Deep breathing, especially in and out through the nose, also reduces high blood pressure, releases tension you are holding on to, and stops the body's fight and flight response to stress.

Add prostate exercises—kegel squeezes—at the same time as deep breathing to get a double benefit. Practice the deep breathing and the kegel exercise while driving or take a minute from the task at hand and chill out this way.

The causes of our stresses can be varied and unique to each of us. Something that stresses you may be balm for someone else. It is all our perspective, not something "out there" causing our stress.

We allow something to be or not be stressful. Seeing the sink full of dirty dishes may elicit a strong negative anger reaction in one and a joyful one in another. It is not the dishes. It's you! One person says, "I can't stand the sink that way," the other sees it as a joyful by-product of a home well lived in with love and family.

Just understanding that you alone are triggering your stress gives you the awareness to catch it in midstream, breathe deep, and let it go.

Learn to Relax

1. Find a comfortable, quiet location that is free of distractions.

2. Now focus on your breathing. Take deep breaths in and out slowly through your nose. Look for areas in your body that feel tense or cramped. Breathe into those spots in your mind. Relax your shoulders. Let go of the tension as you breathe.

3. Close your eyes. Let your breathing become deep, slow, and steady. In and out through your nose.

4. Now imagine the area just below your navel. Breathe deeply into that spot and focus your mind there with every long, slow breath in and out.

5. As an alternative you can focus your awareness to the tip of your nose as you breathe in and out.

6. You will feel very relaxed after just minutes of deep nasal focused breathing.

Stress reduction can include:
- ✓ perspective shifting
- ✓ psychological counseling
- ✓ exercise (this is a no brainer... adopt some form that you like)
- ✓ breathing techniques
- ✓ yoga and pilates
- ✓ time management
- ✓ learning to say "no" to excessive demands on your personal time
- ✓ making optimum choices
- ✓ stopping addictive habits
- ✓ having a pet
- ✓ turning off the TV
- ✓ organizational skills
- ✓ support systems or groups
- ✓ guided imagery and tapes
- ✓ meditation
- ✓ prayer

✓ reading

✓ biofeedback

✓ listening to relaxing music

✓ doing a hobby

✓ contemplation

✓ getting out into nature

✓ self-growth to change a negative perception into positive action

✓ having a steam bath or sauna especially a deep infrared sauna

✓ sitting under a tree or near a waterfall to soak in nature's healing energy

✓ turning off electrical gadgets

✓ create disconnect time from the office

✓ turning off your email program and its beep to action

✓ creating down-time space for loved ones

✓ getting a massage... massage therapy really relaxes

Read some tips from the experts here:

- The Stress Institute [http://bit.ly/r2290b]

- Stress Reduction, Stress Relievers [http://bit.ly/ngHikT]

- Stress Management Health Center [http://bit.ly/n4d75H]

In my life, I have used many of the above techniques at various times. Learning to breathe deeply through my nose has been my foremost action. I have also used listening to self-growth tapes and positive subliminal messages to move me beyond my blocked, stressful state. You may want to check out these powerful stress reduction subliminal message tapes [http://bit.ly/qRtKp1]. They have some free ones you can sample to see if you like them.

Getting deeper insights into what causes your stress will help you find what works best for you. Check out these books and CDs: Stress Reduction [http://tiny.cc/wcrvd]

This simple stress relief method uses subliminal affirmations with soothing sounds to quickly relax you: Subliminal Stress Relief [http://bit.ly/nNiroV]

I was the youngest of my class of 800 students at Harvard. I was 20 and the average age was 26. It was first year of the MBA program, notorious for being the most stressful environment of any college program. After 3 months I was filled with so much stress I had stomach aches, sleep problems, and other nervous symptoms.

I went and saw the counselor. He advised a simple solution. Go running! That's when I took up that activity and it made a huge difference. Combined with a shift in perspective in my mind that failure was impossible, I was able to relax a lot more and thrive.

Meditation, Stress Reduction and Your Prostate

More and more research reveals how powerful meditation can be for your health and well-being and its amazing power to reduce stress. It is worth adopting some form of meditation into your life so you can reap its benefits.

Look at what changes can be measured in the brain after just 8 weeks of meditation:
"Mindfulness meditation benefits and changes brain structures in 8 weeks" [http://bit.ly/qsg9fw]

Meditation may be the Future of Anti-Aging:
- "Meditation may be the Future of Anti-Aging, Part I" [http://bit.ly/n9aQFD]
- "Meditation may be the Future of Anti-Aging, Part II" [http://bit.ly/qmeIht]

Study Shows Meditation Lowers Stress:
- "Body-Mind Meditation Boosts Performance" [http://bit.ly/nyO5BE]

A new study indicates that DNA can be altered through diet, exercise, and meditation. Read this article if you think you are a victim of faulty genes as the cause of your prostate problem:

• "Comprehensive Lifestyle Changes Including A Better Diet And More Exercise Can Lead Not Only To A Better Physique, But Also To Swift And Dramatic Changes At The Genetic Level" [http://bit.ly/pmGNzZ]

Amazon has lots of products on meditation:
- Meditation Downloads [http://tiny.cc/o7eqb]
- Meditation [http://tiny.cc/f3swh]

Free downloads:
• download.meditation.org.au/guidedmeditations.asp [http://bit.ly/o85015]

My favorites:
- www.dreamsalive.com [http://bit.ly/ocgLHt]
- www.mindbodytrainingcompany.com [http://bit.ly/oV6NSV]

High-tech meditation:
I tried these meditation methods over a 2-year period. There were not my style but you may like them. It uses a technology called entrainment to bring you deeper. Warning, they are expensive:
- www.project-meditation.org/community/ [http://bit.ly/qxGQNO]
- www.centerpointe.com

This next program is much cheaper, just as effective, and you only need to do it for 30 minutes. I don't know about you, but I like short and sweet ☺

- www.meditationprogram.com [http://bit.ly/q6Msrq]

And this may be the easiest of them all… effective and very affordable:

- Deep Meditation with Subliminal Affirmations [http://bit.ly/pMlffa]

If you need help with changing your eating habits without being stressed, then do try this download:

- "Develop Healthy Eating Habits" [http://bit.ly/psUDzN],
a natural hypnosis MP3, that will help motivate you to adopt healthy eating habits.

The bottom line is that you do not need any of these helpers. They are all optional. Just focusing on your breathing as described earlier is the foundation for all meditative practices.

I urge you to incorporate some form of meditation and relaxation into your daily life. The rewards are simply too great to ignore this practice. For us men, especially those active in the stressful business world, our prostates will sing their praises as we learn to remove stress from our bodies and minds.

Chapter 18: Prostate Massage

Prostate massage can be a powerful health benefit for the prostate and/or an amazing sexual technique. There are two types of prostate massage:

1. internal prostate massage
2. external prostate massage

By sitting all day, as most men now do, we restrict the flow of blood to the prostate and this is one of the causes of our prostate troubles, especially when combined with all the other factors discussed earlier in the book.

Prostate massage helps nourish the prostate gland by increasing circulation to the area, bringing fresh oxygenated blood flow, thus benefiting many prostate conditions. You can ask your health practitioner for advice on whether prostate massage can be beneficial for you.

Internal Prostate Massage

Prostate massage used to be done regularly by doctors and urologists to remove prostate fluids from the prostate during a digital rectal exam because of its health benefits. Enlarged prostates were often treated with prostate massage. Fluids are released in this way without an erection.

This is also called prostate drainage or prostate milking and is quite healthy for the prostate. It releases stagnant fluids and increases blood flow to the prostate refreshing and invigorating the gland. The process can soften the gland and release tension. It was a standard procedure until about 40 years ago, and then the practice ebbed away.

But it can be done by you or by a partner today. You can use your finger or a special prostate massager for the same purpose specially designed to use your pubococcygeus or PC muscles to apply the right amount of gentle massaging pressure. I much prefer the prostate massager device. They are quite effective. Internal prostate massage works because of the adjacent proximity of the prostate through the thin rectal wall.

• Finger Massage

Here is how to do internal prostate massage with your finger:

1. Make sure you have had a recent bowel movement so your rectum is completely empty.

2. Have a hot shower or bath to get clean or even a sitz bath to relax your pelvic muscles.

3. Make sure your fingernails are very smooth and short.

4. Wear a good quality latex glove (available at all pharmacies).

5. Lie down on your back or side with a towel beneath you.

6. Apply lubricant-KY jelly or equivalent or a natural castor oil **liberally** to your fingers and anal area.

7. Gently press the pad of your middle finger against the anus so it starts to relax.

8. Move your finger gently in a tiny circular motion.

9. After a while slowly increase the pressure always allowing the anal muscles to relax as you then push a bit firmer until your finger starts to enter.

10. It is all about the right angles to find the easiest way in. Your finger should be facing forward some towards your front as you find the way in.

11. Once you get the angle right, it will slide right in an inch or two if you have enough lube.

12. Now just relax and breathe deeply while your body adjusts.

13. You can then very gently massage your prostate through the wall of the rectum by moving your finger in a "come here" fashion.

14. **Being very gentle is essential**, especially if you have a prostate condition because too much pressure can be too much for the prostate and can injure its very delicate internal structure of membranes. So always be gentle, never vigorous.

15. Eventually, you may start to see some fluid escaping your flaccid penis (a few drops or more). It does not matter if any fluid comes out, the massage is still very beneficial as it moves the blood inside the gland. Often after the massage you will excrete some fluid.

16. After 5-10-15 (less time at first) minutes, slowly remove your finger.

• Using a Prostate Massager

Here is how to do internal prostate massage with a Prostate Massager [http://bit.ly/oNPZxk]:

First read what the manufacturer says about them:

> *"The Pro-State prostate massagers are specifically designed for effectiveness and ease of insertion. Once inserted into the rectum, the anal sphincter naturally pushes the Pro-State up toward the prostate gland and the external arm of the Pro-State pushes up against the perineum. Contraction and relaxation of the anal sphincter pivots the Pro-State massager up and down providing a hands free massage of the entire prostate...*
>
> *In addition to massage of the prostate, the Pro-State prostate massagers are the only prostate massagers that provide acupressure therapy on the specific*

prostate perineum point. According to the precepts of Oriental medicine, massage of this acupressure point is beneficial for optimal prostate health and sexual function. The Pro-State prostate massagers combine these massages into one sophisticated method simultaneously, thus providing an effective massage."

Read more about the Pro-State prostate massagers [http://bit.ly/pztwWa].

Prostate massagers are wonderful because they massage the prostate gland automatically while you simply lie there relaxed doing gentle kegel squeezes. The massager is designed to move only as much as those squeezes allow and are specifically designed for this purpose. They cannot slip too far in or create too much pressure by accident because of their great design. Basically you follow the above instructions using the massager instead of a finger. A prostate massage will leave you feeling great.

Prostate Massager Tips

Here are some tips when using the prostate massager:

- ✓ Always make sure you use lots of lube.
- ✓ The angle of entry is important. If you are having problems getting it in, then adjust the angle. When you get it right (facing forwards some) it will slip right in.
- ✓ Once you have it in about a half-inch or so, adjust the angle until it finds the easy way in. When you have it right, a simple kegel squeeze will slide it suddenly all the way in.
- ✓ Now just relax and breathe and adjust to the feeling for a good 5-10 minutes.
- ✓ Now you can begin with simple kegel squeezes very gently, very gently.
- ✓ You do not want to over stimulate especially if you have a prostate condition.
- ✓ Take your time, go slow and be gentle.
- ✓ You may or may not expel some fluids. It does not matter either way. Your prostate will be happy in either case. Often after the massage you will excrete some fluid if none came before.
- ✓ Please do not overdo it, 10-20-30 minutes is plenty of time.
- ✓ Gently remove the device.
- ✓ Wash and clean thoroughly.

A New Electronic Prostate Massager:

An Internal Prostate Massager [http://bit.ly/qpo6zt] is a small electronic device that massages the prostate gently with pulsing waves—and only takes a couple of minutes to do. These battery operated massagers use sonic waves, which help to move congested fluids out of the prostate gland and allow fresh blood and normal fluids to flow.

An Internal Prostate Massager [http://bit.ly/qpo6zt] can be much more efficient than a manual massager, much like a sonic toothbrush—many more massaging movements per minute (up to 40,000) with a noticeable effect in 5 short sessions, according to the manufacturer. Scroll down to order Option #1.

External Prostate Massage

External prostate massage can be done by direct massage of the perineum area or by using a special device.

External Prostate Self-Massage:

1. Use some natural castor oil or almond oil to massage the perineum area while at the same time doing your prostate exercises, squeezing the pubococcygeus or PC muscle. The combination is very powerful and will bring much of the benefit of internal prostate massage.

2. About one inch below the rectum towards the scrotum is a key acupuncture point and is sometimes known as the Male G-Spot because it can stimulate the prostate during sex. It can also be used to stop ejaculation if pressed deeply just before the tipping point. See chapter 21 for information on Sex and the Prostate.

3. Massage gently at first and increase the pressure as you go along. Then massage deeply the G-Spot, all why doing your prostate exercises squeezing and holding with deep breathing.

External prostate massager:

The Prostate Cradle [http://tiny.cc/wcrvd] is a wonderful invention that does the massage for you by just sitting. Highly acclaimed, you will find this device a natural and safe easy way to get the benefits of prostate massage.

Read what the company has to say about it:

> *"After ten years of research and guidance from Medical Doctors the world's first anatomically correct, external prostate massager was created: the Prostate Cradle...*
>
> *The Prostate Cradle was invented by a Certified Massage Therapist who was challenged with prostate health issues. His doctors recommended prostate massage therapy. However, at the time the only prostate massagers available were invasive. Traditional prostate massage involves rectum insertion. He knew there had to be another way!*
>
> *The Cradle provides a revolutionary new way to massage the prostate: Simply sit on it! No movement or rocking is required. Body weight creates gentle pressure for a stimulating massage. The Cradle is not like sitting on a bicycle seat. The unique anatomically correct shape avoids sensitive areas. The Cradle carefully reaches underneath the pelvic arch to massage the prostate and perineum area, also known as the "Male G-Spot."*

Chapter 19: Prostate Exercises

Prostate exercise strengthens the prostate and helps cleanse it of toxins by increasing blood flow through it. After all, the prostate is both a gland that secretes seminal fluids and a muscle that pumps it out for our pleasure (designed with the intent of being successful in procreation). The prostate also removes toxins, protecting sperm and enhancing the chance of impregnating. So exercising the prostate makes good sense.

An added bonus of prostate exercising it is that it helps you control ejaculation and the duration and strength of your erections. Nice bonuses. Sign me up ☺.

Prostate exercise happens by engaging your pubococcygeus or PC muscle. Kegel exercises or pelvic floor exercises are the name used for both men and women to strengthen the PC muscle. It stretches from the pubic bone to the tailbone, supporting the inner organs of the pelvic area and the function of the sphincter muscles (anal and bladder sphincters). In men kegel exercises also help to squeeze the prostate gland allowing more blood to flow through it, helping to cleanse it.

That's why prostate or kegel exercises for men are recommended for treating prostate conditions like enlargement from benign prostatic hyperplasia (BPH) and prostatitis, or inflammation of the prostate. Kegel exercises can also be used for treating urinary incontinence because these exercises strengthen the bladder sphincter.

For women reading this book, kegel exercises will strengthen your pelvic muscles and organs. As a result it will heighten your sensations during sex. Within two weeks you will be able to squeeze tight your vagina muscles. I will leave it to you to imagine the pleasurable benefits of this skill for you and your partner!

Do you know how to squeeze your PC muscle? It's real simple. Just squeeze your stop-pee (and stop-pooh) muscle next time you are urinating to stop the flow completely. That's what you want to exercise, your PC muscle. Just tighten all the muscles around the scrotum and anus. It automatically engages the prostate and you are on your way.

You can now do this exercise several times a day anywhere: while sitting, driving, walking, talking, or now while you are reading this book! Squeeze, hold, release. That's it. The world's easiest exercise and perhaps also the most beneficial! And only you know you are doing it! To get the most benefit from it, you need to do sets. You can vary:

✓ the speed of the squeezes from slow to fast,

✓ the duration of the holding time,

✓ the number of repetitions, and

✓ the number of times during the day you do sets.

Beginner Level:

1. Breathe deeply while doing the exercises, remembering to clench only the PC muscle.
2. Squeeze and release quickly 10 times. Do 3 reps with a 10-second break between them.
3. Squeeze and hold for 10 seconds. Do 3 reps with a 10-second break between them.
4. You've just done one set. Repeat for a total of 3 sets for the day.
5. Repeat this process every day for 1 to 2 weeks.

Intermediate Level:

1. Breathe deeply while doing the exercises, remembering to clench only the PC muscle.
2. Squeeze and release quickly 20 times. Do 3 reps with a 10-second break between them.
3. Squeeze and hold for 20 seconds. Do 3 reps with a 10-second break between them.
4. You've just done one set. Repeat for a total of 3 sets for the day.
5. Repeat this process every day for 1 to 2 weeks.

Advanced Level:

1. Breathe deeply while doing the exercises remembering to clench only the PC muscle.
2. Squeeze and release quickly 30 times. Do 3 reps with a 10-second break between them.
3. Squeeze and hold for 30 seconds. Do 3 reps with a 10-second break between them.
4. You've just done one set. Repeat for a total of 3 sets for the day.
5. You can do a mix-up: squeeze 30 then hold one for 30 seconds.
6. Repeat this process every day for 1 to 2 weeks.

Master Level:

This is a whole body exercise that strongly squeezes your prostate and stomach muscles at the same time. The breathing is advanced yogic breathing.

1. Breathe deeply, ideally in and out through the nose while doing the exercises.

2. You are going to squeeze not only the prostate with PC contractions but the whole body at the same time and in particular the stomach muscles.

3. Bend your legs into a semi crouch, legs hip width apart, hands leaning on your knees, arms straight, fingers splayed downwards.

4. Arch your back upwards like a cat, bum out and up, small of the back arched head up while

5. Breathing in deeply through the nose.

6. Then, come upwards into a quarter crouch, with knees still bent a bit. Your back then bends a bit into a concave rounded position, as hands move up to mid-thigh level, arms straight, head downwards.

7. Breathe out powerfully through your nose from the base of your diaphragm.

8. Clench your PC muscle and at the same time lift it upwards and pretend there is a lemon inside your tummy and squeeze all the juice out of it pulling your tummy deeply inwards towards your spine.

9. Tighten (contract) every muscle in your body while pulling up on your kneecap muscles, thigh muscles engaged, and holding all the squeezes, energy moving upwards.

10. Hold for 10 seconds then release back down to the start position (see Step 3). Breathe in through the nose and repeat Steps 3 to 10 of the exercise.

Note: If your stomach muscles are not strong already, then 10 reps is way too many, not that you won't be able to do them but 2-4 hours later your stomach will be in agony. Start with 3 reps and work your way up to 10 over a couple of weeks.

Remember to do your prostate exercises every day. These are especially easy to do when you are waiting at traffic lights or watching TV. Put those down times to good use and your prostate will sing its praises!

Chapter 20: Exercising

Any writer who talks about good health has to urge readers to take up exercising as a key component of turning your health around or maintaining the gifts of good health.

Well this writer is no different! If exercise is not already part of your lifestyle, then get with it. You can't become healthy and be sedentary. You know it! Add exercise and movement to your life and your prostate will be happy.

We were born to move our bodies every day. We all know that we need to add exercising into our daily routines for weight and health benefits.

Our sedentary lifestyles impact our prostates directly. It is crucial to add movement throughout the day to counteract the effects of so much sitting time. Read this excellent article about the importance of movement: Why Movement Trumps Exercise [http://bit.ly/q8ugNZ]

Enough about that! I will share some tips with you that I have gleaned over the years of doing these sports: running including 3 marathons; swimming; biking; hiking and mountaineering; climbing; skiing—all types, especially back-country telemarking; ultimate frisbee (football with a frisbee); and yoga and tai chi.

Tips

- ✓ Do something you love.
- ✓ You can get in shape for a sport by doing body exercises (that use your own weight rather than dumb dumbbells).
- ✓ Learning how to breathe properly while moving is extremely important.
- ✓ Training with bursts of intensity is far more beneficial than steady pacing.
- ✓ Varying routines prevents injuries.
- ✓ Stretching also helps avoid injury.

By doing something you love, exercising becomes enjoyable rather than a burden. Training so you can do your sport then becomes the motivator.

Bodyweight exercises have been proven to be one of the best ways to train because your own body weight is best for you, rather than using machines that target a specific muscle. You get much more benefit and utilize more natural muscle groups doing bodyweight versions.

It is also far cheaper, totally portable, and always ready to go!
Push-ups are an example of a bodyweight exercise. Squats and pull-ups are two other good examples. Matt Furey is the master of these forms of exercise.

Matt Furey, if you have never heard of him, became the first Westerner to win the world Kung Fu championship in China. Bodyweight exercise is how he trained. Matt has written many books on how to exercise. His Combat Conditioning [http://bit.ly/rfl0j8] book is the basis for his training. Just doing several of his exercises will exhaust you in just a matter of minutes.

Matt Furey is not only a top trainer but also inspiring motivational writer and speaker. Don't let his looks distract you. He is totally flexible and capable of doing exercises you can only dream about at this stage!

The methods in Matt Furey's book, *Combat Conditioning: The all natural idiot-proof way to get into the best shape of your life* [http://bit.ly/rfl0j8], changed me for the better. I was able to spend far less time getting fit with amazing results. As an example, I play ultimate frisbee (sort of football with a frisbee), a stop-start-run fast-offense-defense game that I play with others many years below my 63 years at the time of this writing. I can't recommend his techniques enough.

What is so good about them is how fast you can do them. It is not like spending an hour at the gym. You start where you are and add more as you can. Matt Furey explains it all. The big bonus for many is the weight-loss and muscle gain that happens.

About 15 years ago I read a book that changed my life. It was called *Body Mind and Sport* [http://amzn.to/oDdSBY]. The most important part of the book was how to breathe while exercising. I had heard of various techniques while running but nothing like this.

The author, a doctor and elite competitive ironman triathlete, described how to breathe in and out through your nose in a special way that I have mentioned in this book. The results are simply amazing. Your breathing slows to about half the rate while at full tilt, your heart slows and strengthens, and you have such power. He performed better while training less. His buddies all wondered what new drug he was on!

After learning the breathing, about one week later I did a tough 15-km race up and down steep hills. I was able to do great in the race all while keeping the deep, slow breath.

Basically, you breathe out from your nose with power from deep down in your belly. This empties you fully so when you breathe in you get maximum oxygen. All must be done with your nose. He explains why and how in great detail.

I use it now while playing ultimate or when I'm skiing something steep. The powerful out-breath enables me to make intense turns with balance. The breath does it—deep and intense and focused. Like doing yoga in action

For more info, read this book: *Body, Mind, and Sport: The Mind-Body Guide to Lifelong Health, Fitness, and Your Personal Best* [http://amzn.to/oDdSBY] But be careful of the diet section. You know more from here how to test what is ideal for you.

Deep breathing is so important because most men, by the time they are just 50, may have lost as much as 50% of their lung capacity compared to their youth. Lung capacity predicts health and longevity. So you gotta move and expand your lungs. It doesn't have to take long. Read on dear reader...

The latest exercising breakthroughs derive from intense bursts of speed rather than the old method of LSD—long slow distance. It mimics our heritage of stop-run-stop to escape saber-toothed critters!

LSD in runners has had tragic consequences of some runners dying at the finish line. The explanation of long slow distance training is simple. Your heart and lungs shrink to become more efficient! Just the opposite of what you would expect.

High intensity exercises create an oxygen debt that triggers metabolic processes that increase lung capacity over time. The opposite happens with low intensity duration activities like running distances. They negatively affect lung capacity unless you add high-intensity interval training. These force the lungs to expand.

When you run at bursts of speed or train with bodyweight exercises, you force your lungs and heart to expand. The more you do over time, the more your capacity expands.

You go full tilt (walk, run, ski, swim, jump, hill or stair sprints—whatever your pleasure) for 30 seconds. Then you stop or walk slowly for a couple of minutes while your heartbeat recovers to normal. Then you do it again for a total of around 5 times. That's it! Done for the day in just 10 minutes!

But you do want to learn more, especially if you are a couch potato who is just starting. You can read expert advice here from Dr. Al Sears: PACE Training [http://bit.ly/nP9ftg]

Varying your routines strengthens you. The same, old routine becomes stale. Be sure to alternate exercises, sequences, and days that you do your routines and add variety.

And add some form of stretching like yoga or Matt Furey's *Combat Stretching* [http://bit.ly/qQOEIY].

I like yoga sun salutations. They are a superb combination of bodyweight exercise and stretching. Do them in batches of 12. Here is a simple version to watch that you can follow: "Yoga For Beginners" (on YouTube) [http://bit.ly/mPQszj]

For a more advanced version, do not put your knees to the ground as you go from downward facing dog to upward facing dog or cobra. You are then doing a Matt Furey Hindu push-up.

Rebounders are one great fun exercise device. They have many added health benefits: increasing vigor, enhancing digestion and elimination, and toning the endocrine system. The bouncing directly activates the lymph system, and it benefits your prostate thus removing toxins from the body.

- ReboundAir [http://tiny.cc/rv92s] is an excellent brand with top reviews
- Cellerciser [http://tiny.cc/loi1k], which folds also has high reviews

Of course a simple skipping rope will do the same trick. Both are lots of fun. At the very minimum add walking to your life. And add 30 second bursts of power walking at full tilt every now and then. The rewards are huge! You'll lose weight, feel great, and help heal your prostate.

Exercise! Make it part of your life. It will reduce stress and weight, calm your emotions, and help you feel good. Your prostate will love ya.

Chapter 21: Sex and the Prostate

I saved the best for last!

Men! Inform yourself now and start adopting some of the ideas in this book. Not only will you be benefiting your prostate, but also your overall sex life and vitality can only improve as a consequence.

It's a win-win for you!

You see, your prostate is the gateway to sexual fulfillment, and sex is very good for your prostate. Since it is also a muscle, exercising it by ejaculating makes it pump and stay healthy. So regular sex is good for your prostate while abstinence can lead to a build up of more and more toxins.

Remember what we said about how complex the male sexual/reproductive system is? It is not just about a penis and gonads! Simply put, the prostate is the key to maximum sexual pleasure. Having a healthy prostate makes it possible to have great sex into your senior years.

While its main function is to produce fluid that becomes part of the semen, during orgasm muscle contractions squeeze the prostate, which pumps fluid into the urethra to transport the sperm out the penis. A very pleasurable event! That's the technical part. Advanced sex practice and secrets utilize the energy potential of the prostate to achieve sexual heights that most men don't even know about, let alone master.

In the last sections on prostate exercises and massage, we talked about how important it is for your prostate health to exercise your prostate by doing Kegel or prostate exercises.

When you next do them, feel your perineum muscles as you squeeze and release. Actually touch them all the way from the scrotum to the anus and see how strong they are (or can be!). Now find the acupuncture spot about half way between them. If you press in with your finger at this spot and move it a bit until you find the exact spot (you'll know), then you have got it right! This is the external male G-Spot. The internal G-Spot is the prostate itself that you can reach with a prostate massager or your finger or your loved one's through the rectal wall.

The external male G-Spot is a crucial sex tool. You can use it to control ejaculations by pressing it firmly before the point of no return. This way you can fall back from just before the peak and extend sexual orgasm, which can be separate from ejaculation. In advanced practice, it is possible to *injaculate* rather than ejaculate. See links below.

Remember that the sperm and semen produced by the testes and the seminal vesicles must enter the prostate through the ejaculatory duct. So squeezing or pressing the G-Spot helps to contain the ejaculate at source until the point of no return or you choose not to ejaculate.

By strengthening the prostate muscles and thereby being able to squeeze tight the perineum muscles to contain the energy in your prostate, and/or by pressing and activating this G-Spot, you can delay and extend sex for a long time. You are using your prostate for maximum sexual gratification this way.

Of course the other benefit of the exercise is to make your erections stronger. Muscle is muscle and exercising a muscle strengthens it. When you do PC squeezes (kegel exercises), the prostate and the inner penis or "hidden" penis (actually about 1/3 the length of the erect penis) gets stronger as well. You can feel that part of the penis when you have a strong erection... it extends inside the perineum right below the prostate. I guess that is why this pubococcygeal muscle is nicknamed the "love muscle"!

Many ancient Taoist (China) or Tantric (India) sex practices and secrets depend on being able to control ejaculation and develop inner orgasm. Basically, the longer you can build sexual energy without ejaculation, the more intense and prolonged lovemaking becomes, and then you can choose whether to ejaculate or not.

Breath control plays a big part as well in sexual performance. Practicing deep breathing in and out to slow arousal when you find the breath quickening can prolong sex. By focusing on deep breathing, the sexual energy moves up the body and delays ejaculation.

How often should a man ejaculate? Depends on your health, your age and stamina. If you find yourself weakened, then you are coming too often. The goal is to move the energy through sex and to become rejuvenated. You can have more frequent sex but do not ejaculate if you find yourself weakened. Find your optimum level by how you feel. In advanced sex practice you *injaculate* instead.

The old question, "Is sex good for the prostate?" is easily answered: YES! The key is not to over ejaculate because if you find sex weakening you, you must learn these advanced practices to injaculate or not ejaculate at all, and then you can have sex as much as you want. So learn some of these techniques and keep squeezing your prostate muscles!

Prostate stimulation can produce an exceptionally strong sexual response and intense orgasm in males that are receptive to this sexual technique. In fact, very advanced sexual tantric technique teaches how to control ejaculation by squeezing the prostate at the right moment to achieve multiple orgasms.

Sexual Prostate Massage

Sexual prostate massage enhances erections by allowing extra blood flow into the base of the penis during arousal. The difference is that you now add sexual stimulation to the equation either for masturbating or your partner to stroke you.

   ✓ Either by yourself or with a partner, use whichever method you prefer: finger or prostate massage device (Prostate Massagers [http://bit.ly/oNPZxk]).

✓ Apply lube to the penis and scrotum areas and combine stimulation with the prostate massage. If using a finger wear a latex glove.

✓ It is best to start the prostate massage first for a while, as you want the benefit of the massage.

✓ Once you are ready, **always being very gentle** with the prostate massage, adding the sexual enhancement will result in an incredible prostate orgasm as your whole body feels the stimulation inside and out.

Here are some superb sites where you can learn more advanced skills and insights:

✓ **Multi-orgasms for men:** "Any man can become "multi-orgasmic". It only requires a basic understanding of male sexuality and certain techniques. Most men's sexuality is focused on the goal of ejaculating, rather than on the actual process of lovemaking. Once a man becomes multi-orgasmic he will not only be able to better satisfy himself, but also more effectively satisfy his partner."

"Multiple Orgasm"
www.whitelotuseast.com/MultipleOrgasm.htm [http://bit.ly/q89177]
(Accessed 12 April 2011)

✓ **Sacred spot massage:** "The G-Spot or Sacred Spot of a man is his prostate gland. Tantric philosophy considers the G-Spot a man's emotional sex center. Massaging the man's prostate releases tremendous amounts of emotional and physical stress."

"Sacred Spot Massage"
www.whitelotuseast.com/SacredSpotMassage.htm [http://bit.ly/nOCZJg]
(Accessed 12 April 2011)

✓ **Tantra 101:** "Always remember to breathe! Breathing is such an important part of Tantric sexuality. The deeper you breathe the more you'll be present in your body and out of your analytical mind, and the more you'll both feel! Now this may sound far fetched. What does deep breathing have to do with pleasure? Well follow the logic here. Tantric masters know that the deeper you breathe the more relaxed you get. The more relaxed the body gets the easier the blood flows, the more blood goes throughout your body especially to the skin and underlying tissue, the more receptive the nerve endings are to pick up the stimulation."

Lamborne, C.T. "Tantra 101 - Not Just For Men"
lovenectar.com/Tantra_Article_Tantra_101_NotJustforMen.php
[http://bit.ly/niX1o6] (Accessed 12 April 2011)

✓ **Tantric Ejaculation Mastery:**

"Ultimate Ejaculation Mastery teaches you to separate ejaculation from orgasm by infusing your whole body with that glorious energy. When you learn the orgasm mastery formula, you can avoid the contractions that initiate the emission of semen. When you're super turned on, you can still have those pelvic muscle contractions that feel so wonderful. That's what

causes a dry or energy orgasm, a long series of slow pleasurable spasms with a rush of energy without ejaculating. I call these inner or implosive orgasms because you pump the energy back inside, circulate it over and over again, and reach higher and higher peaks."

Pokras, Somraj. "Tantric Ejaculation Mastery" www.tantra.com [http://bit.ly/oXM5SJ] Click on Tantric Techniques >>>Articles>>>Tantric Ejaculation Mastery (Accessed 16 April 2011)

✓ Tao of Sex 1:

"The fourth benefit of the Deer Exercise is that it builds up sexual ability and enables the man to prolong sexual intercourse. During "ordinary" intercourse the prostate swells with semen to maximum size before ejaculating. During ejaculation, the prostate shoots out its contents in a series of contractions. Then, sexual intercourse ends. With nothing left to ejaculate, induce contractions, or maintain an erection (energy is lost during ejaculation), the man cannot continue to make love. But, if he uses the Deer Exercise to pump semen out of the prostate in small doses, pumping it in the other direction into the other glands and blood vessels, he can prolong intercourse."

"The Deer Exercise for Men" www.nine3.com/DeerMan.html [http://bit.ly/ooLsTK] (Accessed 10 April 2011)

✓ Tao of Sex 2:

"In Taoist sex traditions, the man has his orgasm without ejaculating. He injaculates, instead. By pressing an acupuncture point located halfway between the anus and scrotum, the ejaculation can be reversed into an improved orgasm and the semen is recycled from the full prostate and reabsorbed into the blood. This point is known as the Jen-Mo acupuncture point or the Lion...

When the Jen-Mo point is pressed just prior to an anticipated ejaculation, the energy goes up into the body through the meridians which originate at this point, instead of going out of the body as it does during ordinary ejaculation.

Done in this way, the man still feels the pleasurable sensations which come with the pumping of the prostate, and he still experiences an orgasm. He continues to press this point until the orgasm, or "injaculation", is complete...

With depression of the Lion, it may take as long as five minutes to empty the prostate. This results in a five-minute long orgasm!"

"Injaculation vs. Ejaculation: Prolongation of arousal and longevity" www.nine3.com/Magic.html [http://bit.ly/nzjL8O] (Accessed 21 April 2011)

✓ Becoming a Masterful Lover:

Want to learn sexual mastery and how to give women incredible orgasms? David Shade tells you in simple language and explicit techniques what and how to do it. Unbelievable material, but he is convincing! His goal is to teach that giving women exquisite pleasure is the ultimate in male sexual pleasure and connection.

David Shade is "America's Renegade Sex Expert" who had the courage to go outside the boundaries of conventional wisdom to find the things that really work and work very powerfully to give women incredible pleasure. As a result, he has improved the sex lives of tens of thousands of couples worldwide.

You can get a free CD that explains his insights here:
The Secrets of the Masterful Lover [http://bit.ly/nY70DO]

That section was fun! May you be blessed with great sex!

Chapter 22: Final Message from the Author

Life can be a real challenge at times. Having a severe prostate problem can push you to the edge.

My hope in writing this book has been to give you the courage to meet your tests with the faith that you can succeed and overcome them.

The road can often be very bumpy. You can climb up a long hill only to find that you must drop down again as if no progress happened.

Healing is a journey with many ups and downs along the way. You will feel moments of elation and intense hope, as well as bouts of despair and fear. Step back and see yourself moving through time and space. Realize that the whole path is sloping upwards. Every setback is a chance to test to see what went wrong. Now you can correct course. The lows are not as low, and the destination is closer. The results, your improving condition, confirm you are well on your way to a healthy prostate.

You may become discouraged, but know this: the crisis and hard challenges will pass. You will come out from the darkness. You will find the light and will heal. Just keep forging ahead.

With this book, you have been gifted a toolbox that I never had. You will find the right implements in it to speed you on the way. Each one of you will find your own special tools to get the job done. All you need is an open mind and the willingness to allow your body wisdom to light the way and heal itself. One day you will find yourself healthy, happy, and healed with a Healthy Prostate.

I thank you the reader, for in writing and sharing I have learned so much. The teacher learns from the students. This work has helped me to crystallize my thoughts, focus my message, and share my blessings.

It has been an inspiration for me to write this book. I truly thank all those practitioners who have helped me in my healing process. I have learned some pearls of wisdom from you all that have helped me get here.

Each of us builds on the labors of those before us. We could not be where we are individually or as a society without those prior efforts. Thank you, thank you, and thank you again! May your returning health warm your soul on your life's journey.

Wellness, Longevity, and Laughter

Let's end on an up note!

Your prostate journey passes through many stages from crisis to progress, from highs to low, from setback to headway, from despair to hope, and lots in between. I have found during the hard times to realize that "this moment will pass," and this helped me endure the tough moments and days. If I can find some lesson or glean an insight, then I can use those times to correct course. I can be a slow learner, so sometimes I end up failing again! Eventually, I get wiser, and those tough times do pass.

I have discovered that the healing journey can take time. It may seem that the magic bullet of a pharmaceutical or a surgery is the better way to go. Whenever I had those thoughts I realize that it is too simplistic, for poisoning the body or cutting something out is just not the natural way to heal.

> *"Regaining your health is not about applying a magical quick fix; rather, it is a reconstruction process that affects every part of your life... It would be very simplistic to assume that a few vitamin pills, a new wonder drug, an operation, or even an alternative medical treatment could, in the spur of a moment, undo the effects of many years of neglect.*
>
> *The body may have had to endure much strain from not receiving proper nourishment or sufficient sleep and exercise for years on end. You can find the key to bring balance into every aspect of your life by starting to take responsibility for your own health."*
>
> Moritz, Andreas   *Timeless Secrets of Health and Rejuvenation*
> [http://amzn.to/nmUh4Y]

Remember we are coded to heal if we do the right things. If you clean your cut and keep dirt out of it, then it will heal by itself with a minimal amount of care. Healing your prostate is the same. It will take time but you will get there.

The additional benefits of this approach cannot be underestimated!

✓ Your whole health and well being are improving at the same time because you are treating your whole body with optimum diet and lifestyle habits now.

✓ You are thus benefiting your overall wellness and longevity, adding energy to your life rather than being depleted by invasive techniques.

✓ You lose weight as a by-product of the changes you are making.

✓ Your stress load is reducing, as you start to see results and your lifestyle becomes more grounded and centered.

✓ You learn new skills like meditation or exercising methods.

- ✓ As old doors close you find new ones opening you could never imagine. (If you had told me 8 years ago that I would be writing an extensive book on prostate health, I would have thought you were over the edge and in need of a good kick to wake you up!)

My prostate has been a hidden blessing to me. It has allowed me to discover what is most important to me in this short, sweet, and very challenging life that we are given to pass through in a very fast blink of the eye!

Love of family and friends, enjoyment of the outdoors and the magic of nature, growing fresh food, watching the apple blossoms open each spring with their promise of an apple to follow in the fall, catching a deer nibbling and looking at me peeing off the deck before I see her—I would not trade these for all the success of the business world. I would never have believed this in my younger years when driven by and for money and "success" as the primary objective in life.

Prostate challenges have honed me to a sharper edge of discernment for what is truly important. I would not exchange the now, for it is perfect as is, with all of its rides! I just have learned to float more gently, perhaps with the blessing of a bit of grace and laughter.

On a further up note, let us remember the joys and benefits of laughter for its wonderful ability to instantly erase tensions and stress, for its soothing joys and heartfelt glee. Laughter, perhaps the best medicine of all for what ails you!

Here are just a few of the many benefits of laughter:
- ✓ Laughter is fun, especially the uncontrollable kind! Can you remember the times it brought you to tears and you were begging the laughter to stop because it was so unstoppable and all encompassing?
- ✓ Laughter lowers stress levels
- ✓ Laughter boosts immunity
- ✓ Laughter exercises the heart
- ✓ Laughter reduces pain
- ✓ Laughter helps you maintain a positive frame of mind
- ✓ Laughter reduces muscle tension

To read many more benefits, go here: "Laughter is the Best Medicine – The Health Benefits of Humor and Laughter" [http://bit.ly/nIIbi1S]

May laughter fill your days!

I wish you all the joys of this life and hope that you have learned some valuable insights on your journey to a **Healthy Prostate**!

Blessings to you dear reader!

Ron Bazar   August 6, 2011

The greatest pee of my life...

Ah the good old days of youth! Strong prostate and powerful bladder.

How could I know that decades later the opposite would happen to me.

Here's the story of the greatest pee of my life...

The year was 1976 in March. We were in Peking China still under Chairman Mao's rule where everyone wore the same bland communist outfit (the Mao suit). It was called by that name Peking ever since the West came to China in the 1800s. It changed to Beijing in the late 70s.

We were in intense contract negotiations for the distribution rights to all of China's ginseng manufacturers for the territory of Canada and the United States. I was CEO and President of The Ginseng Root Of Life Company Ltd. I was there with my business partner, Managing Director, Peter Vizel. We were only 28 and 27 years old.

At the table were their negotiation team of translator, political watchdog, the CEO of the Head Office of the China National Native Produce and Animal By-Products Import and Export Corporation as well as the Directors of the three main branches that produced ginseng in China, the Peking Native Produce Branch, the Tientsin Native Produce Branch and the Dairien Native Produce Branch.

The contracts being negotiated were for many millions of dollars. At that time, this trading corporation was in the top five of the largest Chinese trading companies.

They sat on one side of the table (6 of them) and we on the other.

We had been at it for hours that day. It was already 1:30 in the afternoon and we had been drinking copious amounts of jasmine tea that are constantly offered, drunk and refilled during that time. They were also offering the obligatory Double Happiness Brand of Chinese cigarettes!

"Ah, Mr. Bazarrr, tsigarette?"

"No thank you," I said.

"Tsigarette?" "Tsigarette?" offered across the table with big smiles and a cigarette pushed forward from the pack during particularly tense moments...

...until you had to take one and light up with the zippo lighter we used to light their smokes with the flourish zippo snap opening and lighting from years of experience lighting other smokables back home... (They just loved that zippo, as none were available those days in China during Mao's regime.)

(It took me several years to kick the smoking habit after that trip).

By now the amount of bladder pressure was enormous, as breaking for a pee break was unthinkable—the first to go would lose face. That is why the tea was constantly being offered and toasted to drink, so we would crumble first.

And drink we had done, copious amounts... since 9 am!

They are masters of these games, of course, but we knew we could not succumb first. So we smiled, drank, and toasted them in equal measure throughout the long morning into the early afternoon.

The impasse was broken finally at 1:45 pm when the idea was presented to stop for a lunch with the offering of going to the famous, yet closed to the public, giant restaurant in the Summer Palace. They opened it just for us. (Of course this was pre-planned by them). In this way we could suspend the contract talks and break for a bathroom visit without either side loosing face.

Ah! What a pee! Never had I gone like that! Standing there at the urinal and going, going and going seemingly forever in a bliss of the longest pee on record!

And lunch was even better, a twelve course banquet. Each of us had 3 personal waiters! One just for the refilling of the highly potent Maotai* for all the toasting to Canada-China friendship!

But that is another story!

* Maotai has been used on official occasions in feasts with foreign heads of state and distinguished guests visiting China. It is the only alcoholic beverage presented as an official gift by Chinese embassies in foreign countries and regions. It received additional exposure in China and abroad when Zhou Enlai used the liquor to entertain Richard Nixon during the state banquet for the U.S. presidential visit to China in 1972. It is one of China's official state banquet wines and claims to be one of the world's three best known liquors (together with whisky and cognac) and is therefore presented to all official guests of state.

Product Appendix

Appliances & Equipment & Supplies

- Alcohol Prep Pads [http://bit.ly/qaLEJ9]
- Aquasana [http://bit.ly/peKByu]
- Bath Dechlorinators [http://tiny.cc/xd3vp]
- Berkey Water Filters [http://amzn.to/pvpDYp]
- Best seller and inexpensive external catheter #1 [http://bit.ly/oaKjsB]
- Best seller and inexpensive external catheter #2 [http://bit.ly/nYIypQ]
- Cellerciser [http://tiny.cc/loi1k]
- Champion Juicer [http://amzn.to/oOzhJF]
- Comfortable Bicycle Seats by Spiderflex [http://www.spiderflex.com]
- DribbleStop - Urinary Incontinence Clamp [http://bit.ly/n9CQOI]
- Lidocaine [http://tiny.cc/hqyu6]
- Office and Home Air Purifiers [http://www.airpurifiers.com]
- Other Internal Catheters [http://bit.ly/oLfTcM]
- Other Prostate Cushions [http://tiny.cc/5yqfw]
- Perfect Pendulums [http://bit.ly/m7J913]
- Pro-State Prostate Massagers [http://bit.ly/pztwWa]
- Prostate Bicycle Seats [http://tiny.cc/mqor9]
- Prostate Cradle [http://tiny.cc/wcrvd]
- Prostate Cushions [http://prostate-cushion.com]
- Prostate Massager [http://bit.ly/oNPZxk]
- Prostate Treatment Device for Prostatitis and BPH [http://bit.ly/oniKLH]
- ReboundAir [http://tiny.cc/rv92s]
- Sitz Bath Commode [http://tiny.cc/1jp9i]
- SpeediCath Coudé Intermittent Catheters [http://bit.ly/r5qZev]
- Spongy Wonder Bicycle Seats [http://www.spongywonder.com]

- Sprouters [http://tiny.cc/lym2r]

- The SEAT® (Bicycle seat) [http://bit.ly/qYJ3v7]

- Top of the line external catheter [http://bit.ly/phxJph]

- Urinary Catheters [http://1.usa.gov/oGOwzu]

- Water Distillers at Amazon.com [http://tiny.cc/7lvc1]

- Whole House Chlorine Water Filters [http://tiny.cc/1n41c]

- Xylocaine Ointment Tube [http://bit.ly/niVyUT]

Books & CDs

- A Healthier You from the Inside Out [http://bit.ly/paM9v7]

- Ageless Body, Timeless Mind: The Quantum Alternative to Growing Old [http://amzn.to/nkEzy0]

- Alternative Cancer Treatments: Books [http://tiny.cc/47u6b]

- Ayurvedic Healing, 2nd Revised and Enlarged Edition: A Comprehensive Guide [http://amzn.to/okRlD4

- Body, Mind, and Sport: The Mind-Body Guide to Lifelong Health, Fitness, and Your Personal Best [http://amzn.to/oDdSBY]

- Cancer Is Not A Disease - It's A Survival Mechanism [http://amzn.to/rbKt9l]

- Combat Conditioning: The all natural idiot-proof way to get into the best shape of your life [http://bit.ly/rfl0j8]

- Deep Meditation with Subliminal Affirmations [http://bit.ly/pMlffa]

- Disconnect: The Truth About Cell Phone Radiation, What the Industry Has Done to Hide It, and How to Protect Your Family [http://amzn.to/ok6ILa]

- Fasting-The Ultimate Diet [http://amzn.to/mVP3K3]

- Free Meditation Downloads [http://amzn.to/qM8f0f]

- Invasion of the Prostate Snatchers: No More Unnecessary Biopsies, Radical Treatment or Loss of Sexual Potency [http://amzn.to/oxkJl8]

- Know Your Fats : The Complete Primer for Understanding the Nutrition of Fats, Oils and Cholesterol [http://amzn.to/oTm9XB]

- Master Cleanse ebook 1 [http://tiny.cc/6ecfr]

- Master Cleanse ebook 2 [http://tiny.cc/nmv7s

- Meditation [http://tiny.cc/f3swh]

- Nourishing Traditions: The Cookbook that Challenges Politically Correct Nutrition and the Diet Dictocrats [http://amzn.to/nB9irS]

- Outsmart Your Cancer: Alternative Non-Toxic Treatments That Work (Second Edition) With CD [http://amzn.to/pW2sot]

- Prostate Health in 90 Days: Without Drugs or Surgery [http://amzn.to/qEGzzg]

- Stop Making Cancer [http://bit.ly/nbAJB5]

- Stress Reduction [http://tiny.cc/wcrvd]

- The Amazing Liver & Gallbladder Flush [http://amzn.to/qls7Te]

- The Complete Idiot's Guide to Fasting [http://amzn.to/q40d1v]

- The Liver and Gallbladder Miracle Cleanse: An All-Natural, At-Home Flush to Purify and Rejuvenate Your Body [http://amzn.to/oNIlta]

- The Miracle of Fasting: Proven Throughout History for Physical, Mental, & Spiritual Rejuvenation [http://amzn.to/oF6F3c]

- The Miracle Results of Fasting: Discover the Amazing Benefits in Your Spirit, Soul and Body [http://amzn.to/ngcCmx]

- The Natural Prostate Cure [http://amzn.to/r7ib38]

- Timeless Secrets of Health and Rejuvenation [http://amzn.to/mRERca]

- When the Body Says No [http://amzn.to/r4a5ic]

- Wild Fermentation: The Flavor, Nutrition, and Craft of Live-Culture Foods [http://amzn.to/q29P2N]

- Zen Macrobiotics for Americans [http://amzn.to/o0Hpps]

Cleansing Kits & Detoxifiers

- Colonix [http://tiny.cc/yijc5]

- Far Infrared Saunas [http://tiny.cc/ydp2o]

- LL's Magnetic Clay Bath (heavy metal cleanse) from LifetimeHealth [http://bit.ly/ooQYzP]

- LL's Magnetic Clay Baths [http://bit.ly/qBYtQe]

- PectaSol Chelation Complex [http://bit.ly/quLgxF]

- Sambu Elderberry Cleanse [http://tiny.cc/doyet]

- Swanson's French Green Clay [http://bit.ly/q4zcS6

Household Products

- AlwaysEco Pest Control Products [http://bit.ly/pUvdzT]
- Orange TKO [http://amzn.to/rgC6Jv]
- Organic Household Products [http://tiny.cc/qzyg4]

Organic Bodycare Products

- Dr. Bronner's Bodycare [http://tiny.cc/wpqzs]
- Organic Bodycare Products from Amazon [http://tiny.cc/0ppl4]
- Perfume & Cologne [http://bit.ly/n5AiVp]
- Sunscreen [http://bit.ly/q4RSxq]
- Tongue Scrapers and Cleaners [http://tiny.cc/trzk6]
- Zinc Oxide Sunscreen [http://tiny.cc/trzk6]

Oils, Foods, Teas, Herbs, and Supplements

- "Ancient Minerals" Magnesium [http://tiny.cc/rsaqa]
- Avocado oil [http://tiny.cc/ajyjo]
- Ayurstate - from India Herbs [http://bit.ly/q13kAw]
- Ayurstate for Prostate Care – from Amazon [http://amzn.to/pJA5hi]
- Bell Prostate Ezee Flow Tea [http://bit.ly/rrZEnr]
- Beta Sitosterol [http://tiny.cc/s5f73]
- Black Currant Oil [http://tiny.cc/z8u0x]
- Borage Oil [http://tiny.cc/cbjfo]
- Brassica Tea [http://bit.ly/qyXuxo]
- Castor Oil [http://tiny.cc/8v3sf]
- Chia Seeds, organic [http://tiny.cc/8v3sf]
- Chinese Herbs for Prostate [http://bit.ly/r4kBjW]
- Chinese Prostate Pills [http://bit.ly/nuuu7f]

- Chinese Prostate Supplement [http://bit.ly/nFvNXP]

- Cod Liver Oil [http://bit.ly/py6nHA]

- Ellagic Acid Extract [http://bit.ly/orB5qH]

- Ellagic Acid Supplements [http://www.ellagicdirect.com]

- Ellagic Ultra [http://www.vitapurity.com]

- Ezekiel Cereals [http://tiny.cc/00x15]

- Evening Primrose Oil [http://tiny.cc/z2p6i]

- Fish Oil Omega-3, organic [http://tiny.cc/yq2uh]

- Ghee [http://www.pureindianfoods.com]

- Green Pastures Blue Ice Royal Capsules [http://bit.ly/njtFp8]

- Green Superfoods [http://tiny.cc/afu5f]

- Highest Quality Cod Liver Oil [http://bit.ly/py6nHA]

- Kokoro – Natural Progesterone Cream [http://bit.ly/osi1Zg]

- Manuka Honey [http://tiny.cc/git1i]

- Mother Nature Prostate Formulas [http://bit.ly/qyhZrV]

- NatPro – Natural Progesterone Cream [http://bit.ly/oEFRTH]

- Melatonin [http://amzn.to/pfsq4E]

- Men's Formula [http://bit.ly/qEcGyG]

- MyGest - Progesterone Cream [http://bit.ly/quzte2]

- Neoprostate [http://bit.ly/nVifzC]

- Organic Maple Syrup [http://tiny.cc/vkyus]

- Organic Miso [http://tiny.cc/0uqbt]

- Prostate Dr. – Native Remedies [http://bit.ly/qyIRWj]

- Prostate Protection – A holistic approach to prostate health [http://bit.ly/pLwY7F]

- Prostate Supplements at Amazon [http://tiny.cc/3244d]

- Prostate Supplements at Roger Mason's site [http://bit.ly/mZn72T]

- Prostex [http://tiny.cc/u2c3a]